# EVERYDAY AYURVEDA
# *for* Women's Health

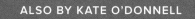

# EVERYDAY AYURVEDA
# *for* Women's Health

TRADITIONAL WISDOM, RECIPES, AND REMEDIES FOR OPTIMAL
WELLNESS, HORMONE BALANCE, AND LIVING RADIANTLY

## Kate O'Donnell

PHOTOGRAPHS BY CARA BROSTROM

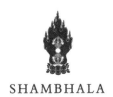

SHAMBHALA

Shambhala Publications, Inc.
2129 13th Street
Boulder, Colorado 80302
www.shambhala.com

Cover and interior design: Rita Sowins / Sowins Design

9 8 7 6 5 4 3 2 1

First Edition
Printed in Malaysia

Shambhala Publications makes every effort to print on acid-free, recycled paper.
Shambhala Publications is distributed worldwide by Penguin Random House, Inc., and its subsidiaries.

Library of Congress Cataloging-in-Publication Data
Names: O'Donnell, Kate (Ayurvedic practitioner), author. | Brostrom, Cara, photographer.
Title: Everyday Ayurveda for women's health: traditional wisdom, recipes, and remedies for optimal wellness, hormone balance, and living radiantly / Kate O'Donnell; photographs by Cara Brostrom.
Description: First edition. | Boulder, Colorado: Shambhala, [2024] | Includes bibliographical references and index
Identifiers: LCCN 2023011378 | ISBN 9781645471684 (hardback)
Subjects: LCSH: Women—Health and hygiene. | Medicine, Ayurvedic. | Medicine, Ayurvedic—Formulae, receipts, prescriptions.
Classification: LCC RA778 .O33 2024 | DDC 613/.0424—dc23/eng/20230502
LC record available at https://lccn.loc.gov/2023011378

This book is dedicated to Shakti,
the force of creative power.
May we always remember she lives in us,
as in all beings.

# Contents

Recipe and Practice Lists  viii

Foreword by Dr Claudia Welch, Doctor of Oriental Medicine  xi

Author's Note  xii

Introduction: Luminosity, Ayurveda, and Women's Health  xv

## Part One: Foundations of Ayurveda for Women  1

1. Hormone Balance: A Holistic Perspective  3
2. Reenvisioning Your Body: Ayurveda Basics of Form and Function  9
3. Reclaiming Women's Anatomy in Ayurveda  23
4. Celestial Bodies: Influence of the Sun, Moon, and Planets  47

## Part Two: Aligning with the Rhythms of Nature  53

5. Dinacharya: The Ayurveda Daily Routine  55
6. Sleep and Evening Routines  63
7. Optimizing Digestion and Metabolism  67
8. Detoxification and Rejuvenation: Practices for Essential Balance  78
9. Lunar Rhythms for Health and Evolution  89

## Part Three: Finding Balance through the Seasons of Life  103

10. Navigating Principles: Money, Family, Desire, and Dharma  105
11. Healthy Menstruation  119
12. Managing PMS and Menstrual Imbalances  131

13. Fertility Enhancement and Pregnancy Prevention  149
14. Pregnancy and Childbirth  159
15. Self-Care for the New Mother  167
16. Perimenopause  178
17. Menopause  187
18. Longevity and Healthy Aging  199

## Part Four: Kitchen Medicine  209

19. Therapeutic Spices and Herbs  211
20. Herbal Infusions  217
21. Digestives and Culinary Spices  228
22. Women's Health Tonics  239
23. Medicinal Meals and Condiments  262
24. Nourishing Treats  300

Appendix A: Healing Practices  314
Appendix B: Food Therapeutics Reference Charts  330
Appendix C: Bibliography and Resources  333
Acknowledgments  336
Notes  337
Index  338
About the Author and Photographer  350

# Recipe and Practice Lists

## THE RECIPES

### SPICED WATERS AND DIGESTIVE MIXES

Basic Cooked Water  230
Essential Spiced Water  231
Ajwain Water  232
Cooling Coriander Water  233
Soothing Rose Sweet Tea  234
Cooling Fennel Soft Drink  235
Essential Spice Mix  238
Sweet Rose Masala  236

### HERBAL INFUSIONS

Nourishing Herbal Infusion  218
Cooling Herbal Infusion  220
Refreshing Phanta Infusion  221
Cleansing Herbal Infusion  222
Raspberry Leaf and Nettle Brew  223
Triphala Tea  224
Cool-the-Flash Tea and Spritz
   with Rose and Sage  226
Double-Duty Sage and Salt
   Deodorant Spritz  225

### WOMEN'S HEALTH TONICS

Basic Almond Milk  240
Basic Coconut Milk  241
Homemade Flax Milk  242
Best Medicinal PSL
   (Pumpkin Spice Latte)  244
Date Shake  243
Sexy Cacao  249
Moon Milk  247
Golden Mind Milk  248
Longevity Bone Tonic  253
Moringa Green Drink Three Ways  250
Aloe-Pom-Cran Tonic  254
Pomegranate Lime Mocktail  255
Raspberry-Ginger Secret Smoothie  260
Strawberry Rose Smash  259
Raisin Mantha  261
Chyawanprash Herbal Jam  256

### MEDICINAL MEALS AND CONDIMENTS

Creamy Coconut Breakfast Kichari  264
Yogurt Rice with Pomegranate
   Seeds  265
Warming Wheat Soup  268
Red Rice Kanji  271
Spiced Barley Soup  269
Essential Mineral Vegetable Broth  272

Yellow Dal Supreme  273

Chicken Soup with Coriander and
 Lemon  276

Lotus Root Curry  279

Every Body Dal  280

Spicy Black Gram Soup  281

Beets and Barley Stew  284

New Moon Kichari  286

Umami Kichari  288

Beet Love Two Ways: Gingered Beet
 Soup and Herbed Beet Pickles  289

Warm Arame and Kale Salad  292

Pumpkin Seed Cilantro Pâté  293

Carrot and Green Bean Palya  294

Mixed Greens Chutney  297

Sesame Crunch Chutney  298

Triple Mineral Gomasio  299

### NOURISHING TREATS

Black Sesame Balls  303

Date Honey  305

Almond Cardamom Diamonds  306

Rasala Medicinal Yogurt  311

Kate's Tahini Treat  309

Hibiscus Rose Cordial  312

## THE PRACTICES

### PRACTICES FOR HEALTHY ARTAVA AND APANA

Herbal Sitz Bath  316

Yoni Steaming  318

Castor Oil Packs  318

Breast Massage  320

### PRACTICES TO SUPPORT HORMONAL BALANCE

Nadi Shodhana (Alternate
 Nostril Breathing)  321

Sitali Cooling Breath  323

Abhyanga (Oil Massage and Dry
 Brushing)  323

Moonbathing  327

### PRACTICES FOR MIND, SLEEP, AND MOOD

Shiro Abhyanga (Head Massage)  328

Sama Vritti Ujjayi (Rhythmic
 Breathing)  322

Herbal Bath Ritual  329

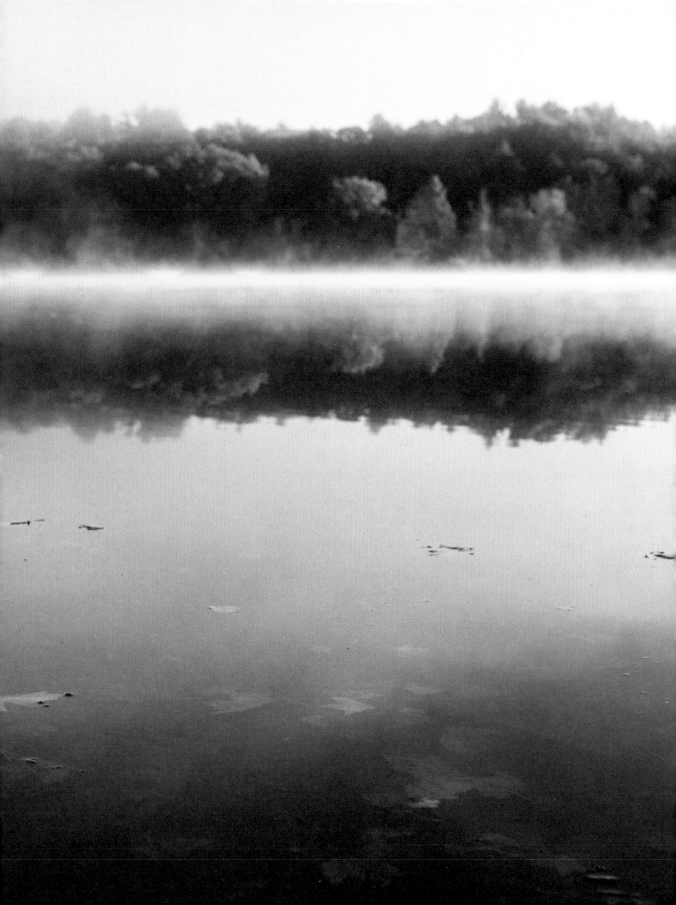

# Foreword

I've recently been contemplating the difference between two Sanskrit words that can both be translated as "truth" yet have a curious difference. Each relates to health in general and women's health specifically.

*Satyam* is that underlying, unquestionable truth or oneness behind the variety and differences we perceive all around us.

*Rtam* is the rhythm (a closely associated and similar sounding word) and order assigned to that truth.

In the macrocosm of the world and universe, we witness this order and rhythm in the change of seasons (*rtu*); in the progression from dawn to midday to dusk to starry night and back to dawn; in planetary orbits, movements of galaxies, and rotations of the globe; in the pitter-patter of rain and the gentle falling of snow; in the migration of birds; in the growth, maturation, death, and dropping of plant seeds; and in innumerable other large and small natural phenomena.

In the microcosm of a woman's body, we see the rhythm of the onset of menarche, the menstrual cycles, the time frame of pregnancy, the arrival of menopause—the secretion and depletion of hormones as their quantity changes measurably from minute to minute, day to day, month to month, decade to decade. As no two days of the lunar cycle look the same, no two days of a woman's monthly cycle look the same. All these phenomena reflect the order and rhythm of truth.

In the modern world, we have become distant from natural rhythms. We have constructed worlds wherein we indiscriminately eat foods grown in or out of season, without knowing where or how they are grown and processed. We manipulate or supplement our hormones with synthetic ones. We can't sleep at night and are tired during the day. We aren't sure when we are hungry, and we consult the latest advice on how much water to drink. We don't know when to be active and when to be passive. It is harder than ever to know what is true and what is truth.

By returning to and contemplating the rhythms in our lives, matching our habits and activities with the times of day and seasons, we not only have the potential to regain or maintain personal health and hormonal balance, we also have the side benefit of developing, nurturing, and stabilizing our relationship with truth itself by witnessing and aligning with the order and rhythm of truth. What greater call might there be in these turbulent times?

*Everyday Ayurveda for Women's Health* is a deft guide and comfortable companion to help us return to this relationship. Kate O'Donnell helps us learn to refine our senses and become better attuned to the natural macrocosmic and microcosmic order and rhythm of truth.

*Dr. Claudia Welch, Doctor of Oriental Medicine*

# Author's Note

It's such an interesting, challenging time to write a book on women's health. Concepts of sex and gender are being deconstructed, which leaves us somewhere in the middle of finding an inclusive, effective, and concise language in which to communicate about the reproductive system. There's a lot of Ayurveda language to absorb without getting confused with strait-laced English. Here's how I address this.

First, what if the reproductive organs aren't reproducing in this lifetime? Throughout this book, we will call the reproductive organs "generative organs" and "the generative system." We address many of the generative meanings a life cycle can express, whether through procreation or other manifestations of creativity.

We might have once said "female reproductive organs." What if a person with a uterus and ovaries isn't aligned with all the other assumptions tied to the word *female*, and what if a person doesn't intend to reproduce with these organs? That's why we will call them generative organs. I may use the term "women's health" but not to be exclusionary. By this I mean people who need to care for ovaries and a uterus; who undergo menarche, menstruation, and menopause; who have the organs that gestate and birth babies; and who wish to consider the health and integrity of this generative system. If you have these organs but don't identify as a woman, I hope this information reaches you in a sensitive and beneficial way.

As for assumptions surrounding the words *female* and *woman*, in this book I often use the word *lunar*. Many rituals and routines support lunar energy, the counterpart to solar energy, which is traditionally assumed to be male. As you will learn, in the Vedic view, these two energies are the grand dichotomy within humans; their balance is the key to health and happiness, and their meanings go beyond gender.

Lunar energy—naturally receptive, cool, and soft (the opposite of the active, hot, and intense qualities of solar energy)—was always considered by the ancients to be a "feminine" quality. Interestingly, Eastern images of gods and enlightened beings sometimes appear androgynous to symbolize the balance of the two energies. This is what we are all after: a balance of naturally coexisting polarities in our beings. All people are an amalgamation of solar and lunar energies; however, modern cultures, especially in the West, seem to have been leaning far into solar energy for a long time. This has had ramifications for our health. Most of us of any sex or gender would be wise to take stock of this and cultivate lunar qualities in our bodies and energies as an effective path to maintaining health and longevity. Our nature may also require the cultivation of solar energy. My intention is to provide the language and tools to help you observe changes, recognize imbalances, and preserve your inborn, essential balance.

You may find more Ayurveda anatomy in chapter 3 than you were looking for! You don't need to learn it all to use this book, however. I have taken care not to use the Western scientific language for generative parts when I can avoid it. The beautiful thing about using the Ayurveda language for our bodies is that words are visualizations accompanied by felt sensations. I provide a new language that you can own and experience, which empowers you.

The ancient Ayurveda texts discuss menstrual health as the most important aspect of a woman's physiology, due to her central purpose of procreating. I have chosen not to have children and to cultivate a different sense of dharma, so you can imagine this gives me pause. I can see, however, that there are golden nuggets here about care of the generative system that supports optimal physiology to take women *anywhere* they want to go in life. Rather than discount the male-centered worldview of these texts, I share this information in practical and embodied ways to support the organ system that weaves through the core of our bodies and supports a womb space of potent energies.

We have spent too long feeling confused by complicated language about our bodies. I hope you find this book a living, intuitive manual that you come back to over and over.

Communication requires language, and we are navigating this evolving landscape together. I hope our conversation helps you reenvision your body in profound ways. My intention is to keep it simple, yet in-depth enough to illuminate what you need to mine the truth of what your body is telling you, learn wise choices, and own your healing path. Let's get the conversation going.

Kate O'Donnell

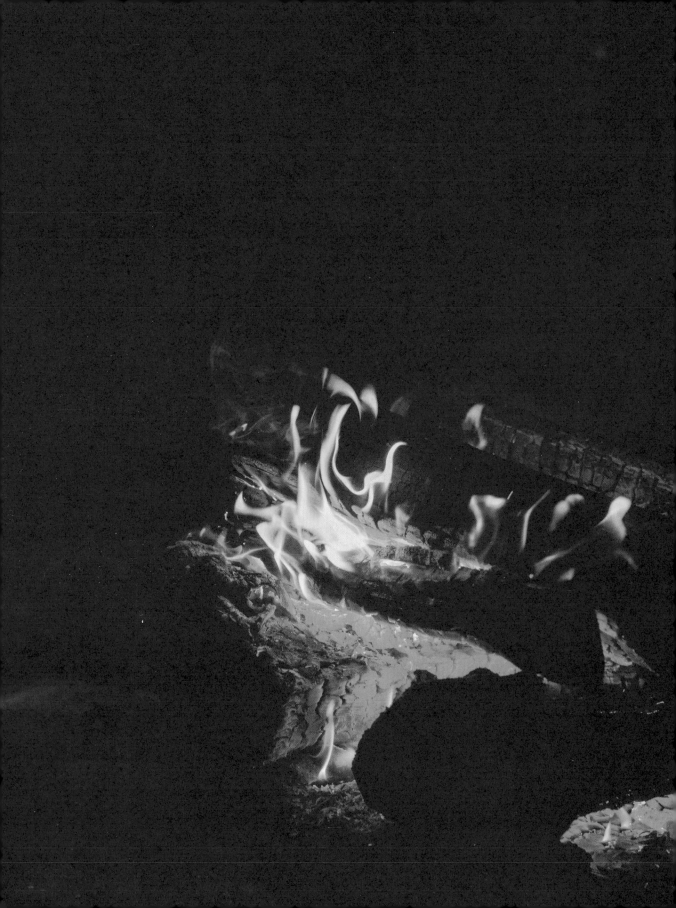

# Introduction

## LUMINOSITY, AYURVEDA, AND WOMEN'S HEALTH

Ayurveda, an ancient system of medicine, reminds us of so much we already know to be true but perhaps forget in the busy flow of day to day. We forget that we are luminous bodies, that our tissues are built from medicinal foods, forged by fire into vessels that hold love, intention, and the capacity to create. At the center, we are bright. When we tend to our inner flame by eating well and preserving the fires that glow and fuel our minds, hearts, and connections, we are radiant. I want each of us to feel connected to our inner fire and to know ourselves as celestial objects on earth. We are magical, as all life is magical.

Luminosity is born of a subtle metabolizing process governed by *tejas*, the energetic essence of the fire element and metabolic activity. Tejas is a glow of embers, not a raging flame. It is the heart of heat and the source of luminosity. Tejas is the luster in our skin and eyes, and that which brings ideas to light.

How do we tend to our intrinsic brightness? Fire and burning embers are disturbed by wind and smothered by lack of space. In a subtle context, wind is daily activity and mental activity. Wind is motion. Space is the ability to spread and expand. This expansion is essential for women. We are expansive and must allow ourselves time and space for the digestion of food, experience, and emotion. We must learn how to slow down when we need more space and to soothe the winds when they become unruly.

We can recognize the signs of unruly wind: lying in bed while our minds race, waking up in the night with many thoughts that won't stop, being unable to sit still or be quiet, or feeling afraid of time alone. We can learn to think of these disruptions as *vata* imbalance—more on that later. The pace of daily life tends to be too fast. Many women take on too much, support too many, and push too hard. Preserving one's inherent radiance and tejas is a practical endeavor that involves establishing personal boundaries and integrating self-care with the care of others.

When activity is in harmony with one's capacity for movement and change, the fires are balanced. Prioritizing time and space for digestion, reflection, and expansion yield the most profound expression of health. The feeling of being in the flow with life, in a state of dharma, is magical.

Many tools in this book balance our natural movements in body and mind: when we eat, sleep, restore, and cleanse. I also share a cosmic road map for life, both spiritual and practical. The practices and deeply nourishing recipes support tejas, while new lifestyle rhythms ensure there is time and space for the fires to burn steadily.

# HOW TO USE THIS BOOK

I am not trained in Western medicine, nor am I a doctor of Ayurveda. I have studied Ayurveda and Yoga in the United States and India for twenty-five years. I have more experience receiving Ayurveda medical care than its Western counterpart, and I understand my own (female) body through the language of Ayurveda. In this book, I offer an experiential language for and perspective on women's bodies, as well as foods and practices that connect you to inherent healing abilities.

As a practitioner, I have witnessed many women manifest in different stages of life. I notice patterns, gather citizen data, and observe bodies. Women are building a trove of women's wisdom. *The Everyday Ayurveda Book of Women's Health* and my interpretation of Ayurveda perspectives are my contribution.

The information in this book can be used in tandem with Western modes of care and as an alternative viewpoint. I encourage you to foster a relationship with a Western medical provider for routine care. As you observe your body through an Ayurveda lens and follow some of the practices in this book, you will know *your* normal and be able to spot when something isn't right.

I do not offer medical advice in this book, and I am careful not to confuse the Ayurveda perspective with Western diagnostic terms when possible. For example, you will not find Ayurveda "cures" for conditions in this book. What you will find are lifestyle rhythms and a knowledge of healing foods, herbs, and spices that will transform your body into a balanced, naturally detoxified, and nourished environment for your mind and spirit. When things go out of balance, it is not your fault. This is the way of bodies: we are each imperfect. If you are seeking agency in the healing process, this book gives a broad view of a woman's life span and is a guide for consistent self-care that shifts disease trajectories.

This book has four parts. Part one offers a background on Ayurveda, its history, and its foundational principles, such as the five elements and three *doshas*. This part also aligns the modern view on hormones with Ayurveda language and describes the generative system from an Ayurveda perspective.

Part two is full of self-care practices: how, when, and why to do them. I offer a broad view of Ayurveda's health maintenance techniques, and you need never push yourself to "do it all." Trying to do everything in this book would be exhausting! Attempting to do self-care perfectly can be a source of stress and make imbalances worse in the long run.

Part three covers the changes and transitions the generative system undergoes through the stages of life. Our bodies and hormones, as well as our desires and values, may shift and affect our health, our lifestyle choices, and our sources of personal power. Ayurveda perspectives, practices, and remedies for stages of menstruation, fertility management and pregnancy, perimenopause, menopause, and longevity are all covered.

Part four is chock-full of recipes for meals, tonics, and herbal preparations to support the unique needs of women's bodies. Be empowered to sample the recipes freely and forge medicinal connections with your food. You don't need to understand every concept in the book to use the recipes, though as you dive in deeper, over time, the efficacy of the formulations will make more and more sense.

This is the kind of book you will keep coming back to. You don't need to read it cover to cover to benefit. Take your time as you let the information sink in, and make a recipe or two in the meantime.

## THE ORIGINS OF AYURVEDA

Ayurveda (pronounced "EYE-yer-VAY-da") may be the oldest continuously practiced health system in the world, dating from two thousand to five thousand years ago. The earliest information on Ayurveda is contained in the *Rig-Veda*, a body of orally transmitted ancient Indian scripture. The Vedas are believed to have originated from the *rishis*, sages in deep states of meditation.

*Ayurveda* is loosely translated as the "science of life." *Ayur*, or "life," has four parts: the physical body, the mind, the soul, and the senses (sight, hearing, touch, smell, and taste)—contrary to the Western model, which focuses mostly on the physical body. Ayurveda looks at the whole person, using diet, biorhythms, herbal medicine, psychology, wholesome lifestyle, surgery, and therapeutic bodywork to address the root cause of disease. While Western medicine excels at resolving acute situations, Ayurveda excels as preventive medicine.

It recognizes that every human is a microcosm (a small part or reflection of) the macrocosm (the big picture or universe). Our minds and bodies are made up of the same elements that make up everything else around us; we are moved by the same forces that move the oceans, winds, and planets.

In my practice working with women, imbalances seem to occur and reoccur due to the choices we make, the values that drive us, and the vantage point from which we observe and engage in our lives. Our guiding principles are a huge factor in how our lives, even our health, manifest. According to the ancients, one of the biggest problems for humans is the compulsion to know ourselves as nothing more than a body. I want us to look to a sense of interconnectedness, on a soul level, as a prerequisite for healing. I want us to reach for a healing modality in which nature is our teacher, where the phases of the moon, the wind and rain, and our very life energy (the brightness at the center) are the guiding principles.

The most fascinating thing about women's health is how our bodies are obviously linked to natural forces. Our actions reinforce this truth. Feeling in sync is both a philosophical and a practical endeavor.

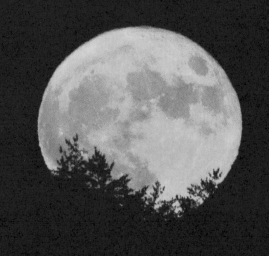

# PART ONE

# FOUNDATIONS *of* AYURVEDA *for* WOMEN

The first time I traveled to India, I didn't have a sense of how far I was from home until I saw the moon. That night, it was a fingernail moon, at an odd angle. It was hanging *sideways*. My jaw dropped, and I stared at the white sliver in the sky. I wondered at how I had traversed the planet to reach this vantage point. Same sky, same eyes, same moon—different place. When the moon turned upside down, my sense of place shifted, and my sense of self expanded. I was taking in not only where I stood, but also how that spot was a tiny point on a cosmic globe. Imagine how visions of the night sky have enriched the consciousness of humans for millennia. What kind of realization might it hold for you?

As my love of India propelled me into the study of Ayurveda, I found the tools of this cosmic science to be surprisingly down-to-earth. It's all about yoking the body to the cosmos through nature's rhythms. Rather than (or in addition to, depending on your proclivities) navel-gazing, we scrape tongues; take stock of poop, pee, and sweat; and eat a seasonal diet. In this physiological integration lies a spiritual integration. Finding Ayurveda was everything I had been seeking: a practical path to self-evolution.

In part one, I share Ayurveda's view of the body, hormones, and generative system, as well as the integration of cosmic factors with our energy bodies.

# 1

# Hormone Balance

## A HOLISTIC PERSPECTIVE

Balance is the central theme in Ayurveda and comes up in relation to women's hormones. Because the interrelated system of hormones in the female body is so complex, it's difficult to pin down why hormones go awry. In Ayurveda, balance is a clear system of checks and balances between the qualities of matter: building and lightening, like anabolic and catabolic energy. This law of thermodynamics is applied to all substances and activities in Ayurveda. What if we applied it to hormones?

The tricky thing is that classic Ayurveda texts don't discuss hormones. With the invention of more advanced measurement techniques, hormones became a research topic only in the early 1900s. We have to look at the roles of hormones in the body and then extrapolate their links to Ayurveda.

Hormones and the endocrine system essentially rely on communication. Certain glands and organs, like the thyroid and pancreas, release chemical hormones directly into the bloodstream. Hormones are messengers that move around the body, triggering and regulating growth, fertility, and metabolism.

Hormones are produced by organs (kidneys, pancreas, ovaries, testes) and by glands (thyroid, pituitary, pineal, hypothalamus, and more). These are the hormones familiar to most of us:

**Reproductive hormones.** Estrogen, progesterone, and testosterone
**Stress hormones.** Adrenaline and cortisol
**Growth hormone.** Human growth hormone (HGH)
**Metabolic hormones.** Insulin and thyroid-stimulating hormone (TSH)

To keep it simple, we will focus on two pairs of opposites: stress and sex hormones.

Hormones maintain balance in bodily functions like growth and metabolism. Modern Ayurveda considers hormones to be subtle forms of *agni* (fire), which governs all transformation and digestion. These subtle messengers do not exist as individuals, but in relationship to each other. Here, the language of hormones can be problematic from a holistic viewpoint. It is difficult to understand hormonal changes in the context of the entire being. Environment, stress, exposure to chemicals, even primal factors such as how we breathe or whether we feel safe, may all influence the original message the body sends to stimulate glands to make or withhold hormones.

What triggers the production of hormones, where, and why, is extremely complex. Zeroing in on a single chemical and regulating it—with a synthetic hormone, for example—does little to address the root cause of a hormonal imbalance. In Ayurveda, a causative factor will continue to make trouble if it goes unrecognized. Imagine trying to plug a leak when the gasket itself is broken.

Hormones influence digestion, sleep, and reproduction, and these functions are interconnected. For example, eating late at night affects sleep. Ayurveda tells us this is because it engages the *pitta* dosha, which is active and hot and opposes the qualities of sleep which is slow, cool, and stable. Western science tells us that digestive enzymes will interfere with the release of sleep hormones—same message, different lexicon.

If we look at sleep problems and other factors of pitta dosha, we may recognize that daily actions have been firing up pitta for a long time, leading to eventual sleep problems. Taking melatonin would just treat the symptom. Ayurveda looks at our daily food intake and sleep flow to reveal the factors that are aggravating pitta, then slowly introduces calming and cooling activities and substances to counteract the imbalance.

While it can be helpful to focus on details, Ayurveda invites us to look at a bigger picture. The good news is that you may find this perspective simpler to understand and easier to work with in your own life.

## THE TWO PLAYERS IN ESSENTIAL BALANCE

The two components of essential balance have many names: *langhana* (lightening) and *brmhana* (building), or *ha* (solar) and *tha* (lunar), as the hatha yogis described; yang and yin, respectively, according to Chinese medicine; catabolic and anabolic by Western names. These basic energy opposites are present in body, mind, planet, and cosmos—get-up-and-go and mellow-down energies. Each influences the mind, blood, glands, and emotions with their qualities: light, hot, and dry versus heavy, cool, and moist. Throughout this book, I use the terms *lightening* or *reducing*, and *building*, as well as *solar* and *lunar*, to describe this duality.

Enjoying solar activity in the daytime and lunar activity at night, for example, is a path of balance. Like increases like, and opposites balance. At its most basic, essential balance and all its fruits are attributed to the right amount of reducing and building. So simple, yet so difficult to maintain. Culturally, solar energy is favored, and modern life tends toward productivity, activity, and stimulation. Introducing lunar energies is a big part of healing.

# AYURVEDA, SEX HORMONES, AND STRESS HORMONES

Hormones tend to have solar or lunar qualities. Some hormones, like adrenaline, speed things up, whereas others, like melatonin, slow things down. If we apply the concepts of reducing and building energies to the hormones associated with women's health, we end up with (surprise!) a basic duality between sex and stress hormone balance.

One of my teachers, Claudia Welch, Doctor of Oriental Medicine, trained in both Ayurveda and Chinese medicine. She is the author of a groundbreaking book, *Balance Your Hormones, Balance Your Life*. In this book, she simplifies stress and sex hormones as yin and yang and describes hormonal imbalance as a systemic imbalance of the two. Her book is a must, a deep dive into her comprehensive research and clinical findings.

Here are the basics:

- Stress hormones are yang—lightening/catabolic, stimulating, and motivating
- Sex hormones are yin—building/nourishing, calming, and grounding

These two groups of hormones and their qualities are always in relationship and are wired to balance naturally. But today's catastrophic levels of stress are interfering with our sex hormones. Read on to see how Dr. Welch explains this and why it matters.

## THE SKINNY ON STRESS

Stress hormones, mainly adrenaline and cortisol, are secreted by the adrenal glands in response to stress. They stimulate and motivate the organism to get out of harm's way. They are secreted together, but adrenaline is responsible for short-term response and cortisol for longer-term. Adrenaline gives you a burst of energy and is eliminated from the bloodstream quickly. Cortisol affects the metabolism and the release of sugars into the blood, and it supports tissue repair. This hormone helps the body hold up in adverse conditions for longer periods. Cortisol sticks around in the bloodstream and can irritate the tissues and organs. Cortisol is released when the body perceives a threat as a stressful situation that is long-term, such as working on a dissertation, as a long-haul migration—a prehistoric stressor. Our cortisol stores are tapped. Stress hormones are also secreted in response to mental stressors, which may be where a lot of our imbalances are generated. When we perceive "adverse conditions," a lot of the time the adrenal glands keep sending cortisol. If we were on that prehistoric migration, the body might need this constant metabolic stimulation, but sitting at the computer all day, all year? Not so much. Signs of a cortisol imbalance are having a sensitivity to loud noise, being easily startled, having a strong and imbalanced startle response, feeling jumpy, and sweating excessively.

Chronic stress means the body doesn't get an opportunity to rest, digest, and dissipate old cortisol from the blood. Over time, this leads to many imbalances, including weight gain, depression, and thyroid dysfunction. Because cortisol increases sugar in the blood, it is linked to the "spare tire" pattern of weight gain often associated with menopause. (Adrenaline and cortisol are not the only hormones secreted for stress, but I am keeping it simple and sticking with the big two.)

## THE SKINNY ON SEX HORMONES

The two dominant sex hormones for women are estrogen and progesterone, estrogen's balance buddy. Estrogen is produced in the ovaries until menopause, when production shifts to the adrenals and many other locations, namely the fat tissue, in smaller amounts. Estrogen can be found in every tissue of the body. Think of estrogen as the builder: it provides juicy qualities, builds the uterine lining, and lends moisture to the skin and generative tissues. Since estrogen's agenda is to build, it needs to be opposed by its buddy progesterone. Too much unopposed estrogen can cause water retention, weight gain, fibroids, and fibrocystic breasts.

While both estrogen and progesterone are builders, progesterone is lighter and warmer than estrogen, so it provides a balance. In the menstrual cycle, for example, estrogen builds the uterine lining; as progesterone increases and body temperature rises during ovulation, it stabilizes the growth and opposes estrogen's building. This allows the uterine lining to mature and provide a field for a fertilized egg. As the end of the cycle arrives, progesterone drops, causing a release of menstrual blood.

Progesterone keeps estrogen levels healthy. But is also acts as a building block for estrogen: it can convert into estrogen when necessary.

## THE STRESS–SEX HORMONE CONNECTION

A body will always prioritize survival over reproduction. The stress response is a response to danger, whether real, anticipated, or imagined. The body's natural habit of prioritizing stress hormones over sex hormones can be strained over years in what Dr. Welch calls "the bucket syndrome." The bucket of sex hormones gets robbed by the bucket of stress hormones, as progesterone shape-shifts into cortisol to supplement the never-ending demand. There is a hole in the bucket: any of the fixes we apply—healthy fats, herbs, or synthetic hormones—will flow out of the hole to fuel stress hormone production until we address the stress, thereby plugging the hole.

Just as progesterone and fats are building blocks for estrogen, they are building blocks for stress hormones as well. Stress steals all the resources. Couple that with a natural decrease in sex hormones after the age of thirty-five, and women need to have a reckoning with stress factors.

Juicier sex hormones act as a stress buffer in our twenties, but we may feel more anxious or less physically, emotionally, mentally, or spiritually resilient as we get into our forties.

Signs of increased stress hormones and depleted sex hormones include fertility problems, increased perimenopause symptoms, irregular periods, weight gain, mood swings, inflammation, and mental or physical burnout.

## Stress Busting

Certain rejuvenating foods and herbs can be used to provide building qualities to oppose the hot, intense nature of stress, but they must be used in tandem with stress reduction or the underlying cause goes unchecked. Working with the rhythms described in part two will address stress, but the following are fundamental principles to consider about how stress manifests.

**Investigate stress.** Some of it is real, and some is perceived. We spend a lot of time worrying about things that haven't happened yet or never will. Stress is a process, not a circumstance.

**Learn to observe first and react later.** A stress trigger happens. . . . Pause. Breathe. This creates the opportunity to respond differently. Moving through life on stress autopilot keeps us from getting to the bottom of what's driving the process.

**Get to the heart of what makes you tick.** The opposite of this is what makes you sick. Intention setting, taking stock, and digging for our deepest desires in life are central for women's agency.

Tectonic shifts in how we *do* life, prioritizing health and happiness, are best undertaken with a sound foundation of routine, ritual, and realization. All this is explained in this book.

## BALANCED LIVING: A PRACTICAL PATH

The Ayurveda way is juicy and full of life, with an essential balance of nature's duality at its core. When you are in a time of full steam ahead, prioritize time for filling thy cup. Consider indulging when digestion is strong rather than when someone else thinks you should, and choose each day's exercise routine based on how much energy you can spend. The body knows what's best, and it's telling you. Listen. Trust. There is a time for everything: enjoy, indulge, work, rest, rejuvenate.

The approach to balanced hormones in this book is threefold:

1. Provide the qualities that support hormonal balance through diet, body therapies, and herbal medicines that can be digested and assimilated well.
2. Move toward integrating daily, seasonal, and lunar rhythms that balance rest, satisfaction, and meaningful work.
3. Nestle each day in a larger context of your stage of life; be present with motivation and value and cosmic influences.

Sometimes it can feel like the world is moving so fast that you'll get lost if you slow down. That is just stress talking. Every healthy choice you make advocates for a balanced way of being in the world.

# 2

# Reenvisioning Your Body

## AYURVEDA BASICS OF FORM AND FUNCTION

The information in this chapter underscores how we look at women's cycles, diets, and stages of life. The building blocks of bodies are the same as those of all matter: the five elements. A human body, like everything in the cosmos, has all five elements working together. The body's elemental composition determines your constitution, or personal makeup of the functional compounds called doshas. The elements, the doshas, and the qualities they all bring to your body make you, *you*.

Ayurveda categorizes the medicinal properties of substances by their elemental composition and their qualities. For example, milk is oily and moist, and lettuce is light.

All substances also contain all five elements: a carrot contains space and gasses, the heat of the sun, and water, while its structure—hard and fibrous—is made of earth. Starting this chapter with the physical factors of how elements manifest in your body and in foods is a tangible first step.

We start with the basics of a body: five elements, three doshas, and twenty qualities. The qualities move us into how to use substances, practices, and lifestyle rhythms to foster essential balance.

## THE BODY AND THE FIVE ELEMENTS

In Ayurveda, all matter is composed of the five elements. Different combinations of these elements make up the variations of form in the universe: a rock versus a cloud, milk versus a carrot, and me versus you.

- Space (also called ether)
- Air (also called wind)
- Fire
- Water
- Earth

Take a few moments to consider where and how each of these elements contributes to your body.

**Space:** Every body has lots of space in it—usually filled with food, acid, fluid, and waste products.

- The digestive tract (from the mouth to the anus) is a long, cavernous tunnel.
- The uterus is designed to hold and release.
- The ear is a delicate organ in which sounds bounce around.
- Bones are porous, hard tissue yet hollow and filled with marrow.
- The skin, our largest organ, is exposed to the qualities of space all the time.

**Air:** Anywhere there is movement, there is air. Space is passive, while air moves around. Anywhere there is space, there will be air. You can feel air on your skin and see it moving the clouds across the sky, but it is not the sky itself.

- Respiration is the movement of air in and out of the nose or mouth.
- Passing gas and belching are movements of air out of the intestines and stomach, respectively.
- The cracking of joints is the sound of air moving out from the spaces between the bones.
- Menstruation, ovulation, and their downward flow require the movement of air.
- The fluctuations of the mind and attention are subtle forms of air movement.

**Fire:** On earth, anywhere there is heat, fire is there: a hot spring, a lightning bolt, a forest fire. The fire of the sun warms the earth, as it does the human body. The core of the earth is fire, just as the human core—the stomach and small intestine—is. All heat in the body comes from fire.

- The stomach and small intestine have hot acids and enzymes.
- The blood, including menstrual blood, is red hot.
- The metabolism "cooks" and refines food with heat.
- Some hormones, such as adrenaline, cortisol, and progesterone, are hot. (Think puberty, PMS, hot flashes, or pregnancy.)
- The function of the eye requires fire. Consider how your eyes can get hot, red, and dry if you overdo it looking at the computer or TV screen.

**Water:** Water covers the planet in rivers, oceans, the cells of plants, and humans. Our bodies are about 60 percent water, and we are filled with liquids.

- All the mucous membranes covering the digestive tract, the eyes, and the sinuses rely on water.
- Water is the basis of the lymphatic fluid flowing through the body.
- Blood contains water.
- Digestive juices contain water.
- The synovial fluid lubricating the joints is the water element that keeps the joints "juicy."
- Saliva is water flowing into the mouth for the first stage of digestion.
- Water supports the juicy aspect of the body, which results in fertility and creativity.
- Estrogen, composed of water and earth, provides moisture to the body, as with cervical fluid.

**Earth:** In nature, earth is anything solid: soil, rocks, trees, and the flesh of animals. This is the solid structure of the body—all the meaty stuff.

- Adipose tissue (fat) is insulation.
- Muscle fiber is the earth element holding the skeleton in place.
- The bone tissue (not the hollow center) that comprises the structure of the skeleton is also the earth element.

Ayurveda views the human organism as a microcosm of the whole universe. When we eat a carrot and transform it, absorbing and assimilating its elements into our tissues, the body takes the water, earth, and other elements of the carrot and incorporates these elements into our own structure, thus linking our bodies to the world.

## THE THREE DOSHAS: HARDWORKING BUT FINICKY

Most people who have heard of Ayurveda have heard of the doshas. These are the functional compounds that arise naturally when the five elements come together in three distinct combinations in an organism. *Dosha* means "that which is at fault." But doshas aren't a problem until an imbalance has been lingering. These energies maintain health when they are in normal states and damage the body if they are in abnormal states. It is more important to understand how to maintain balance than it is to dwell on doshas as the bad guys in the body.

There are three doshas, known as *vata* ("that which moves"), *pitta* ("that which transforms"), and *kapha* (literally, "mucus"). Each performs a specific function in the body and manifests as a recognizable grouping of qualities.

### The Doshas and Their Elements

Vata (that which moves): Space and air

Pitta (that which transforms or digests): Fire and water

Kapha (that which lubricates): Earth and water

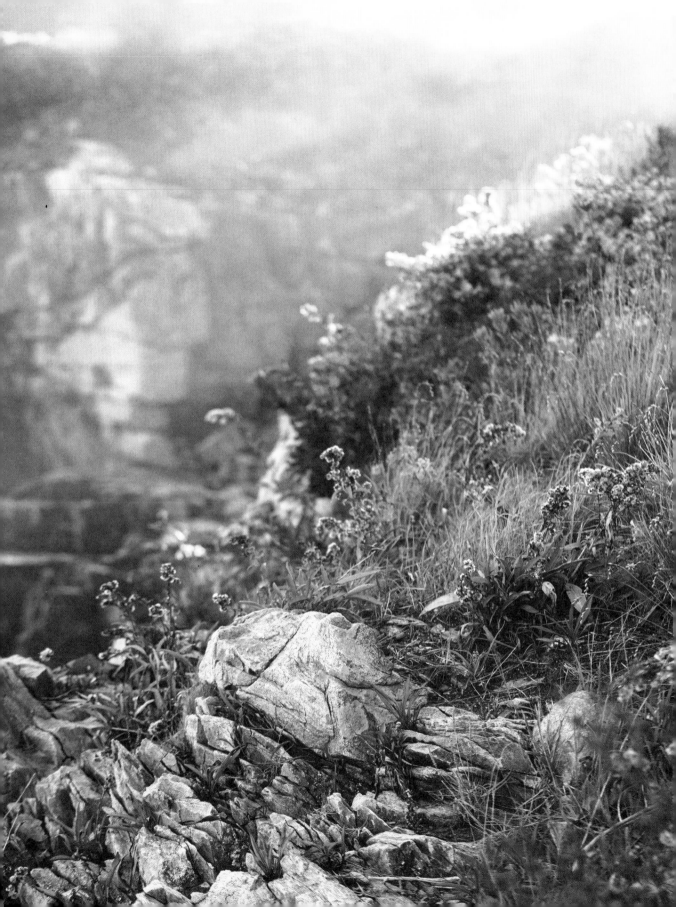

Each of these doshas has sites where it is more prevalent and governs local functions. There are generally early signs in these sites or functions that alert us of an abnormality, such as an increase in gas, anxiety, acid indigestion, poor appetite, menstrual irregularities, or congestion. If a body naturally has more of certain elements, some symptoms may be more familiar than others. If the trajectory of an imbalanced dosha does not shift, the abnormality can eventually cause damage.

Each of the doshas is present in the generative system. Vata circulates through the organs and governs periods, pitta provides heat and red blood cells, and kapha builds the uterine lining and ova. In part three, we discuss how the doshas can affect the menstrual cycle and how they manifest in different life stages, such as pregnancy and menopause.

Knowing the role of the doshas in the generative system—the qualities they provide, the functions they govern, and the basic signs and symptoms of imbalance—can help you monitor your body. This, in turn, can help you make diet and lifestyle choices to support the health of your system. This is where your agency lies: look beyond the symptom to the qualities that are causing it, and you'll have the opportunity to create balance.

## ESSENTIAL BALANCE: REDUCING AND BUILDING QUALITIES

Felt sensations are the key to unlocking knowledge of what your body is telling you and what to do about it. Qualities are involved in any imbalance. For example, acid stomach often arises from drinking too much coffee, a hot, acidic substance in a stomach that is already hot. You might balance this by shifting to a beverage like coconut water or almond milk, both of which are cool and soft.

Qualities are the language we use to talk about food, such as milk being moist and oily and crackers being dry. Once you learn to feel qualities, you will be ready to heal intuitively. (We learn how qualities manifest in foods in part four and in the generative system in chapter 11.)

The basic principle of duality, as we saw in chapter 1, is that our world is made up of coexisting opposites. Like increases like, and opposites balance each other. Toss a damp towel into the hamper, and everything around it also dampens. Hang damp laundry in the hot sun, and it dries. The knowledge of elements and qualities, in yourself and your environment, is the all-access pass to healing.

The qualities, or *gunas*, name the different attributes inherent in all substances. A rock is hard, and a cloud is soft. Chili peppers are sharp, and avocados are smooth. There are ten pairs of gunas with opposing attributes. They describe our world through comparison: it's hot or it's cool; it's sharp or it's smooth. All these pairings represent nature's system of checks and balances that is present in all things, including the human body. When there is an excess (or depletion) of a quality or group of qualities, imbalance can occur.

Ayurveda encourages balance by introducing qualities opposite to those promoting the imbalance and reducing like qualities. For instance, in winter you might enjoy a bit of spicy food to warm you up, but avoid it in summer when the environment is already warm. The same may be true of reducing heating foods during the warmer phase of the menstrual cycle. All the substances and experiences used as medicine (plants, meats, fruits, minerals, and activities) have an effect on the body which is experienced as one or more of the qualities. For example, spicy food makes you feel hot and sweaty; the effect of spicy food is heating and oily. Watermelon makes you feel cool and refreshed; the effect of watermelon is cool and light.

The qualities are divided into two opposing categories: brmhana, or building, and langhana, or lightening. Building increases tissues, whereas lightening reduces them.

- **Building qualities are anabolic.** They build mass and nourish the tissues; encourage moisture; and strengthen, ground, and stabilize the body, ova, mind, and nerves. Healthy reproductive juices result from well-digested building qualities. Examples are comfort foods that make the body feel warm, cozy, and safe, such as warm milk, root vegetable soups, meats, and hot cereals.
- **Lightening qualities are catabolic.** They reduce mass, the tissues, and excess water and mucus, and they put a spring in your step. Reducing foods are cleansing. They lighten up heavy periods and oppose tissue growth. Lightening foods feel refreshing and energizing. Examples of light foods are steamed vegetables with lemon, bitter greens, berries, clear soups, and ginger tea.

# Twenty Gunas: The Ten Builders and Their Opposites

To ground the qualities in experience, the following chart provides characteristics of each guna, examples of foods and activities where each guna is present, and signs to recognize each guna in the body, as well as potential symptoms that could signal its excess.

| GUNA (PAIR) | CHARACTERISTICS | FOODS | ACTIVITIES | SIGNS & SYMPTOMS |
|---|---|---|---|---|
| HEAVY | Dense, solid | Cow cheese, fatty meats, saturated fats, | Sedentary activities | Heavy periods; fibroids |
| LIGHT | Airy, fluffy | Broth, greens, berries, watery vegetables | Vigorous exercise and meditation | Low-flow periods or amenorrhea; difficulty sleeping |
| SLOW | Sedate, relaxed | Fried foods, beef | Overeating, oversleeping, sedentary, slow yoga | Dull type of period pain; fibroids and cysts |
| SHARP / INTENSE | Cutting, clears sinuses, increases appetite | Wasabi, vinegar, pepper, ground ginger | Vigorous exercise, doing math or trivia games | Frequent periods, hot and painful periods, hot flashes |
| COOL | Calm and refreshed | Cilantro, cucumber, lime, coconut, cool drinks | Swimming in cold water, drinking iced water, catching a chill | Feeling cold, especially during period and menopause |
| HOT | Flushed, acidic, fiery | Chilis, citrus, coffee, pepper | Smoking, hot yoga, sunbathing | Heavy or long periods, hot flashes |

| GUNA (PAIR) | CHARACTERISTICS | FOODS | ACTIVITIES | SYMPTOMS & SIGNS |
|---|---|---|---|---|
| OILY/ UNCTUOUS | Viscous, moist, greasy | All oils; foods containing natural oils, such as nuts, fish, seeds, olives | Oil massage, Castor oil pack | Pimples, acne, oily skin and hair |
| DRY | Brittle, hard, thirsty | Corn, large beans, barley, caffeine, crackers | Travel, especially on planes; wind; dry brushing | Light periods; possible skipped ovulation; vaginal dryness |
| SMOOTH | Polished, soothing, soft | Avocado, ripe mango, banana, slippery elm | Taking a bath, swimming, even breathing | Easy elimination; soft skin, hair, and nails |
| ROUGH | Dry, coarse, crunchy | Corn chips, coarse flours, raw vegetables | Jogging in the cold | Dry skin and hair, light periods, skipped periods or ovulation |
| DENSE/ SOLID | Thick, heavy, opaque | Meat, cheese, gluten, dates | Sedentary, using a weighted blanket | Dull period pain, uterine fibroids and cysts, fibrocystic breasts |
| LIQUID | Runny, diluted, aqueous | Broth and soups, tea | Sweating, steaming | Loose stools, copious menstrual flow |

| GUNA (PAIR) | CHARACTERISTICS | FOODS | ACTIVITIES | SIGNS & SYMPTOMS |
|---|---|---|---|---|
| SOFT | Mushy, supple, moist | Mashed potatoes, Brie cheese, baked squash, fruit compote | Gentle yoga, oil massage, yoni steaming | Smooth skin, hair, and nails |
| HARD | Stiff, dry, tough | Corn nuts, rye crackers, very crisp apples, grains and beans that aren't fully cooked | Competitive or aggressive forms of exercise, extreme cold weather | Sharp period pain; spotting before menstrual cycle, back pain |
| STABLE | Safe, comfortable, steady | Meat, dairy, miso, nuts, oils, salt | Staying in one place, following a routine | Regular periods; few perimenopause symptoms |
| MOBILE | Active, restless | Spicy foods, raw foods, juices, bubbly water | Traveling or relocating | Racing thoughts, irregular periods |

| GUNA (PAIR) | CHARACTERISTICS | FOODS | ACTIVITIES | SIGNS & SYMPTOMS |
|---|---|---|---|---|
| CLOUDY/ SLIMY/ STICKY | Adherent, glutinous, hard to get rid of | Cream, cheese, white bread, yeasty beers | Taking prescription drugs, spending too much time indoors | Clogged pores, brain fog, heavy painful periods, fibroids and cysts, polycystic ovary syndrome |
| CLEAR | Transparent, unclouded | Cucumbers and watery vegetables, broths, herbal teas, plain water | Deep breathing, meditating, spending time outdoors | No period pain, easy conception |

| GUNA (PAIR) | CHARACTERISTICS | FOODS | ACTIVITIES | SIGNS & SYMPTOMS |
|---|---|---|---|---|
| GROSS/BIG | The physical body, the material world | Building foods, such as meat, wheat, and dairy | Overeating, grounding | Heavy periods, fibroids and cysts |
| SUBTLE/ MINUTE | The energy body, breath, minute channels like blood vessels | Bitters, fresh herbs, spices, greens | Yoga, breathwork, healing arts, and meditation | Feeling ungrounded |

## QUALITIES AND DOSHAS

Each body has a unique physical makeup. There is no one-size-fits-all approach in Ayurveda; instead, acceptance of the elemental makeup of your body and how to work with this truth brings optimal wellness. One person moves fast, another slow; one person runs hot, another cold; one woman bleeds more than another during her cycle. Everything in this universe has strengths and weaknesses. Culturally, we often think one thing is "better" than another, but of course, it depends. If we are hiking Mount Everest, the hot type has an easier time. If we are in the desert, the cold person is the lucky one. Knowing our own strengths and weaknesses helps us support our bodies with appropriate diets and lifestyles. We thrive when we understand what is "normal" for each of us rather than following a regimen imposed on us without insight.

The doshas are essentially groups of sensations that, due to their nature, occur together and lend themselves to specific bodily functions, such as the hot, sharp, oily qualities of pitta in the stomach for digestion and the cool, slimy qualities of kapha in the vaginal canal for lubrication. Here I describe the gunas of each dosha, which makes these physiological compounds sensual and recognizable. When you are picturing a dosha, always be sure to imagine its qualities. This will help you understand which dosha is acting on your menstrual cycle, for example. Imagine the qualities of a dosha in the menstrual blood: vata will be dry and constricting, pitta hot, and kapha heavy and dense.

## THE QUALITIES OF VATA

Where there is space, air begins to move, and the compound qualities of space and air manifest as cold, light, dry, rough, mobile, and clear (think wind). Space and air have no heat, moisture, or heaviness.

Think of vata as currents; it ushers food and fluids through the body. There is nothing problematic about the qualities of space and air or their function, but too many vata qualities in the body can dry things out, resulting in signs of imbalance such as gas and constipation, increasingly dry skin, scanty periods, and anxiety.

Healthy vata ensures that the body has
- Consistent elimination
- Free breathing
- Good circulation
- Keen senses
- Regular menstrual cycles

Too many vata qualities may cause
- Gas and constipation
- Cold hands and feet
- Anxiety/feeling overwhelmed
- Difficulty sleeping
- Irregular cycles

## THE QUALITIES OF PITTA

Where there is fire, there has to be water to keep it in check. The resulting compound is fire-water, a liquid, hot, sharp, penetrating, light, spreading, oily, smelly group of qualities. (Think acid and bile.) When you chew food, pitta moves in to break it down, liquidize it, metabolize it, and transform it into red blood and tissues. There is no problem with that, unless of course your insides get too hot or too sharp, which can result in signs of imbalance such as acid burps or reflux, diarrhea, infertility, or inflammation.

**Healthy pitta creates**

- Good appetite and metabolism
- Steady hormones
- Sharp eyesight
- Comprehension
- Good complexion (glowing skin)

**Too many pitta qualities might cause**

- Acid indigestion/reflux
- Dysmenorrhea (painful menstruation)
- Red, dry eyes; the need for glasses
- Tendency to overwork
- Acne, rosacea
- Irritability

## THE QUALITIES OF KAPHA

Only when you add water to sand does it stick together. The earth element requires water in this same way to hold the body together. Kapha is like glue: cool, liquid, slimy, heavy, slow, dull, dense, and stable. This group of qualities provides density in the bones and fat, cohesion in the tissues and joints, healthy ova, and plenty of mucus so we don't dry out. If the body becomes too heavy and too sticky, it can result in signs of imbalance such as loss of appetite, slow digestion, congestion, weight gain, fibroids, and fibrocystic breasts.

**Healthy kapha provides**

- Strong body tissues
- Well-lubricated joints and mucous membranes
- Hearty immune system
- Robust menstrual blood
- Fertility

**Too many kapha qualities might cause**

- Weight gain
- Water retention
- Sinus or lung congestion
- Lethargy and sadness
- Uterine stagnation and painful periods
- Cysts and fibroids

## LOCATIONS AND FUNCTIONS OF THE DOSHAS

Each of the doshas has its own territory and specific roles in the body. Kapha predominates in the head, lungs, and stomach; pitta in the midsection; and vata below the waist. It is important to note that *all of the generative organs are within vata territory*. This makes the vata dosha the most likely instigator in imbalances of the generative system.

**Vata (pronounced "VA-tah")**, the energy of movement, is most prevalent below the navel, specifically in the colon, rectum, bladder, uterus, ovaries, thighs, lower back, and legs. It is responsible for elimination, urination, menstruation, ovulation, and circulation, as well as the activity of the sense organs.

**Pitta (pronounced "PITT-ah")**, the energy of transformation, is most prevalent around the midsection, specifically the stomach and small intestine, and in the blood. It is responsible for digesting and absorbing food; making red blood cells and menstrual blood; supporting healthy cognition, eyesight, and hormonal secretions; and maintaining the warmth and complexion of the body.

**Kapha (pronounced "CUP-hah")**, the energy of cohesion, is most prevalent in the head and chest, as well as the upper stomach and fatty tissues. Kapha also makes up the eggs, sperm, and reproductive juices. It is responsible for maintaining the physical structure and immunity of the body; supporting the memory; and providing moisture in the stomach and mouth, sinuses, lungs, joints, and generative tissues.

## PRAKRITI: THE NATURE OF THE BODY

The body's constitution or makeup of the elements, called *prakriti*, is like DNA and is inherited mostly from one's birth parents. Doshas can fluctuate, but the baseline of the body, its intended state of being, has been set. People who are "tridoshic" have an even balance of all three doshas and generally enjoy better health. Those who have one or two primary doshas may be likely to experience imbalances of those same doshas.

Prakriti determines the qualities prevalent in your body and how you react to certain foods or activities. For example, a kapha type can expect heavier, moister qualities, which may manifest as a heavier menses or more viscous menstrual blood, because kapha is dense and sticky. People tend to fixate on knowing their constitution, but the qualities are actually how to balance the body.

# 3

# Reclaiming Women's Anatomy in Ayurveda

Imagine that you were never given language (no labels) and had only the tool of observation to understand life. We take many things for granted about our bodies, like "menstrual cycles are twenty-eight days," because they are explained to us. We have been taught that *explaining* is the pinnacle of understanding, when in fact there is so much knowledge we already *feel* about our bodies and more we can uncover through observation and experience.

Ayurveda invites us to see everything anew, to learn an experiential language. The words to describe the body are all things we feel, like heat and cold, moisture and dryness: wisdom filtered through experience and simmered to an intuitive essence. Once you have the tool—embodied language—you can qualify *your* experience of *your* body and get to know *yourself* through this lens.

In sharing and insisting on our use of Ayurveda's language for generative anatomy, my mission is to empower you with a new way to perceive this aspect of the body. These organs, systems, and functions are all integrated parts of one sacred package: YOU.

We do not need to throw out the centuries of knowledge gained by Western science, but we want to get it working with Ayurveda. Pairing Western science and Ayurveda provides a model that makes sense without using exclusionary language and instead using words that can be experienced. In this chapter, we begin with a crash course in the sexual organs and functions. You don't have to memorize the Sanskrit terms to gain understanding, and there's no harm in jumping ahead to part two if you just want to start exploring healthy lifestyle routines and come back to all this later.

Ayurveda terminology has so much inherent meaning that you may find the concepts simple to integrate. Many Sanskrit anatomical words are visualizations, whereas many English anatomical terms feel clinical.

For example, try replacing a word like "fertility" with *shukra*, which is the essential generative ingredient, the refined end product of our food that produces the immunity cream of life. Something present at any stage of life that is created at the intersection of food, metabolism, and vitality.

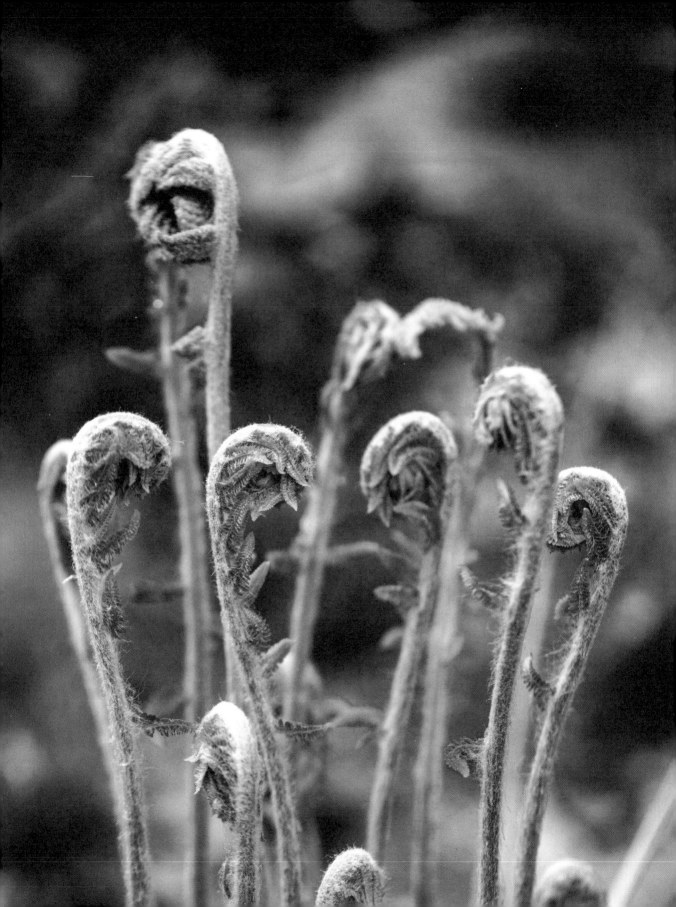

# THE MAP OF THE YONI

I started calling my vagina a yoni in college, upon hearing it from other women in my circle. According to the Oxford English Dictionary, *yoni*, with roots in the Sanskrit and Hebrew languages, means "the vulva, especially as a symbol of divine procreative energy conventionally represented by a circular stone." According to Merriam-Webster's dictionary, *yoni* is "a stylized representation of the female genitalia that in Hinduism is a sign of generative power and that symbolizes the goddess Shakti." Yoni describes a symbol, one that is revered as a goddess and a creative energy center, not the anatomical generative organs.

While Western science provides a detailed, compartmentalized view of the organs in female anatomy—ovaries, uterus, fallopian tubes, and so on—Ayurveda is always more interested in physiology (what an organ does) than anatomy (what an organ is named). Descriptions in the texts are more functional, which is a systems science view. In Ayurveda, we take a step back and look at the jobs being performed by these organs, how they work together, what's working smoothly and what's not, and observable rhythms and patterns to come to an understanding of what are "normal" or healthy functions and what are abnormalities.

We are looking at the body's systems, which are made up of tissues and channels. Tissues, like blood and bones, are static, whereas channels, like the intestines, are dynamic. First, I have created a broad overview of the types of tissues and channels in the body, and then we will home in on those related to the yoni and the generative system.

## Building Blocks of the Body

As we saw earlier, the physical body is made up of the five **elements**: space, air, fire, water, and earth.

These elements compound into three **doshas**: vata, pitta, and kapha.
The doshas bring their qualities and energies to the body and govern specific functions.
The physicality of the body—its tangible, five-element makeup—is observed as seven different kinds of **tissue**: generative, nerve/marrow, bone, fat, muscle, blood, and plasma.
The seven *dhatus* are the distinct tissue types that maintain the structure of the body.
The final, most refined tissue layer is the generative organs.

## DHATUS: THE SEVEN TISSUES

The seven dhatus are the distinct tissue types that maintain the structure of the body.

Each of these tissue types is made of its own kind of cells: white blood cells, muscle cells, generative DNA, and so on. Each of the tissues is uniform in quality and made of a particular combination of elements. Some of the tissues, like fat, require heavier and denser physical qualities, while others, like bone marrow, are lighter and subtler. Taking in foods that have similar qualities to a dhatu will increase it, while not taking in enough of a certain flavor profile will cause a dhatu to decrease.

Building strong tissues requires the right kind of building blocks. Certain substances have affinities for certain tissues. For example, cow's milk has moist, cool, heavy qualities that resemble the generative tissues. Ghee has unctuous, penetrating, and cooling qualities that balance the heat produced by stress in the nervous system. Where the fertility components—eggs and sperm—are concerned, we look for nutrition that comes from moist, cool, and heavy substances.

The tissue types move inward from the outer body and become increasingly refined. Here are the seven dhatus in order, from superficial to deep: *rasa* (plasma), *rakta* (red blood), *mamsa* (muscle), *meda* (fat), *asthi* (bone), *majja* (nerve and marrow), and *shukra/artava* (generative organs). This is important because your food nourishes the layers in this same order: rasa dhatu receives the nourishment first, digests what it needs, sends along the rest to rakta dhatu, and so on. For the health of the generative tissues (*seventh* down the line), a robust rasa dhatu is the key. If rasa is strong, the generative tissue of shukra/artava is more likely to be nourished.

In this book, we go into great detail on three of the dhatus: rasa (plasma), rakta (red blood), and artava (generative tissues) to cover the physiology of the blood, uterus, fallopian tubes, and ovaries. You can find extensive information on all the dhatus and their nourishment in my book *The Everyday Ayurveda Guide to Self-Care*.

## THE CIRCULATION AND MOVEMENT CHANNELS

A distinctly helpful aspect of the Ayurveda view of women's health is the importance of the circulation of *prana* in the channels of the generative system; this circulation is called the *artava-vahasrotas* (artava, for short). The entire body is composed of a tubular network that carries nutrition, waste, and communications where they need to go. A disruption to the body's state of flow can come from stress, a sedentary lifestyle, injury, or clogging of the channels. As much of the generative system and its organs lie in the lower abdomen, constipation, tight pants, and too much sitting are examples of factors that can disturb flow. Since Ayurveda prioritizes physiology over anatomy and doesn't compartmentalize the physical and the functional, good circulation is key. A healthy diet, regular movement, and periodic detoxing are Ayurveda's tools for healthy circulation in the generative system.

Many yoga postures, breathing techniques, and visualizations are also designed to increase circulation and break up blockages in the *srotas* (channels). Yoga texts also point toward an extremely subtle set of channels called *nadis*, through which energy travels throughout the body. The entire body is connected—physically, mentally, and energetically—through a subtle circulatory network.

## ANATOMY AT A GLANCE

The following table lists all the anatomy terms we use throughout this book. I offer clear meanings here so we can move forward with a common vocabulary, but please remain open to different interpretations of these terms in your future studies or in other books.

### Physical Components of Women's Anatomy

| | |
|---|---|
| RASA DHATU | Plasma, lymph |
| RAKTA DHATU | Red blood |
| ARTAVA DHATU | Classical definition: menstruation; ovum<br>This book: all the generative organs |
| RAJAH | Menstrual blood |
| SHUKRA | Reproductive juice; fertility factor; sperm |
| OJAS | The immune factor; the most refined essence of nutrition |
| YONI | The external part of artava (vaginal opening, labia, clitoris) |

### Functional Components of Women's Anatomy

| | |
|---|---|
| RASAVAHASROTAS | The channel of nutrition that penetrates the entire body |
| RAKTAVAHASROTAS | The channel that circulates the blood |
| ARTAVAVAHASROTAS | The generative system |
| APANA VAYU | The downward-moving aspect of vata |

# WHY NUTRITION IS EVERYTHING: RASA DHATU AND RASAVAHASROTAS

The word *rasa* means "juice"—literally, as in a fruit juice, but also figuratively, as in feeling "juicy." Rasa is anatomically the juice of life, and its channel (*rasavahasrotas*) circulates this juice into all your parts. It is the liquid component of the blood that makes up 55 percent of your blood's total volume, and it is full of nutrition, all the building blocks your body needs. Imagine a tree with no sap or a seedling with no rainwater; that is life without rasa—sagging, dry, and sad. Like sap, this liquid runs throughout the body, providing nourishment to each of the dhatus in turn.

This aspect of the body is what makes a person appear and feel full of life. The clear liquid substance in blood, called plasma, is made up of water, salts, enzymes, white blood cells, and proteins. In Ayurveda, rasa dhatu contains all five elements, mostly water, and its function is to nourish the body. The entire lymphatic system is made up of rasa dhatu, which makes it an important player in detoxification as well as nutrition. It is the only tissue that circulates and penetrates the entire body, which makes it the most important layer to care for. The *Charaka Samhita* tells us that from rasa, "the digestive product of food," is derived "continuity of strength, satisfaction, plumpness, and enthusiasm."[1]

Satisfaction and enthusiasm are more than physical concepts. *Rasa* does not only refer to nutrient juice; the word also means essence, emotion, melodious sound, artistic expression, and aesthetic appreciation. Healthy rasa invokes sweetness, love, and faith—the flow of emotion.

## THE PROCESS OF NOURISHMENT

Let's take a tour of how food becomes rasa dhatu and how rasa dhatu builds the rest of the tissues. Rasa is the essence of a body, and the essence of a food and its ability to nourish us. The word *rasa*, when we talk about food, also means "taste." Taste is one way the body recognizes the elements present in a food. For example, a juicy fruit contains water, and a spicy pepper contains fire. When we taste food, we perceive its essence, its rasa. Here, the digestive process begins; the body receives signals to prepare for what's coming. The stomach secretes water element, and the digestive enzymes contribute fire. Together, these two make the "fire-water" of pitta that digests the food.

In the small intestine, the juice is further refined by enzymes to form *ahara rasa* (literally, "food-juice"). This process from mouth to food-juice takes at least three hours. When this nutritional essence of the food is absorbed into the bloodstream by capillaries in the intestinal walls, you have the precursor for rasa dhatu. This liquid nourishment is further refined and then builds the red blood cells, blood builds the muscles, muscles build the fat, fat builds the bones,

bones build the marrow, and marrow builds the generative tissues. Like an irrigation system, the proteins, carbs, minerals, fats, and vitamins wash into the tissues of the body, and the tissues, in conjunction with the fire element, refine the nutrients further until all the tissues of the body are refreshed and satisfied. Satisfaction is a distinct feeling you can learn to recognize.

This process takes at least a month: building rasa dhatu from food takes five days, then five days each for the remaining tissue layers. These time frames aren't exact but do provide a sense of how long it takes to nourish and rejuvenate the body. Rejuvenation is the result of a steady commitment to nourishment over time.

It's a part of this nutrition story that the importance of how, what, and when we eat becomes paramount. The generative system is the farthest from the source of satisfaction and the first to suffer a deficiency. Proper digestion and nutrition (all of which are described in chapter 7) give you the sense of enthusiasm that results from a healthy rasa and so much more.

According to the *Charaka Samhita*, breast milk and menstrual blood are formed from rasa. For those who menstruate and may breastfeed, rasa dhatu is especially important in maintaining healthy function in these areas. Problems in rasa dhatu will likely show up as disorders in breast milk or menstrual blood, such as low milk production or scanty periods. These two very visible aspects of the body may signal a nutrient deficiency or dry quality acting on the rasa and can send an SOS early on, when imbalances can easily be rectified.

Later in life, rasa is essential to anti-aging factors. The top layer of the skin is a secondary tissue, like menstrual blood and breast milk, which signals the health of rasa dhatu. Skin is the largest organ of the body; it is completely visible and of great significance in Ayurveda for diagnostic as well as therapeutic purposes. (Massage with herbal oils and steams are among the remedies involving the skin that we will discuss in chapter 5.) A robust rasa dhatu will provide clear, soft, smooth skin that has just the right amount of plumpness and moisture. The body naturally dries as we age, and preserving rasa through diet and body therapies can turn back the clock!

Signs of Healthy Rasa
- Smooth, soft skin
- Robust menstruation and lactation
- Enthusiasm
- Good level of energy

## RECOGNIZING IMBALANCES IN RASA DHATU

Rasa dhatu's importance is not only its preservation of youth but also its provision of strong tissues, immunity, and emotional resilience. The qualities of this liquid factor should be cool, oily, a little heavy, slow, and smooth—similar to kapha. Imbalances can occur due to dryness or too much oiliness, stickiness, and heaviness. Too much heat can dry out rasa dhatu, as can excessive worry and stress. Too much sticky, oily food can clog it up.

It is important to recognize problems in rasa dhatu. It is much easier to remedy an imbalance in the first tissue than in the deeper ones. Bone tissue, for example, is much more difficult to fix than plasma. The simple way to look at this is to observe two general causes for imbalance in rasa: brmhana (building) qualities and langhana (lightening) qualities. When the basic balance of catabolic and anabolic energies is off, we can observe signs of overnourishment and undernourishment affecting our nutrient layer. A sticky rasa resulting from too many heavy, oily qualities can manifest as water retention, fibrocystic breasts, body aches, or general lassitude. Taking in too much fried food, liquid, and sweets can bring a person to this state. An undernourished rasa from too many light and dry qualities can show up as unwarranted fatigue, scanty periods, and excessively dry skin and hair. Contributing factors include dehydration; too many raw, light, and bitter foods; dry snacks like chips and crackers; and undereating.

The remedy is always to introduce foods, activities, and therapies that have the qualities you need more of and cut down on those that have the qualities you're displaying too much of. You are what you eat!

Healthy rasa is all about diet and digestion. This tissue is so close to the liquid produced by our food that dietary factors impact rasa most. An essential note: the qualities of rasa dhatu go on to build the other tissues as well, so its dry or sticky qualities can be pervasive. Not only diet (what we ingest) but also how well we digest it is paramount to maintaining balance. Imagine trying to nourish an undernourished person who has a slow digestive fire. Making sure the food we eat is efficiently processed within the body is so important, and keeping a balance in the qualities of our foods ensures tissues don't get too heavy or too light. Maintaining quality rasa hinges on diet and digestion. (You can get the scoop on that in chapters 7 and 8.)

**Recipes to Purify Rasa**
    Cleansing Herbal Infusion (page 222)
    Essential Spiced Water (page 231)
    Moringa Green Drink Three Ways
        (page 250)

**Recipes to Build Rasa**
    Date Shake (page 243)
    Moon Milk (page 247)
    Sexy Cacao (page 249)

# SHUKRA: THE SEXY JUICE

As we have seen, rasa dhatu is the nutritive precursor for the whole body. After being refined by agni at each tissue layer throughout the digestive process, the end product is a superfine essence that is responsible for vigor and strength, called *ojas*. The penultimate product of this refinement is shukra. The word *shukra* is used in two ways. One is to describe semen. The other is a broader concept, which is both physical and subtle. During sexual excitement, fluid secreted from bone marrow is said to ooze from the pores in the bones "like water exuding from a new earthen pot"[2] and then circulate throughout the entire body. Artava is useful in conception, while shukra is responsible for a woman's energy.[3] We might equate shukra to sex hormones and growth hormones in this context.

Imagine a subtle-yet-tangible creative juice at the center of your bones that is released through a desire to create. This is shukra, the sexy juice. This energy can be directed toward the creation of progeny or creative endeavors that feed the soul. In Ayurveda, one branch of medicine is called *vajikarana*, the administration of aphrodisiacs, which are used to build strength and sexual vigor. Vajikarana foods and medicines can be used to rebuild shukra, which is diminished by overwork, age, stress, worry, and too much sexual activity. Shukra is an important place to build a sense of potency and creativity at any stage of life.

(You will find a table of vajikarana foods in appendix B.)

## Shukra and Fertility

I use the word *shukra* to encompass the generative juices in any body. For the purposes of this book, we will use the term *artava* (short for artavavahasrotas) to refer to the female generative system at large, and *shukra*—which is sometimes used to describe sperm, or the srotas of the male generative system—to mean the creativity principle and generative juices.

Artava refers to the whole package of the female generative system, primarily its movement aspects. Shukra is the fertility component, including not only the egg itself but also cervical fluid; vaginal secretions; and sexy juice, the physical essence of one's creative potency.

# OJAS AND IMMUNITY

After the formation of shukra and artava, the very finest remaining essence of our food, refined over and over, is ojas. While shukra refers to sexual potency, ojas is the body's innate immunity, its resistance to disease. Ojas is so important in the Ayurveda view because the path of health is to render the body stronger than the disease. Cultivation and preservation of ojas is an ongoing process.

Like maple syrup boiled down from crude sap, ojas is the nectar of nutrition, and it takes volumes of food and days of digestion to produce a small amount. During the process of digestion and metabolism, a small amount of ojas is released into each tissue layer before the remaining nutrition is passed on to the next layer. This provides immunity and strength for each tissue. The refined end product, which takes roughly thirty days to produce from food, results in ojas for the vitality and longevity of the entire body.

Ojas is unctuous and cool, milk-like. It is depleted by stress and worry, excessive exercise, undernourishment, and basically overdoing it. Ojas is seated in the heart and brain. In Ayurveda, nourishing the heart and mind, as well as the body, is part of a holistic approach to building strength.

Medicinal substances called *jivaniya* (substances that give life and promote vitality) are used to restore ojas; such substances include milk, ghee, and meat-based soup. Ojas is best preserved by lifestyle factors like moderation, getting enough nourishment and rest, and practicing "rejuvenating behaviors" (see chapter 8). Cultivating a lifestyle that preserves ojas is key; practiced in tandem with including vital foods in the diet, it leads to fertility and longevity.

The digestive sisterhood of shukra and ojas—immunity, vitality, and the sense of creative purpose we crave in life—results from a mindful preservation and cultivation of deep nourishment. This process works best with the combined approach of optimizing digestion and nutrition, as well as practicing a wholesome lifestyle (see part two).

### Signs of Good Ojas

- Happiness
- Balanced mental and sensory faculties
- Nourished body
- Strong immunity
- Balanced libido

### Signs of Depleted Ojas

- Weakness, low energy
- Hypersensitive sense organs
- Sallow complexion
- Mental confusion
- Increased dryness, for example dry skin and hair
- Low libido

### Causes of Depleted Ojas

- Anger
- Poor nutrition
- Constant thinking or worrying
- Grief
- Excessive exertion or exercise

### Recipes to Promote Vitality and Ojas

Date Shake (page 243)

Black Sesame Balls (page 303)

Almond Cardamom Diamonds (page 306)

Moon Milk (page 247)

You can also find a table of foods that promote ojas in appendix B.

## BLOOD: RAKTA DHATU AND ITS CHANNEL OF CIRCULATION

The word *rakta* means "red." While what we usually think of as blood contains both rasa and rakta dhatus, it is the rakta that contains red blood cells, and these two parts of the blood have different compositions and functions. This tissue is made up of fire and water elements; it is hot; and its function is *jivana* ("life-giving"), or the oxygenation of the body by red blood cells. These cells are created in the red bone marrow but rely on the nutritive juice provided by rasa dhatu for good production.

Life breath is transported throughout the body by rakta dhatu. A healthy rakta dhatu will result in a zest for life, glowing complexion, robust menstrual blood, and a visible luster, especially to the skin and eyes. Rakta dhatu is closely associated with menstrual blood but is not considered the same substance.

## RECOGNIZING IMBALANCES IN RAKTA DHATU

The composition of this tissue layer, fire and water elements, is so similar to pitta dosha that one is generally going to see pitta problems manifest in rakta. All the foods that aggravate pitta—sour, salty, and spicy substances—are the ones that cause imbalances in rakta dhatu. The tendency is for red blood to get too hot or too oily, which can result in feeling overheated, irritable, smelly, and sticky/sweaty. As rakta circulates close to the skin, it is—in conjunction with pitta—the culprit in a lot of skin disorders. Pitta-type people are those who may benefit the most from moderating factors that heat the body, such as sunbathing, hot yoga, and spicy, oily foods.

The oily quality is an instigator here, as the viscosity of the blood is important to healthy circulation and the maintenance of clean channels. Over time, blood that is sour, hot, or too sticky can begin to alter the state of the vessels it moves through, leading to arthritis, high cholesterol, bleeding tendencies, and liver problems. An increased *quantity* of blood, also due to increased pitta qualities, contributes to hypertension and stress on the heart.

The great news is that rakta dhatu, close in proximity to the postdigestive rasa, responds well to dietary factors. Eating and drinking bitter and astringent substances, such as green veggies and Cooling Herbal Infusion (page 220)—which is packed with blood-balancing herbs—keeps the blood in a balanced state.

Exercise can also improve circulation and induce sweat, eliminating some of the wastes from rakta dhatu. You may notice after drinking too much coffee or alcohol, for example, that your sweat is stinkier, or more acrid. If it clears out in a day or two, great; but if an abnormal-for-you kind of stink is sticking around, this is a sign of rakta dhatu imbalance.

As with rasa, there are two kinds of rakta imbalances: too hot and oily, or depleted. Over-heated rakta often comes from overindulging in alcohol, ferments, spicy foods, or stress. This kind of imbalance can lead to heavy, painful periods and hot flashes. Depletion can be due to a lack of vitamins and minerals due to poor diet or digestion, and it leads to exhaustion and light or skipped periods.

These are a few recipes for balancing rakta. All contain minerals and cooling factors that optimize the qualities of red blood.

Refreshing Phanta Infusion (page 221)

Aloe-Pom-Cran Tonic (page 254)

Moringa Green Drink Three Ways (page 250)

Raisin Mantha (page 261)

# Rajah: Menstrual Blood

Menstrual blood is called *rajah* and has its own channel, which includes the uterus, vaginal canal, and its opening (the vulva). Menstrual blood is considered a different substance than rakta, red blood, but both are nourished by rasa dhatu. Menstrual blood is less viscous than arterial blood and contains less iron and fewer red blood cells. One could say it's less concentrated: it is a combination of blood and endometrial cells.

Ayurveda tells us that it takes an entire month for rasa dhatu to mature and create rajah, and that rasa is converted into semen (shukra) in men and rajah in women. The healthy color of rajah is said to be that of a fruit called *gunja*, which is similar to the color of a holly berry. The amount of menstrual blood varies depending on each person's constitution.

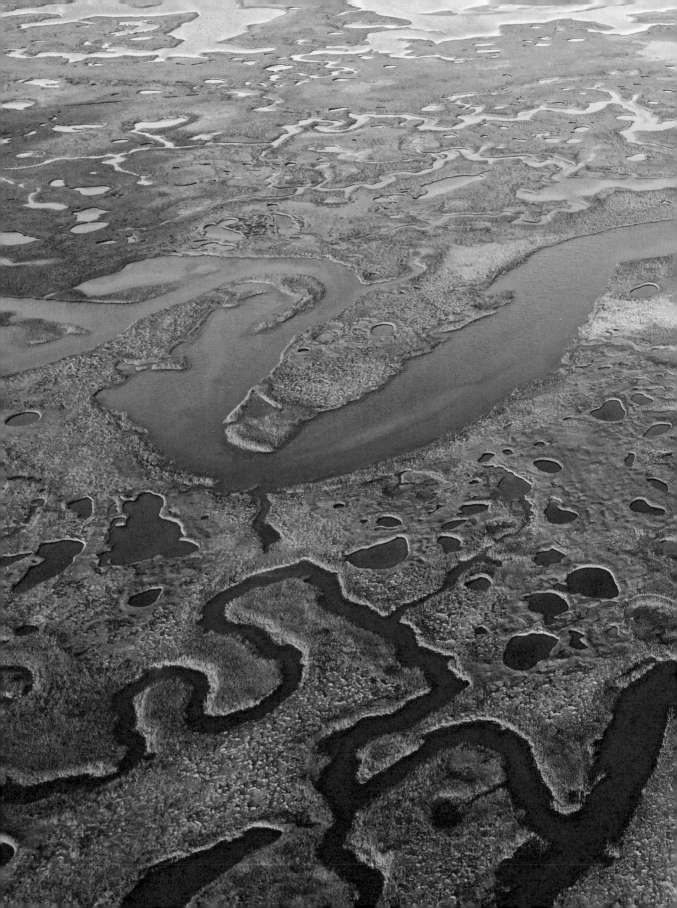

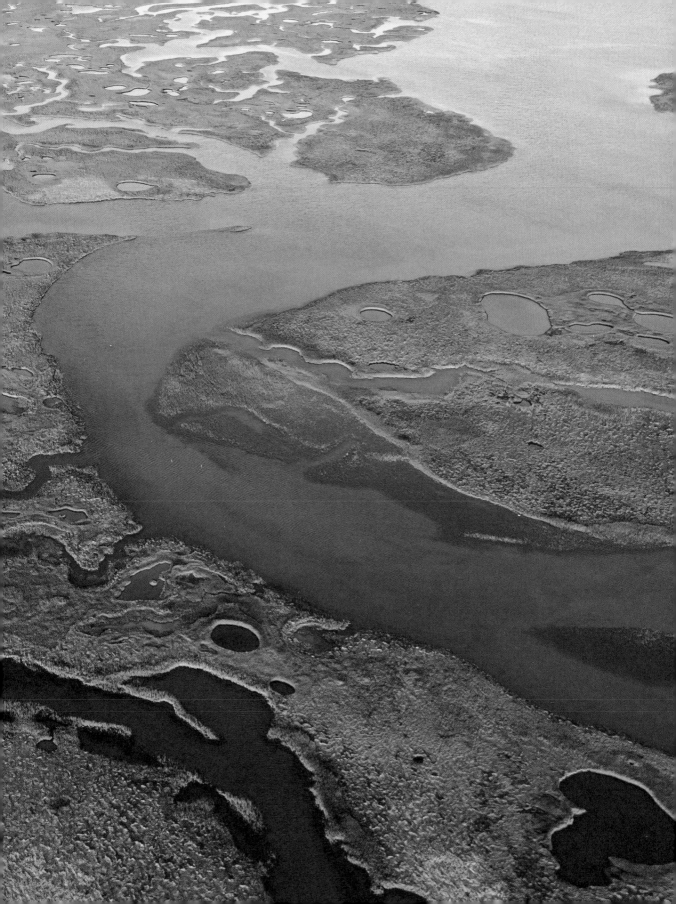

# THE CURRENT OF THE REPRODUCTIVE SYSTEM

The circulation of energy through the pelvic region is a major component of generative health. Information about gynecologic disorders in Ayurveda texts appears among disorders of *vayu*, air and movement. The *Charaka Samhita* states that "the genital organs of women do not get afflicted without the aggravated *vayu*."[4] When we talk about movement, we are talking about vata dosha, and *free-moving prana and all things vata-balancing are the primary healers in women's health.*

Erratic, unstable, irregular vata dosha is most likely to produce problems in the generative system and its functions. There are two major players here: artavavahasrotas and *apana vayu* (the downward-moving flow). When vata is out of balance and begins to affect the generative system, we may see irregular periods, anovulation, dryness, constriction, bloating, low back and pelvic pain, and increased premenstrual and perimenopausal symptoms, including physical, energetic, and emotional manifestations.

## ARTAVAVAHASROTAS: NOURISHING REPRODUCTIVE TISSUE

Artavavahasrotas is rooted in the ovaries and nipples, and the channel passes through all the reproductive organs. The opening is the labia. This channel is responsible for carrying nutrition to build and sustain healthy generative organs, and it also supports the activities of menstruation, ovulation, gestation, and birth. The generative system channel governs flowing actions that happen in the pelvic region: menstruation, ovulation, and birthing, but also urination and elimination. While the uterus, the bladder, and the colon are obviously different anatomical channels, their energetic functions are linked. Blocked energy radiates and can permeate the boundaries between neighboring organs and tissues—for example, low back pain before the menstrual cycle. The spine and the uterus are not physically connected, but they feel intensely linked.

Stagnation of circulation in the generative organs is the most common problem with artava. Energy may get blocked in these organs due to physical causes, like slouching in a chair or wearing tight pants, but also sexual trauma. It's important to proceed with care and gentleness when working with artava. Keeping the energy moving and the nourishment flowing through the generative system is the goal of a lot of healing artava therapies.

# APANA VAYU: THE DOWNWARD FLOW

Circulation in the pelvic region relies on apana vayu. Imagine the artava channels form a river, splitting into smaller creeks that flow to the ocean. Apana moves toward the ocean, and artava is the system of creek beds. Apana is one of the five movement patterns of vata, the one that governs downward flow. The word *vayu*, which means "air" or "wind," signifies that we are talking about the mobile quality of vata, as opposed to its cold or dry qualities. Of all vata's movements in bodies, apana is the ace—and also the one most likely to get out of balance due to the upward- and outward-moving nature of air and space elements.

An imbalance of downward-moving vata often means a deficiency or weakness in the downward flow. Sometimes it can be overactive—which will result in urgent stools, frequent urination, and frequent and heavy menstrual cycles—but due to the expanding, light nature of vata, it is more often weak or blocked. Air and space elements are not dense and full of gravity. To add to this likelihood of upward movement, a majority of daily activity for many modern humans happens above the neck. Imagine how much energy is recruited for the senses in looking, listening, talking, eating, and thinking! Prana is at a premium in the upper body. Couple this with the tendency for many women to hold tension in the abdomen (such as from the constant cultural messaging to have a flat tummy), and over time, the lower regions and their functions can take a hit. Apana vayu is a constant motif in the conversation on generative health.

## APANA AND WOMEN'S NATURAL CYCLES

Apana undergoes natural changes due to menstruation, menopause, and the seasons, and all cycles can cause shifts in one's appetite and digestion, poop, and even mind function and energy levels. Understanding and supporting the natural flows of energy in the body is key to enjoying smooth cycles and transitions. Apana is in charge of the menstrual cycle, and blocked apana is often the culprit in painful cycles. There are many tools to redirect the flow of vata downward. Breath work is especially potent, as breath directly affects the energy body (see appendix A). Foods and herbs can also promote vata's downward-moving action, a process called *anuloma* (see appendix B).

# The Five Vayus

Vata dosha is further broken down into five currents, which perform specific functions in the body. These are known as the *five vayus*. To help place apana vayu in context, let's look at the five currents of vata, and what they do.

**Prana vayu:** Located in the head and heart, *prana vayu* is responsible for respiration and the flow of awareness. Prana moves down and in.

**Udana vayu:** Located in the diaphragm and throat, *udana vayu* is responsible for speech, burping, and vomiting. Udana moves upward.

**Samana vayu:** Located in the area of the small intestine and navel, *samana vayu* is responsible for the movement of food through the small intestine and fans the digestive fire in the stomach. Samana moves horizontally back and forth (imagine the roundabout coil of the small intestine).

**Vyana vayu:** Located in the heart and circulatory system, *vyana vayu* is responsible for the circulation between the heart and extremities. Vyana moves in a circular fashion.

**Apana vayu:** Located below the navel, in the pelvic region and legs, *apana vayu* is responsible for elimination, urination, menstruation, ovulation, birthing, and the movement of energy through the hips into the legs. Apana moves downward.

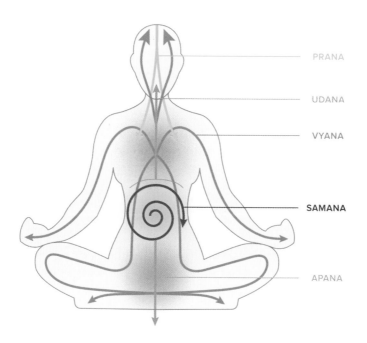

PRANA

UDANA

VYANA

**SAMANA**

APANA

# Practices to Support Apana Vayu

Anything that warms, relaxes, softens, and moistens the lower abdomen, pelvis, and legs will support downward flow. The new moon is the natural time to restore apana, and the lunar rhythms described in chapter 9 have this action at their heart.

Yoni Steaming (page 318)

Herbal Sitz Bath (page 316)

Castor Oil Packs (page 318)

Oiling the Ears and Feet (page 65)

Over the years, I have observed apana vayu to be the number-one factor in maintaining healthy vata and, therefore, overall health for women.

## PRANA: THE PRIMARY HEALING ENERGY

Prana is the inherent life-giving energy; whenever we talk of energy circulating, we are talking about prana. Because, like air, it is characterized by movement, prana is considered the subtle counterpart of vata. They work in tandem. This energy circulates around the body, carried by the currents of vata and directed by the movements of your attention. This means whatever you are thinking about or experiencing through your senses is receiving your prana.

In cases of vata imbalance, the circulation of life energy can be compromised. For optimal health, we must carefully cultivate the smooth circulation of prana. Moderate exercise, quality food, enough rest, good company, and self-love all build life energy; stress and worry drain it. A break in prana's rhythmic circulation can be physical, such as cholesterol blocking an artery or gas trapped in the intestines. However, psychic causes—such as chronic stress, worry, grief, or feelings of disconnection from the body (too much cerebral time)—may be as responsible as physical ones for disease progression.

### PRANA AND THE SENSES

Input from the five senses is a major player in stress; the misuse of the senses is one of the three causes of disease (*trividha karana*). The sense organs are an important part of the subtle body. Even eyeballs and earlobes are infused with prana; with their intimate connection to the mind, they are part of the subtle body. The senses are hardwired to be on alert to protect us and our young from ancestral dangers (tigers, forest fires); in the present day, modern survival instincts are attuned to ever subtler challenges (financial strain, our children's mental health). The senses' persistent pull of the attention outward causes constant stimulation of the nervous system. If this stimulation is not balanced by quiet time, stress and energy deficiency result. Daily self-care practices preserve prana by nourishing and protecting the senses—less stress and more energy!

Like prana vayu, the current of vata that begins at the nostrils and ends at the heart, prana has a close relationship to respiration. Bringing the attention to the breath—the heart of many yoga and meditation techniques—quiets the senses and the mind and nourishes the heart, the seat of prana.

## THE PRIMARY PRANA BLOCKER: SUPPRESSION OF THE THIRTEEN NATURAL BODILY URGES

We suppress bodily urges because we are too busy, too self-conscious, or just not paying attention. Ayurveda says it is the tendency to mess with these natural processes that begins and perpetuates disease. This is a big deal! The body governs its ins and outs with urges like hunger and thirst (in) and burps, poop, and farts (out). Suppressing urges on a regular basis disrupts prana's and vata's flows.

The urges here are human, ever-present, and so important in Ayurveda. There are only two rules:

1. Do not suppress natural urges.
2. Do not forcibly initiate these urges.

Overcoming natural bodily urges with mental effort catches up with you, and eventually the bodily urge will become elusive. Out of the following thirteen physical processes, most people suppress or force at least a few sometimes, if not all the time.

- Farts
- Poop
- Pee
- Sneezing
- Thirst

- Hunger
- Sleep
- Coughing
- Breathing
- Yawning

- Tears
- Vomiting
- Semen

Texts describe the specific imbalances that can result from interfering with each of these urges. There are certainly times when these actions just have to wait, but the less this happens, the better. In many cultures, women, especially, prioritize social codes—such as not farting in public—above their own health.

Suppression of these urges tends to become a habit, steadily disturbing the flow of prana, without us noticing. While menstruation isn't on the list, suppression of any apana vayu functions (such as urine, feces, or farts) contributes to menstrual disorders such as cramping and pain, premenstrual bloating and digestive disturbances, even irregular or absent periods. Vata imbalance from not heeding nature's calls is also a liability in perimenopause and can make symptoms such as hot flashes, mood swings, and digestive changes more difficult to manage.

As women, we must normalize natural functions in ways that may not seem demure. The health we gain from free-moving prana, easier periods, smooth transitions, and inner radiance is empowering—and worth a toot or an extra pee break.

## Help for New Moms

Postpartum is an important time for apana vayu to stabilize, gather energy, and redirect flow. Suppressing any movement of the wind during this time is counterintuitive to healing. New moms may need someone to help them find space for their own potty times, hydration, and meals. Obviously not every urge can be answered immediately when caring for a newborn, but prioritizing normal bodily functions during healing will speed recovery. It's OK to ask for help, even if it's just to be able to use the bathroom.

# Womens' Stories: Healing Apana

This personal story is contributed by Jennifer Kurdyla, an Ayurveda practitioner, yoga teacher, and coauthor of *Root & Nourish: An Herbal Cookbook for Women's Wellness*.

"It only takes a little bit of fertilizer for the grass to grow." That was how my gynecologist explained the diagnosis of "undetectable" estrogen behind the cessation of my menstrual cycle at age seventeen. When I still wasn't bleeding years later, even after allopathic treatments like hormonal birth control, I knew I needed a different approach. Enter Ayurveda. I initially sought a local practitioner for help with my worst symptom: choking pressure moving up into my throat after each meal. In the past, doctors would respond to this with blank stares, but my practitioner knew what I was talking about and could help.

A month-long reset did wonders to reverse this upward flow of udana vayu that had taken over my system, including digestion and menstruation. But it took many years, practitioners, and modalities for me to befriend what was truly "undetectable" in my vata-laden self: apana vayu. I slowly incorporated rituals that embrace the downward-flowing, gravitational gifts of the earth and water elements: daily *abhyanga*, Nadi Shodhana (Alternate Nostril Breath), and Savasana [Corpse Pose]; making (and eating!) ghee with the moon; and bodywork like massage, acupuncture, and pelvic floor physical therapy. Now, I no longer see these restorative practices as "weighing down" my creativity, as I once feared, but allowing me to "flow" easefully with nature, including in regular menstruation.

Nourishing apana vayu continues to allow me to feel worthy of receiving love and taking up space on the earth, which we all need—and deserve—to participate in the creative process of life that flows beautifully, downwardly, from the menstrual cycle.

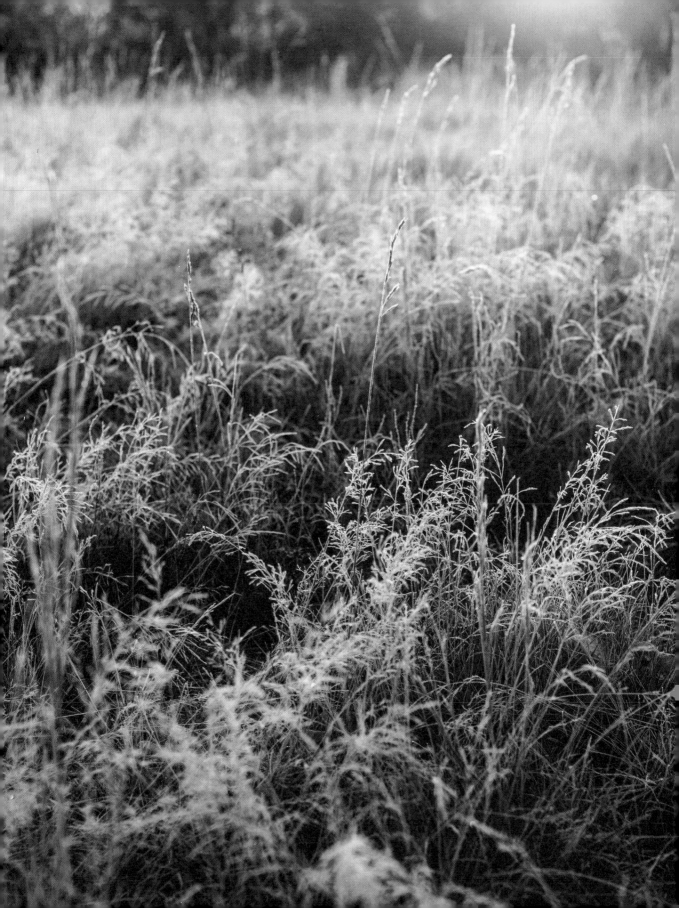

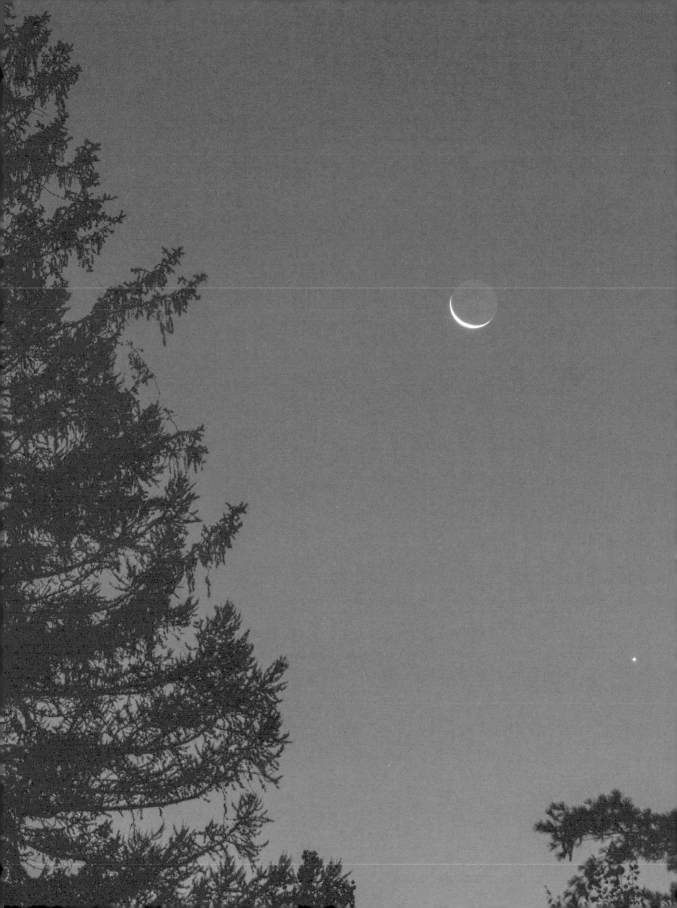

# 4

# Celestial Bodies

## INFLUENCE OF THE SUN, MOON, AND PLANETS

Attuning to the rhythmic influences of celestial bodies can help us channel our energies in cosmic directions. In Ayurveda, the body is not seen simply as its anatomy and physiology. It also references the climate, the age, and the foods available to a person. Individual factors are interwoven with grander scale influences too. Even today, an Ayurveda physician may consult a person's astrological chart before making recommendations.

The sister fields of Vedic astrology, Yoga, and Tantra offer a deeply complex knowledge of lunar practice and ritual. This chapter introduces the concept of celestial bodies as influencers of our health. This book offers just a taste of celestial science, but it would feel like an omission of a distinct women's wisdom not to consider lunar energy. Being in dialogue with lunar rhythms that mirror hormonal cycles reveals the effect the moon has on the subtle body, influencing energy levels, sleep, and moods.

You can practice Ayurveda without ever consulting the heavens, your Vedic astrological chart, or a moon phase calendar, but your understanding of your place in the cosmos will be greatly enriched if you do.

## SOMA AND LUNAR ENERGY

Lunar energy supports a nectar called *soma*, which originates in the pineal gland and is the subtle essence of ojas. Therefore, the moon is seen as a source of building qualities, and the waxing moon is the ideal time of month for activity, fertility, and building immunity as this nectar and its cool, rejuvenating qualities are on the rise. For practitioners of the subtle arts, soma has deep meaning as a nectar of immortality. Its essence is the key to higher states of consciousness. Tapping into the mystic potential of moonlight to rejuvenate the body and mind may be just the thing to curb the heat and inflammation resulting from stress.

Ayurveda texts describe the Adityas, celestial bodies, as astral beings who have great influence over the relationship between humans and cosmos. These celestial beings take on symbolic personalities and energies in ancient myths, and they are centers of influence in Vedic astrology. Planetary, solar, and lunar bodies are big players in the makeup of our universal substratum, and have become, in Vedic lore, symbols of the energies that guide us, drive us, and mire us throughout life.

While modern science remains skeptical about the effects of celestial factors such as lunar cycles on humans, from the view of Ayurveda, it seems illogical to assume a gravitational pull that moves oceans is not also moving us in some ways. In 2017, Nobel Prize–winning research on circadian rhythms normalized the idea of a body clock that is affected by natural forces, such as sunlight. Melatonin, serotonin, and vitamin D absorption are only a few of the molecular functions known to depend on sunlight. The sun and moon influence human endocrine functions, affecting sleep, digestion, detoxification, and ovulation, to name a few. The pineal gland (the site of soma) manages the information from the environment about light and dark, and it regulates sleep and waking by releasing melatonin.

Empirically, the sun and moon affect the earth through both their light and their gravitational pull. The massive sun tethers the solar system with its gravity, pulling the planets toward it and creating a movement pattern in the bodies that surround it. Ocean tides are a result of the moon's gravitational force pulling water toward it. Full moons bring higher high tides and potentially rougher seas. Could there be a connection between the moon and the movements of not only the oceans but our bodies and minds? In Ayurveda's microcosm-macrocosm view, the connection is clear.

A deep dive into research-based studies can seem contradictory and inconclusive. Some note that modern humans demonstrate less influence from solar and lunar rhythms due to the prevalence of artificial light, which allows us to remain active at night and disturbs pineal function. Yet humans have oriented themselves with solar and lunar calendars as far back as we have recorded history.

Living consciously in the flow with the two brightest celestial bodies can help us get that feeling of doing the right thing at the right time. We can take comfort in aligning our lives with the cosmos, which our bodies naturally crave.

## LUNAR RHYTHMS AND MENSTRUATION

Anyone who sleeps at night and is awake in the daylight can feel attuned to solar rhythms (the rising and setting of the sun). Bodies that menstruate, however, have a unique functionality that has been linked to the cycles of the moon since ancient times. Each month, there is a two-week dark fortnight of the waning moon and a two-week bright fortnight of the waxing moon. During the waning moon, the body turns inward for regeneration and purification, while the bright moon is the time to soak up soma and build strength and energy. Just as day and night balance activity and rest, these monthly cycles evoke the essential balance between solar and lunar energies.

There is a vast trove of Vedic science texts on the movements of celestial bodies and their effects. In this book, we focus on attunements that we can use throughout our monthly rhythms, aligning changing energy levels, moods, and subtle appetites to a universal flow. The length of the moon's orbit around earth aligns with the length of a baseline menstrual cycle: twenty-eight days (an average of two measurements—one with respect to the stars and the other to the visual stage of the moon). Whether you menstruate or not, attuning to the moon cycles is a way to communicate with the subtle body.

## INFLUENCE OF SUN AND MOON ON THE BODY

Each day we cycle through a solar and lunar phase. In Ayurveda, the sun and its solar energy is hot, light, and mobile, associated with the fire element. These qualities bring more energy and activity. The moon and its lunar energy are cool, dense, and stable, associated with the water element. These qualities promote juicy tissues and shukra, as well as calm and rest. We might eat lunch at midday to harness the fire element for optimal digestion, and we want to reduce active, hot, and light energies in the evening and promote cool, dense, and stable qualities to settle down at the end of the day.

Going against the grain—for example, by working on a computer at the night and sleeping during the day—undermines the natural rhythm of the body. The body prefers to draw on solar energy for active work, recruiting energy from the cosmos, and to sleep at night, soaking up cool, stable, and restorative lunar qualities. Cool lunar qualities oppose the heating qualities stress brings to the body (refer to chapter 1 on why this is so important for hormone balance).

Each month, we also cycle through a moonlike phase. With the bright fortnight comes more building qualities: the body is juicy and full of nectar, energy moves out via communication and manifestation. During the dark fortnight, attention moves inward for reflection, and the body focuses on letting go, cleansing, and making space. You are likely to notice that you have more energy and might feel more social during the bright moon, whereas you gravitate toward rest when the moon is dark. These shifts are natural and support the kind of balance we all need between activity and rest.

## Hatha Yoga and the Moon

Hatha—*ha* ("sun") and *tha* ("moon")—yoga is essentially the science of balancing these opposing qualities, as in Ayurveda. Observations of lunar cycles, and their impacts on the human energy system, are present in many yoga traditions. Ayurveda texts point toward the significance of the dark and light phases of the moon by suggesting certain activities be favored or avoided during these times, but the details are found among the yoga and tantra texts.

As with Yoga, Ayurveda's model of a human being includes the physical and the subtle, the energy body that is composed of prana and mind. These two aspects of reality, like two tracks for a train, run parallel to and always influence each other. Everything in the cosmos, from our food to our breath to the influence of celestial bodies, is gathered up, thread by thread, and braided into a worldview that is both physiological and metaphysical.

Nadi Shodhana (Alternate Nostril Breathing; page 321) is one simple practice that balances the energy of the two most important subtle channels, the *ida* and *pingala nadis*, which run along the left and right sides of the spine and carry lunar and solar energies, respectively. In a state of balance, the breath will alternate between dominance in the right or left nostril about every hour and a half. This gentle oscillation between the two energy channels supports a most basic and essential balance in the energy body, which is hugely important in keeping the circulation of healing prana balanced as well, since the life energy moves through these channels.

Structural roadblocks such as a frozen shoulder, sinus complications like allergies, or anything that disrupts the flow of the air element in the head, can disrupt this natural rhythm by habitually blocking one of the nostrils. Over time, this inconsistency in the energy movements can lead to imbalances.

# MOON, MIND, AND MOOD

The mind and the body are two strings on the same instrument; the mind is affected when the body is, and vice versa. You might begin to notice if your moods are affected by sunlight, as in seasonal affective disorder. Long periods of rain or northern winters with short days and longer nights affect the mood for many. You may notice that your sleep is affected by a full moon, for perhaps as simple a reason as it is not dark enough for deep sleep.

Whereas the sun is analogous with the body and fire element, the moon is analogous with the mind and water element. The physical body and the pranic body operate like two train tracks, separate but inseparable. The mind's attunement to the moon's energy and the water element may present as feeling "loony" as the full moon pulls on the water element. Lunar energy affects mental pace and attitude, sleep, and ability to focus. Consider the fluctuations during a monthly hormonal cycle: what is caused by hormones, and what is caused by the moon? Do hormones adjust based on lunar phases? Indigenous wisdom traditions generally say yes.

Modern culture tends to promote a solar environment. Productivity is favored; sleep and rest can be fleeting, and the senses are constantly stimulated. What if, each month, you soak up soma when the moon is bright and hold an intention to regenerate around the dark moon? You'll be more active and get more done during the solar phase of a month, while resting more and cooling out during the lunar phase may result in not only better energy and productivity, but also better health overall. And you may even enjoy a mystical, magical attunement to the power of celestial bodies.

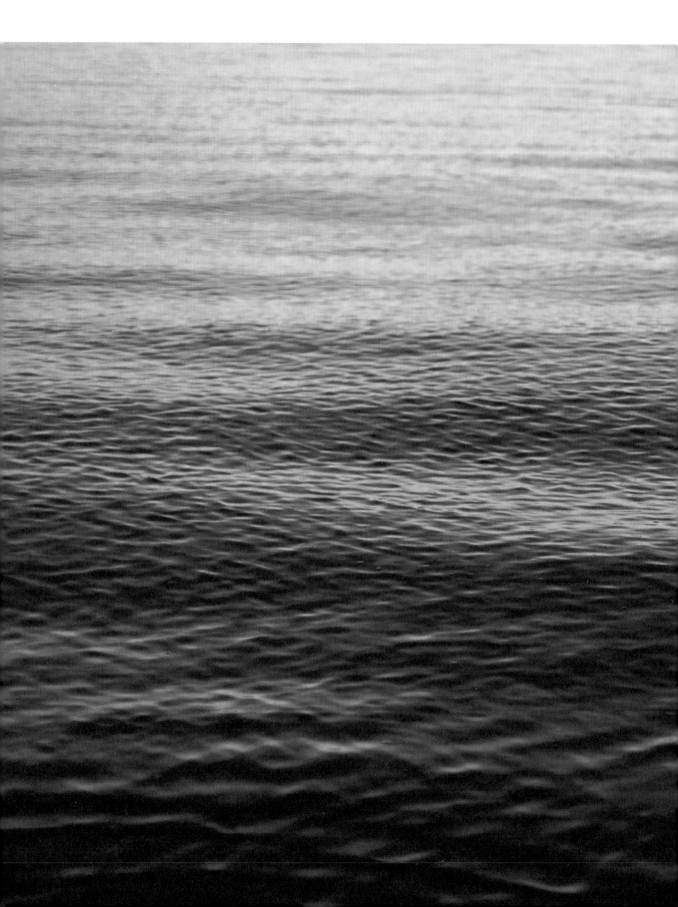

# PART TWO

# ALIGNING *with* *the* RHYTHMS *of* NATURE

The daily and seasonal routines of Ayurveda describe how best to flow with time over the course of a day, a season, and a life span. Working with the flow preserves health; going against it, or ignoring it, promotes disease. This wisdom evolved over many lifetimes; it was born of observing the predictable patterns of change in the environment and the effects these changes have on human bodies.

*Parinama* (change) is the root of aging. The ancient sages realized that although we cannot escape the changes born of time, there are aspects to change that are predictable. Days, months, and a life span have identifiable patterns and therefore predictable effects. The rains come after the dry season; the warmth comes after winter. Bodies are affected by all of the elemental change that is natural: day and night, dry season and rainy season, full moon and new moon. As we dig deep into Ayurveda for women's health, we aren't just focusing on when to eat lunch (though this is essential), we are addressing the rhythms of the cosmos, how they affect us, and the deep sense of balance we can experience when living in sync with universal flow.

The primary flow factor is vata, or that which moves. The generative system is governed by the vata dosha, so nurturing vata is the bedrock of women's health. Working with oil is a primary therapy for balancing the dry, light, rough qualities of space and air, both internally and externally. In addition to keeping a daily routine (which stabilizes the mobile quality), oiling the body quiets vata, allowing the body to restore its natural rhythms. You will see a good bit of oil in many of our healing practices.

In part two, we will move through the daily routine, how to balance elements in the day and night, seasonal considerations for your climate, and ultimately, how aligning with the lunar flow can elevate both health and consciousness. You don't have to read the chapters in order. If one of these topics is at the forefront for you today, get right to it.

# 5

# Dinacharya

## THE AYURVEDA DAILY ROUTINE

Mist rises in the early morning as the rising sun evaporates dew, just as the body rises from sleep, ready to refresh and renew. Along with natural cues, such as sunrise and sunset, the body expects certain changes, like getting sleepy or hungry. *Dinacharya* means "daily routine" and is an essential practice for health. Its routines guide our days so we move in unison with natural cycles and energy sources. Waking, eating, exercising, and sleeping at the ideal times regulates your sleep, digestion, and metabolism, which regulates your hormones. You will feel your energy become more buoyant as you move along with the currents of nature.

Morning cleansing routines ensure the body's most important channels function at top form by keeping the outlets of the channels clear. These practices support clarity in both body and mind, and they feel amazing.

Morning practices are also detoxifying. While the body sleeps, it moves metabolic wastes toward the out channels. It is natural to wake up in the morning and have to pee (and hopefully poop too). There may be some crust in your eyes, perhaps a bad taste in your mouth. Natural metabolic processes create waste, just like a gasoline-powered car releases exhaust when it's running. A few channels are of utmost importance in our morning routines because they expel these wastes to the outside: the mouth, the anus, and the skin's pores. Morning routines purify these channels.

The sense organs are intermediaries between our inner and outer worlds, and starting the day by clarifying the senses will enable us to see, hear, and perceive our world more clearly. This helps us to make better choices and enjoy our bodily experiences.

# A Note for Busy Women

It is not surprising if in reading about ideal daily routines, you feel overwhelmed by the number of people and schedules you are balancing in your day-to-day life. The stage of life called "householding," when there are many demands on your time and energy, may not be the time to adopt this entire schedule. The good news is that managing even *one* of these touchstones consistently can provide rhythm.

Is there a time in your day that is slower—after the kids go to school or when your morning chores are done? For example, you can do self-care after the house quiets down and before the next obligation begins, rather than when the family is running around at the start of the day. Tongue scraping and sipping hot water, however, are *the* routines to do upon waking. Consider keeping a small electric kettle in your bathroom to make hot water, and keep up these two routines undisturbed. If you get this much established, pat yourself on the back and trust that there will be quieter life stages when you can choose to expand your work with dinacharya.

## MORNING ROUTINES AND CARE OF THE SENSE ORGANS

The whole routine can take about 15 minutes once you streamline it over time. If you can, set the alarm a few minutes earlier to relax around these cleansing rituals.

### EMPTYING THE BLADDER AND BOWELS

As soon as you get up, go pee right away, and poop if the urge is there.

Do not check your phone immediately. If this is hard for you, turn off notifications, and buy an alarm clock so you are not tempted to engage with the screen first thing. Avoid multiple snooze settings, especially if it means you will have to hurry when you finally wake up.

If you haven't had the urge to poop yet, it could be because you are running around the house getting ready or thinking about everything you have to do. It is very important to leave time and space for elimination, ideally before eating. Consider spending 5 to 10 minutes simply observing your breath. If that feels like a challenge, try a bit of inspirational reading or relaxed bird-watching. Avoid reading or listening to the news if it agitates you; consume information later. Allow your mind to expand rather than narrow.

## CARE OF THE SENSE ORGANS

Give special consideration to the health of your senses, which are the link between your mind and the world. Clear perception and longevity of the organs themselves are the benefits of caring for the eyes, nose, ears, mouth, and skin. Include the following practices as part of your morning routine.

**Tongue:** Tongue scraping freshens the breath, removes mucus, and stimulates the digestive system. Upon waking, use a stainless steel or copper scraper to remove any mucus coating your tongue. Before consuming any drinks, scrape your tongue five to six times, from as far back as you can get to the tip. Scrape the entire surface of your tongue, *especially* the back. Press gently; do not disturb the tongue tissue. Mucus will likely appear on the scraper, so rinse as needed. When you're done, clean the scraper thoroughly with hot water, wipe it dry, and keep it near your toothbrush. It is not necessary to scrape your tongue at other times of the day.

Follow by sipping a cup of hot water.

**Eyes:** Rinse your eyes well by splashing cool water from the tap over open eyes with your hands four or five times. Follow by blinking several times and rolling your eyes in circles.

**Skin, ears, and nose:** These organs are each exposed to the air element due to sensation, hearing, and respiration, and this exposure affects vata over time. Apply oil to the skin, nose, and ears as part of an oil massage to balance vata. See the sidebar about when to do or not do oil massage. Complete instructions for this type of massage are in appendix A.

| When to Do Oil Massage | When Not to Do Oil Massage |
|---|---|
| • In the morning for detoxification | • After a meal |
| • In the evening to improve sleep and quiet the nerves and sense organs | • When there is ama or indigestion (see chapter 7) |
| • After travel | • During the menstrual cycle |
| • Localized massage for pain relief at any time | • When kapha is aggravated |
| | • When you are sick |

## SHOWER/BATH

Showering (or bathing) in the morning is considered essential for good health. Imagine the innumerable pores on the skin being cleared out after the body's routine overnight detox. If you prefer showering in the evening, that is a good time to use oil massage and showering as a relaxation therapy. Both detoxing and relaxing are beneficial.

Warm water is best on the body for its ability to soften, melt, and remove wastes. The scalp and eyes, however, due to their tendency to accumulate heat are best with cool or even cold water, depending on your climate. The skin should not appear red after showering. Hot showers can be drying; oil massage beforehand protects the skin, and you emerge with a soft, lubricated body. Use natural, moisturizing herbal soaps and shampoos, and avoid fragrances and artificial cleansers. Consider keeping a bit of castor oil in the shower for breast massage (see appendix A).

## What about Cold Showers?

Heat is softening, while cold causes contraction. Exposure to cold and wind are lightening therapies, and warm oil is building and nourishing. Where there are slow, heavy, or stagnant qualities, cold-water showers and baths can invigorate. Do not use oil in conjunction with cold therapies.

## SUNLIGHT FOR HORMONAL BALANCE

Hormones, the messengers of the body, respond to nature's rhythms. In Ayurveda, hormones are a subtle form of agni (fire element). Fire governs the eyes, the "digestion" of light, and the activity of the pineal and pituitary glands to some extent. Exposing the body to natural light and reducing unnatural light supports hormonal balance, or optimal agni function. For example, darkness promotes melatonin production, so sleep comes on after the sun goes down. Many female hormonal imbalances are affected by unnatural lighting, such as screen use late at night or a lack of natural light. A simple daily routine such as regularly getting sunlight at a similar time of day is a way to signal the messengers to do the right thing at the right time.

Enjoy a 15- to 20-minute daily "sun bath" at the same time of day, as many days as possible. In general, it is best in the morning to invoke agni. In cool, northern climates in winter, this is best done when the sun is strong, during the pitta time of day, from 10 A.M. to 2 P.M. Take your hat off and expose your forehead and the front of your scalp to the sun (but keep your ears covered in the cold). In hot climates, do this in the early morning, when the sun is not at its peak. You may still need to cover your head and just let your eyes receive the sun.

You can also sunbathe indoors by sitting in a patch of sun. Watch where the sun falls in the midmorning hours in your home or workplace. Stake out a seat in the sun for a part of every day.

## *RITUCHARYA*: SEASONAL SHIFTS

With a shift into the crisp autumn air, one may begin to notice lighter periods and drier skin, hair, and generative tissues, seemingly all of a sudden. Rather than feeling confused by the changes, note how through the Ayurveda lens, this increasing dryness of the body in autumn makes complete sense. We can shift our daily practices accordingly to increase moisture. When viewed in a larger context of qualities and seasons, applying moisture to balance dryness is as natural as watering a houseplant.

Observing the qualities in changing seasons is an excellent place to learn how heat and cold, moisture and dry air affect you. Awareness of the annual cycle allows us to view the changes in our bodies in relationship to the bigger picture of nature's changes. Shifting food and self-care practices with the seasons then becomes a part of essential balance.

*Rtu* means "season" in Sanskrit and can be traced back to a root meaning "the order of things." An understanding of the order of doshas, their qualities in an annual cycle, and how these affect us alerts us to shift our routines with the seasons. The doshas and their qualities fluctuate. For this reason, you may notice seasonal shifts in the qualities of your periods and the timing of your cycle. Imbalances may tend to arise during a certain season. What follows is a breakdown of the qualities of seasons in different climates and methods for naturally keeping doshas in seasonal balance.

> Hot weather has reducing qualities, such as light, intensity, and mobility, that weaken the body. Cool weather is building in nature with heavy, stable, and dense qualities that strengthen the body. Too much reducing or too much building causes imbalance, so essentially, changes in the diet or daily routine are intended to maintain a balance of reducing and building, in tandem with the qualities present during annual cycles.

## SEASONS AND QUALITIES

Every place on earth has its own seasonal flow based on whether the planet is tilting toward or away from the sun. A temperate environment may have four seasons, while a tropical locale may have two. It could take a year to observe how the environment you live in affects your qualities. Keep track of dry skin, water retention, congestion, digestive changes such as loose stools (more likely in hot weather), and constipation (more likely in cold or dry weather). Begin to notice these signs in the body as manifestations of qualities. Consider whether these qualities are matching up with seasonal changes. It takes time, but patterns will emerge.

Winter is the vata time of year, and postmenopause is the vata time of life. If you are dry and run cold, this time of year will likely require more warming and moistening qualities. If you run hot, this time of year may feel refreshing.

Summer pitta is the hot time of year, and the fertile years are the pitta time of life. If you run hot, this time of year will require more cooling. If you run cold, this may be an easy time for you.

Spring is the kapha time of the year, and prepuberty is the kapha time of life. If you often feel heavy and moist, springtime will require more cleansing qualities. If you are dry, you might feel some relief during the cool, rainy season.

## THE BASICS OF WORKING WITH SEASONAL QUALITIES

Here are a few things to consider about changing your routines according to climate and season. A little bit of seasonal shift in diet and activities creates a smooth annual cycle.

### In Hot Weather

- Favor sweet, bitter, and astringent tastes.
- Avoid things that heat the inner body, such as alcohol, ferments, spicy foods, and acidic fruits and vegetables such as oranges and tomatoes.
- Enjoy lighter foods such as legumes; rice; quinoa; coconut; juicy, sweet fruits; and fresh, cooling vegetables like lotus, cucumber, and zucchini.
- Drink cooling spiced waters and herbal infusions with ingredients like cardamom and hibiscus.
- Exercise during the early morning hours, before it heats up.

### In Cold Weather

- Favor sweet, sour, and salty tastes.
- Enjoy foods that build the body such as wheat and oats, urad dal, meat (if you eat it), root vegetables, bananas, dates, and sugarcane.
- Enjoy a moderate amount of foods that warm the body such as ferments, warming spices, cashews, pickles, citrus fruits, and olives.
- Drink warming spiced waters with ingredients like cinnamon and ginger.

- Sleep a little more.
- Exercise a little more.
- Practice oil massage at least once per week. Follow with a hot bath.

### In Humid or Rainy Weather

- Enjoy foods that dry and lighten the body such as barley, corn, millet, and legumes.
- Favor foods that purify rakta dhatu such as prunes, berries, and greens.
- Avoid too much moist, heavy food such as dairy, potatoes, fried foods, and sweets.
- Favor dry brushing over oiling.
- Exercise a little more.

### In Dry Weather

- Enjoy foods that moisturize the body such as sesame, dairy, almonds, ghee, and olive oil. If you don't get enough good fats, you may begin to notice dry stools or dry skin.
- Use moistening herbal infusions with ingredients like licorice, marshmallow, and slippery elm.
- Favor oil massage, including oiling of the ears and nose.

Remember the qualities *you experience in your body* are those that are true. Although you may have learned that the rainy season aggravates kapha, if you feel dry instead, stick with your moistening foods and practices. Self-observation is the key. And remember, any small seasonal shift you make with the practices listed here is money in the self-care bank!

# 6

# Sleep and Evening Routines

The key to mastering a restorative sleep routine is knowing there is an ideal time for it: between 10 P.M. and 2 A.M. Sleeping, on an empty stomach, during these hours ensures the body's ability to harness the energy of pitta and use that heat and penetrating quality to cook out toxins. A lot of organ cleansing and regeneration happens during this time. In the wee hours of the morning, undisturbed by food and sensory input, the body focuses on pushing toxins to the channels of elimination. The timing of sleeping and waking makes all the difference in supporting the body's ability to get rid of waste and to rest deeply.

To support this daily detox, 9 or 10 P.M. is the ideal time to begin slowing down, disengaging from work and screen time, and preparing for sleep. Staying awake past 10 or 11 P.M. will compromise the body's detox time. Sleeping and digesting do not go well together. Eating a heavy meal after 8 P.M. requires digestion during sleep, when agni in the stomach is low. Allowing for at least two hours between food and bed will ensure healthy digestion, sound sleep, and routine detox.

There's good sleep and bad sleep. Good sleep happens naturally at night, between sundown and sunrise. Not-so-good sleep happens in the day and can be the result of exhaustion, disease, depression, or overeating. Sleeping in the daytime increases kapha, which may result in low agni, congestion, sluggishness, and weight gain. In cases of exhaustion—physical as well as mental—sleeping during the day may be necessary for a time. Those with weak constitutions and the elderly may enjoy a healthy habit of daytime napping.

## The Myth of Night Owls

According to Ayurveda, there are no human "night owls." Nature rules, and humans sleep at night. When you are working night shifts, are caring for a baby, and encounter other unavoidable factors that hinder sleeping at night, you can maintain health with a consistent schedule, including self-care practices and rhythmic sleep cycles that follow a daily clock. The key is to be consistent.

# TOO LITTLE SLEEP

Most people suffer from a lack of sleep rather than an excess. Ayurveda texts define causes and management for a lack of sleep, which is said to occur in those with vata imbalance, the elderly, and the overworked. In some cases, texts say, it is simply part of a person's constitution to suffer from lack of sleep.

Here we cover basic sleep hygiene, and we'll go into more details about sleep interrupted by hot flashes in chapter 16.

## Causes of Lack of Sleep

- Excessive cleansing of the body
- Fear, anxiety, anger
- Uncomfortable bed or sleeping quarters
- Suppression of sleepiness
- Dry food (too much raw food, popcorn, crackers, etc.)
- Workaholic habits
- Changes in sleeping time (jet lag)
- Use of screens after 8 or 9 P.M.
- Consumption of rich food at night
- Consumption of too much alcohol

## Practices to Improve Sleep

- Eat dinner two to three hours before sleep.
- Consume moist, grounding foods, such as milk, ghee, whole grains, soups and stews, and calming herbal teas.
- Try a head massage and/or foot massage before bed. Simply applying a small amount of oil to the crown of your head and making small circles on your scalp with your fingertips can improve sleep.
- Be sure the place you're sleeping is not too hot or cold and smells pleasant. Apply a dab of lavender oil on your temples.
- Take a 15- to 20-minute sense break between 2 and 6 P.M. to calm vata.
- Think positive thoughts. Remember your achievements, give thanks, and visualize picturesque places.

## OILING THE EARS AND FEET FOR VATA MANAGEMENT

Ayurveda texts recommend oiling the ears and feet to calm vata. Keep a small container of sesame oil by your bed and massage a tablespoon into the crown of your head, your ears, and the soles of your feet nightly. Rub a few drops of oil onto the entire ear and the bones behind the ear with small circular motions, and slide your fingertips into the ear cavern to coat with oil.

With both hands, rub each foot lengthwise along the soft part of the sole, then side to side. Spend a little extra time rubbing the sensitive area beneath the ball of the foot using circular motions. Gently stretch and oil the toes. Wear a lightweight pair of socks to bed to protect your sheets. As a bonus step, use castor oil to soften calluses.

## HERBS FOR SLEEP

Incorporate infusions, hydrosols, and essential plant oils that quiet the nerves such as rose, lavender, jasmine, and sage into your nightly routine.

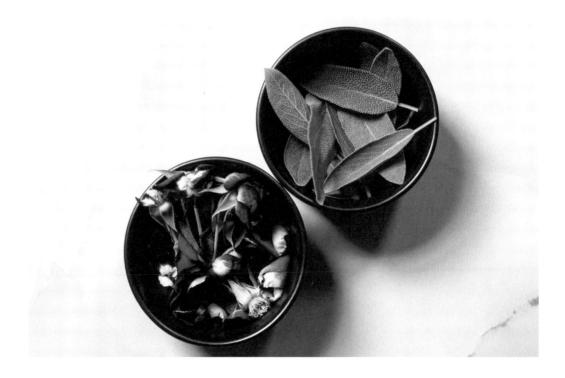

# Calming Brews

These recipes contain calming herbs and can be used near bedtime to quiet the mind, help you fall asleep, and support staying asleep.

Golden Mind Milk (page 248)

Nourishing Herbal Infusion (page 218)

Raspberry Leaf and Nettle Brew (page 223)

Moon Milk (page 247)

Cool-the-Flash Tea and Spritz with Rose and Sage (page 226)

In my experience, the most common problems affecting sleep are going all day without resting the senses, lack of a sleep routine, the use of screens at night, and suppression of the natural urge to slow down. It's OK to feel tired! If the day has been very stimulating, expect it to take some time to wind down. Good sleep hygiene goes on all day, not simply at bedtime. If you lie down in bed and experience racing thoughts, it is likely these recommendations can help you sleep better. The mind needs time to absorb the day's events before bed. Eat a warm and easy-to-digest dinner, massage your feet with oil, and turn off all screens before 10 P.M.!

While these recommendations are practical, your relationship with sleep can be philosophical. Prioritizing sleep is very important. If you do have high stress, keeping the mobile quality balanced so it doesn't interrupt sleep can mean making some paradigm shifts. In our culture of solar energy, putting rest first can feel like going against the grain, and a two-hour slowdown ritual at night might feel indulgent. When there is vata imbalance, however, elaborate measures to support sleep is completely natural—and necessary. If your stage of life does not allow this kind of time, follow any of the recommendations you can, and improve the quality, if not quantity, of your sleep.

# 7

# Optimizing Digestion and Metabolism

Your body's health, stamina, and luster begin in your stomach. Healthy rasa from balanced digestion nurtures your skin, menstrual blood, fertility, immunity, and luminosity. Food is sexy, food is shukra, food is life. This chapter shows that how we think about food is the key to overall healing and that strength, inner radiance, and luminosity all result from deep nourishment, a state of body that is cultivated with love and acceptance over time.

Making food *medicinal* is as much about your relationship to food and eating as it is about understanding the qualities of different foods and how to prepare them. Ayurveda texts address both of these aspects, and in some passages, nourishing the heart is mentioned right alongside physical nourishment, especially for those who are postpartum, pregnant, or intending to conceive.

Food nourishes the spiritual heart in many ways. One of the first points my doctor taught me about food in Ayurveda is that homemade food is always preferred to "outside food." This is because the energy of preparation decides the ultimate purity and nourishing quality of the food. Putting energy into preparing food, and into your kitchen and dining space, in simple ways truly makes the food more satisfying and its nutritional benefits more available.

Ayurveda texts describe the vessels food should be served in, even the attitude and dress of those serving the food, and point to a general sense of ambiance and gratitude. There are so many ways to bring the sacred into the dining experience—and many of them are free.

Somewhere along the way, modern culture changed the idea of food into little more than fuel, a slowdown in a busy day, or an antagonistic influence on the body. Food is so much more, a fundamental relationship for nourishing your blood, womb, and self. In your mission to choose and source foods that nourish, prepare them with care, and sit down to enjoy them is a reclamation of the sacred nature of food and self-nourishment.

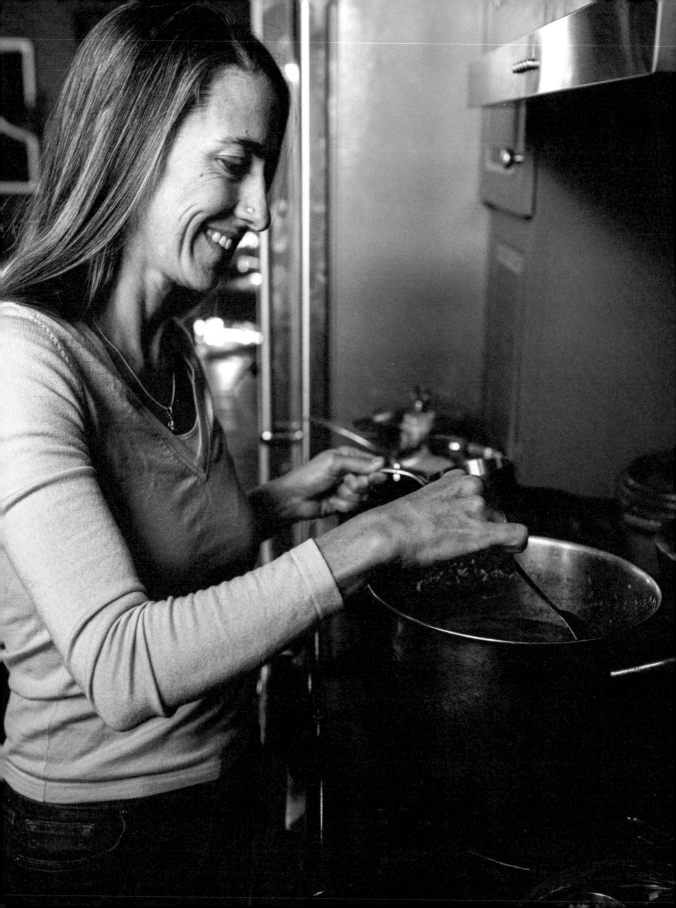

# AGNI: DIGESTIVE FIRE

Agni (pronounced "UG-nee") is fire, one of the five elements. In digestion, *agni* refers to *jathara agni*, the fire of the stomach. Keeping the digestive fire strong is your number-one priority. If you have the correct amounts of water, fire, space, and food in the stomach, you should digest food well. This means the stomach makes a nice ahara rasa, food-juice that supports ojas, artava, menstrual blood, skin, and breast milk. This food-juice is the building block of healthy generative tissues.

After the fire element "cooks" and liquifies food in the stomach, smaller metabolic fires get to work, breaking down fats and proteins, metabolizing, absorbing, and making body tissues (like fats, muscles, and sexy juice) from the rasa. The food you eat becomes your body, and how the food is rendered into resilient tissues is decisive in the integrity and radiance of the body. The mother agni in the stomach governs the smaller metabolic fires, and the same rituals and rhythms you use for good digestion generally support metabolism as well. When agni is burning strong, toxicity is not allowed to lodge in the tissues; rather, it is broken down and eliminated. In this way, good digestive fire keeps the body free of ama, undigested matter, which gunks up the works, weakens the system, and promotes imbalance.

The jathara agni in the stomach builds like a little campfire. You must have kindling to get it started. If you put too much wood on it, the fire is smothered. If you don't give it enough wood, the fire can't burn strongly to create light and warmth.

Smothering the fire by overeating is a common cause of low agni. It's easily remedied by skipping a meal to allow the fire to build up again (except in the case of eating disorders or unsteady blood sugar levels). Anytime you feel a loss of appetite, this indicates a low digestive fire and is a good time to skip a meal.

Poor digestive fire gives rise to many of the imbalances of rasa and rakta that we discussed in chapter 3, causing the quality of the blood to become too sticky or too dry because of poor-quality ahara rasa in circulation. Sound digestive fire is central to being well nourished enough to support the demanding functions of a woman's body—not only for monthly regeneration of blood, but also subtle factors like one's creative drive.

# Know Your Digestive Fire

Knowing your fire requires a deep dive into the center of your body. Get familiar with the fire in your stomach by noticing when you are hungry and what your hunger feels like. Observe that there is the hunger of the stomach and the hunger of the tongue. The tongue wants stuff that tastes good, while the stomach wants stuff that will build rasa.

To tell the difference, ask yourself, *Is it only chocolate that sounds good right now, or would I get excited to eat a homemade soup?* Getting to know your digestive fire can really be that simple!

## SPOTLIGHT ON SNACKING

Snacking interferes with digestion. Imagine cooking rice but adding half of the rice to hot water at the beginning and adding the rest after 10 minutes of cooking. Your final product will be half overcooked and half undercooked. This is what happens to ahara rasa when you eat food before digestion of the previous meal is complete.

Snacking seems to happen for two reasons:

1. We are too busy or too overwhelmed to sit and eat a meal.
2. We are eating for a reason other than hunger. This could be emotional eating, as well as feeling low energy or sleep-deprived and looking for a pick-me-up.

Snacking has become a cultural (and consumerist) habit. Eating small bits of food—usually those that don't require warming up, such as nuts, chocolate, chips, and the like—seems easier in the moment than cooking. What is not easy is managing the far-reaching effects of poor digestion that inevitably result from snacking.

Sitting down to eat proper meals, and not eating in between, is also a habit. Shifting from the latter to the former requires time, effort, discipline, and care. You have to care enough about your health to prioritize nourishment. Snack happens! When nutritious food is accessible, snacking is often a result of poor planning. Deep nourishment is not something to let slide.

**Try this:** Take a week to experiment with how much breakfast you need to get you through until lunch without snacking. Once you get this balance consistent, which may take a month or more, you can start observing the space between lunch and dinner. Of course, if you work a very physical job, like landscaping or construction, you may need to eat more often. However, stick to meals and avoid grazing. Know that it may take you six months or more to feel comfortable eating meals and not snacking.

## Late Afternoon Crash

It is natural to feel an energy crash between 2 and 6 P.M., when vata starts to accumulate from the mobility of the day. Many reach for caffeine, sugar, or snacks during this interval. Try a short rest instead. Whether it's a quiet walk outside, 10 minutes of meditation, or a catnap, this rest allows your senses to regenerate and refresh, leaving you less likely to crave stimulants to keep up in the afternoon.

## HOW TO EAT: BEST PRACTICES, HOW MUCH, AND WHEN

How we eat is often more important than what we eat. You might have a carefully chosen, lovingly prepared meal, but if you eat it in the car or at the computer, your digestion and assimilation of the meal are compromised.

Food habits and routines are not about perfection. Following health-giving food practices *most* of the time is better than pushing too hard to follow the rules *all* the time. When your digestive strength is optimal, you can get away with some indulgence when the time is right! "Practice" so you can enjoy good health and good food. Pleasure is an important aspect of eating in Ayurveda and not to be forgotten. Take care to temper your occasional indulgences with good digestive practices, and keep the sacred nature of food and self in the picture.

**Slow down.** Eating when you are truly hungry and eating slowly enough to sense when you begin to feel full are the best care you can give your digestive fire.

**Practice gratitude.** Just as you would take care to listen to a friend in need, take care to notice food. When your body smells the food, it begins to prepare the appropriate enzymes for the food it recognizes. Before it is even in your mouth, the process of digestion has begun! Engage your senses by looking closely at, smelling, and feeling the qualities of the food. What are its colors and textures? Make a practice of taking a few moments to take it all in before you eat.

**Sit down when eating.** Eating standing up does not allow proper downward movement of digestion. In addition, you will probably notice you have better awareness of your portions when you sit down to eat.

**How much to eat.** The ancient texts of Ayurveda suggest that "two parts of the stomach should be filled with solid foods, one part by liquids and the remaining one part should be kept vacant for accommodating air."[5] The amount of food you can hold in your cupped hands is a good measure to go by.

Drinking liquid is an important part of each meal. The ideal drink is warm water, plain or with lemon, or a spiced digestive tea such as Essential Spiced Water (page 231). Drinking from a small cup that holds 6 ounces or so will suffice. Drinking a lot of water less than 30 minutes before a meal, or less than two hours after, will dilute the digestive juices. The right amount of liquid will make a nice ahara rasa.

**When to eat.** Eating at the proper time of day decides whether the food will be well digested or not. A burger at noon is preferable to a salad at midnight. The digestive fire is strongest between 10 A.M. and 2 P.M., the pitta time of day; therefore, make lunch your largest meal of the day. Eat light at night.

**How often to eat.** Remember that digestive fire is like a campfire. If you keep putting wood on it, the flames will be smothered. If you wait too long to add wood, the fire will die down. Most of us are in the habit of eating too often. The fire never gets to come to full strength because it always has something new to digest. The practice of not eating between meals allows the fire to grow (see the next section on following nature's meal rhythms).

**With whom to eat.** When eating in company, take a moment to feel gratitude for each other and the food, and pause to take it all in. There is nourishment everywhere in a shared food experience—not just in the substance, but in the energy of preparation and the connectivity of relationships.

# Celebratory Meals

A *lot* of my community members report stress around celebrations that center around food because they are working on balancing digestive fire, and a large, complicated meal is something they aren't yet ready for. Bringing a dish to share that you know you digest well ensures that you will get what you need from the gathering and frees you to have smaller portions of the rest.

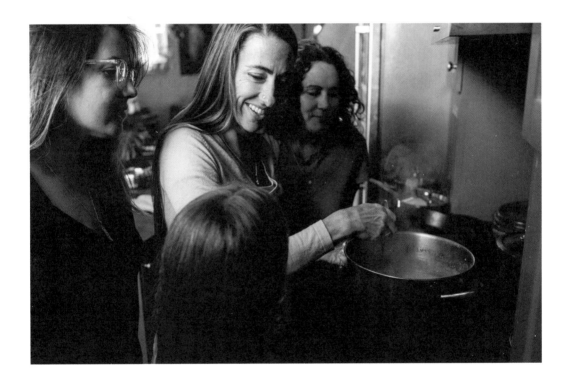

# FOLLOWING NATURE'S RHYTHMS FOR DIGESTIVE HEALTH

The following meal rhythms harness the heat of the digestive fire, which mirrors the sun as it warms up and cools down each day. The most potent time for digestion is around the sun's zenith. Keep in mind that cold weather usually increases your digestive fire and appetite, and you may find your meal flow changes with the seasons. Appetites also change with stages of life, and our bodies need less food as we age. Shifting from three meals to two may help manage metabolic changes with menopause and aging. First, find a three-meal-per-day option, then a two-meal flow.

## BREAKFAST

Before noon, the fire has not yet reached its peak, and a light breakfast is recommended to ease into the day. However, if you are awake early or exercise before breakfast, you may find your morning meal needs to be more substantial. Eat enough to get you through to lunch.

## BIG LUNCH

As the sun reaches its peak after noon, pitta and its power of digestion is high. Lunch is the ideal time to eat the most food or the most complex foods, such as fats and proteins. It is also the time for eating a treat, but have it as dessert and not between meals.

## SUPPER

The word *supper* is similar to the word *supplement*. This light evening meal is to supplement if you didn't get enough food earlier in the day. If you are in the habit, as many are, of having a family or social meal at night, do yourself a favor by being sure to eat a nourishing lunch, so you will be less tempted to overdo it in the evening, as the digestive system is winding down for the day. Remember that family and social meals can be more about the precious time spent with loved ones than about the food. Shift the focus to being nourished by the company you have, and you will feel satisfied by a lighter meal.

Eating dinner two to three hours before bed ensures that you will fall asleep without food still in your stomach. This will allow your organs to do some cleanup while you rest, rather than work through that late dinner. As in all things Ayurveda, it's what you do habitually that counts. It's fine to have late meals sometimes, but as a habit, eat lighter and earlier—especially if your metabolism has slowed down with menopause.

## THE TWO-MEAL FLOW

Another daily rhythm, one that works well in hot weather, is to eat two meals per day: a bigger meal in the late morning before it's too warm and one as the day cools down. In many hot-weather countries, there is a siesta, or rest, in the afternoon and a late dinner after sunset when it is cool. In Northern regions, summer sunset may be as late as 9 P.M., so eat your second meal around 6 P.M. if you plan to get to bed early.

**Simple Version:** Eat more food in the earlier part of the day. It digests better.

## TOXINS AND BUILDING AMA

When food doesn't break down completely due to less-than-ideal food choices or eating practices, and/or stress, ama develops. This is a thick, sticky, leftover substance that sits in the stomach and smothers the digestive fire, precipitating more ama from future meals. This result of incomplete digestion can dull and slow the mind as well as the body.

If these factors continue for a while, ama begins to travel from the stomach, via the rasa and rakta dhatus, and gunk up the channels of circulation and nutrition, organs, and other body systems. Anywhere there is a weak spot, ama likes to stick around, as in the case of joint inflammation or chronic congestion. Once ama is in the tissues or channels, metabolism slows down. This systemic situation can be responsible for the common complaint of "brain fog." Ama exacerbates many PMS symptoms and may be a player in the development of polycystic ovary syndrome (PCOS). It takes years for ama to accumulate, and the processing of long-standing ama will take months of consistent digestive practices; in some cases, it may require the help of an Ayurveda professional.

Addressing early signs of buildup (listed in the checklist on page 76) by modifying food choices and habits, or undergoing a detoxification period, can clear ama out. The remedy is to stoke digestion of the sticky, leftover substance. **Important note:** Clearing ama from the digestive tract is way easier than clearing it from the deeper tissues. Get to know the signs from the check-list, and if you've been experiencing a number of them for a year or more, seek out a practitioner who can help you, or consider visiting a *panchakarma* center for a residential intervention that takes three to four weeks. (See the resources in appendix C for trustworthy centers.)

## WHAT CAUSES AMA?

Ama is caused by a poor diet, an imbalance in digestive fire, and the stagnation of wastes (think back to the suppression of urges we discussed in chapter 3). Unresolved emotions and experiences can also promote physical stagnations that lead to ama formation. Ayurveda texts are very clear about avoiding mealtimes when you're angry or anxious to reduce the production of ama. Imagine how variable your appetite becomes during extreme stress, and consider replacing a complicated meal with one of the tonic recipes from chapter 22 to provide nourishment while giving your body space to digest emotion when needed.

The body can handle some stress, or some poorly digested food, from time to time. If you really want that tub of popcorn at the movie theater, enjoy it (and head in with an appetite). Take care not to repeat it tomorrow. When poor habits become the norm, compromised digestion can get serious.

## Ama Checklist

If you *consistently* experience several of the following, you might have ama buildup:

- Opaque, white coating on the tongue that doesn't scrape off
- Heavy feeling in the stomach or back of the throat
- Bad taste in the mouth, bad breath
- Chronic congestion
- Grogginess after meals
- Heavy, sticky, stinky stools
- Stronger than usual body odor
- Lymphatic congestion (swelling such as swollen breasts before periods, bloating after meals)
- Constipation and/or diarrhea
- Low libido
- Mental confusion (brain fog, especially after eating)

## REMOVING AMA

When you follow best practices for digestion, more often than not, your body will process ama, you'll have fresh breath, your digestive fire will burn brightly, and you will feel that your food digests and metabolizes well. You may begin to notice a tendency for your tongue to develop a thick, white coating when you eat certain foods or eat late at night. Look for this when you scrape your tongue in the morning, not right after eating. This tips you off to what's not working and is a great place to start giving your agni some TLC. (For more on tongue scraping, see page 58.)

## Ama, Inflammation, and Rasa

Ama circulating in the rasa dhatu has its own signs and is not uncommon. In my experience as a practitioner, it can be linked to what Western medicine calls inflammation. Ama from poor digestion enters rasa dhatu first, and compromised food-juice is absorbed through the small intestine into the bloodstream. The opposite of ama—which is cool, heavy, and sticky—is fire. As the body turns up the heat to "cook" the ama out of the system, you may begin to experience excess heat, swelling, and body pain—all signs of "inflammation." Autoimmune conditions, rooted in inflammation in Western medicine, are often rooted in long-term ama in Ayurveda.

If you are experiencing chronic signs of autoimmune disorders, seek further evaluation. If you are experiencing early signs of inflammation, and you feel your digestion isn't working very well, it's worth checking in with an Ayurveda practitioner for a protocol for processing ama. Ayurveda techniques to improve digestion also work well in tandem with Western treatments to ensure the process doesn't start up again later due to the same digestive weakness.

## Ama and Undereating

In cases of undernourishment, whether intentional or due to malnutrition, the body may begin to exhibit signs of ama. Undernourishment, and binge eating (eating too much and then too little), cause agni imbalances that lead to ama over time. In these cases, fasting will not improve digestion. Better to establish a dedicated practice of regular meals, served warm, moist, and nicely spiced. For more on easy-to-digest nourishment, see part four.

# 8

# Detoxification and Rejuvenation

## PRACTICES FOR ESSENTIAL BALANCE

One spring the potted thyme plant I keep indoors in winter underwent a transformation. Once I moved the plant outside again, all of the greens died back, and it sent up tiny, tender new shoots. Over a week or two, the new shoots expanded with leaves larger and brighter than the winter stems. The thyme plant was reborn. It was an inspiring sight to witness the instinct for renewal and to feel it mirrored in myself and my community, as the warmer weather mobilized minds and bodies with fresh energy and ideas. Most growing things on this planet balance a period of full steam ahead with a time of cleansing, and women are no exception. In Ayurveda, allowing space and time for these transformations is a part of basic self-care.

Your period is a natural time of detoxification, a superb example of cyclic cleansing, and the lunar rhythms described in chapter 9 support this. However, with an increase in endocrine-disrupting chemicals (EDCs) in a lot of the products women are exposed to—cosmetics, household cleaning products, even conventional feminine hygiene products—supporting detoxification is more important than ever. These "reproductive toxins" are chemicals that have an affinity for the generative organs; cause hormone disruptions; affect the uterus, ovaries, and breasts; and can even affect a fetus. Ayurveda-style cleansing improves agni, honing subtle metabolic function, which optimizes your body's natural detox mechanisms. It is an amazing skill to learn and integrate.

This chapter provides a how-to home cleanse, but it is important that you understand the context of how and when to use this tool, or cleansing can be harmful and vata aggravating. Doing a home cleanse is not always necessary, and the ideal scenario is for the body to get rid of wastes consistently, doing a mini-detox every night. Going to bed by ten and eating a light dinner is one of those important routines that sets us up for a nightly detox between 10 P.M. and 2 A.M.

I teach that cleansing can also be a clearing of old habits, energy patterns, or messy desk space. The point is to slow down enough to take stock of your daily rhythms, your diet, and your dinacharya practices and see how they are serving you. Are there qualities in need of balance?

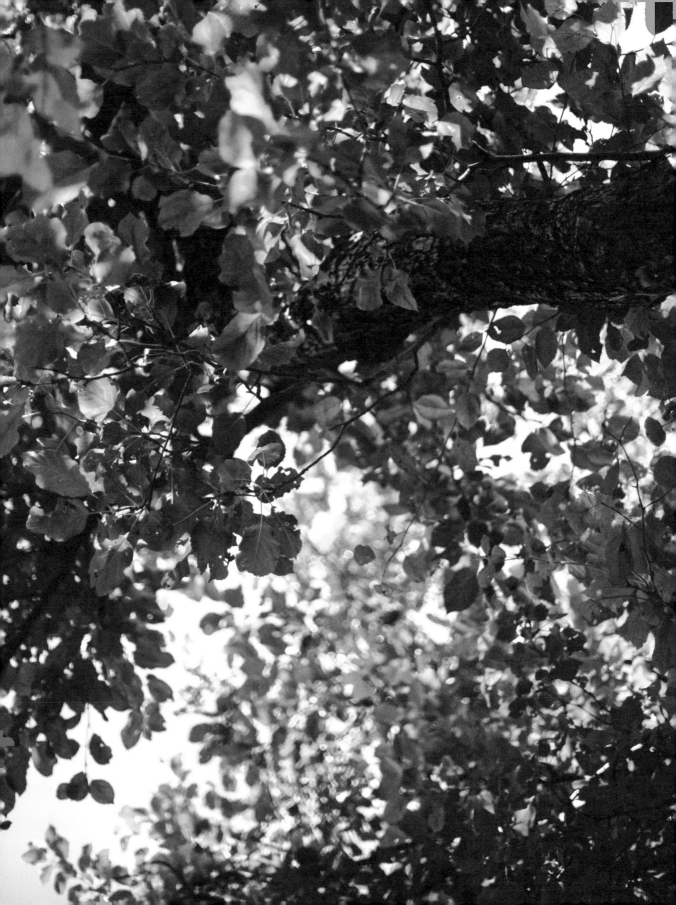

## DEFINITION OF *CLEANSE*

The Ayurveda concept of cleansing is used as a prerequisite for nourishment, and the two together maintain essential balance. Placing detoxification into a complete context with rejuvenation, understanding why and when we might need them, and when we do not, gives us a golden tool for cultivating health.

Take a long view, and imagine yourself doing purification about once every year. Some years it may feel appropriate to "go big," and other years the program may be shorter or quite moderate. More is not better, and timing is everything. When you do not feel strong—when you are a caretaker, very busy, or under a lot of stress—is a good time to go easy. At another moment in your life, you may find that you have more freedom or that you can recruit friends and family to help you carve out time to retreat and go deeper into self-purification. Addressing qualities as they present in your body is of utmost importance. More targeted approaches for different stages of life are discussed in part three and can be layered with the basic home cleansing guidelines.

When we talk about "doing a detox" or "doing a cleanse," it often doesn't mean *shodhana* (cleanse) in the traditional sense. I like to be careful when I use these terms, because it's one of those wellness trends that can be overdone. People just love to "detox," whereas the concept of receiving deep nourishment is truly the hard part for many. It seems this is a result of a cultural favoring of solar qualities, the active, sharp, and intense side of essential balance.

Detoxification is essentially the process of langhana (lightening). Light foods and body therapies that draw out toxins later need to be balanced with a reintroduction of grounding foods and therapies. Then cleansing is always coupled with essential rejuvenation through nourishing foods, medicines, and therapies. The *Ashtanga Hrdayam* says that "Rasayana (rejuvenation) given to someone who has not completed cleansing first is like trying to dye a dirty cloth." This means the tissues will not soak up the nutrition or medicine. They need to be prepared to receive it first.

Healing substances such as herbal milk or ghee will work better after a light diet, when the body will absorb the carrier fats and their medicines easily. Taking an herbal milk after a burger and fries is likely to overload agni. So it's helpful to think about cleansing as a practice that works in tandem with rejuvenation. The nourishment that follows cleansing is often the whole point—especially so when we are working with artava dhatu.

# MODERN BODIES AND TRADITIONAL PRACTICES

The ancient texts were written in times and places where undernourishment was more common than overnourishment. Doctors with whom I study today make amendments to the traditional knowledge for bodies that are overnourished. Perhaps the long-term changes have to do with industrial farming practices, the fact that poor-quality food is more accessible, or the indigestibility of processed foods leading to excess fat (especially trans fats) and clogging of the channels. Such a discussion is beyond the scope of this book.

What we don't know yet are the full effects of the chemicals that surround us via our household cleaners, toiletries, cosmetics, dyes, packaging, pharmaceuticals—the list goes on. Endocrine-disrupting chemicals, commonly found in plastic food containers, are especially problematic, because they disrupt how hormones are made or directed in the body by mimicking them and binding to receptors on cells. This is another aspect of the modern environment that was not present in ancient times as it is today and another good reason to consider periodic cleansing as part of a healthy rhythm.

We need to expand how we think about cleansing and look at purification on many levels. The fundamental importance of the task is not only to "purify" but to maintain an essential balance of lightening and nourishing qualities in life over time. For those who are strong and working with imbalances that haven't yet lodged in the tissues, home cleansing is an excellent annual regimen to consider. A five- to seven-day cleanse can give the body a chance to eliminate doshas and their qualities that may be causing problems. You can assist this by introducing opposite qualities through foods, herbs, and therapies. A longer period can target deeper healing and is best undertaken with guidance.

You may have heard of *kichari*, Ayurveda's healing food. This mixture of rice and mung beans with spices and ghee is said to be good for all body types and will not cause any imbalances. Eating this "monodiet" for five to seven days (or even three) allows you to eat enough food to undergo a cleanse without losing too much strength and without creating imbalance by going too deep too fast. Slow and steady is the way of the home cleanse. The simple diet is how we allow the digestive tract, the major pathway for elimination of toxins, to get rid of stuff that doesn't need to be there, and how we help agni to grow bright and take care of ama. You can emerge feeling fresh and with a good appetite for healthy foods.

## PREPARING FOR CLEANSING

Keeping the person stronger than the disease is the best approach to staying well. Best results come when you've laid solid groundwork. Sliding back into suboptimal food and daily routines soon after a detox can "retox" you to a greater degree than where you started, because your tissues want to soak up what's coming in. The agni gets sensitive with any change in diet, and this also requires a careful reintegration of more complicated foods over at least a few days. Be prepared to prep with healthy habits beforehand and go slow to reintegrate.

Someone with zero body fat or scanty periods should not lose weight in the name of a seasonal health regimen. For this person, undertaking a cleanse might look like not eating junk food, eating only foods that nourish the body, and focusing on building qualities. This allows the body to clean up. But it also requires a focus on nourishment and the preparation of good food, possibly more than three times daily. Home cleansing requires cooking, grocery shopping, sitting down, and eating.

A big problem I see often is that people want to take on a cleansing diet but keep the same rigorous lifestyle. Rest is an essential aspect of Ayurveda cleansing. If the attention and senses are going outward all day, this activity requires nourishment, so kichari alone may not cut it. The inner channels, which may indeed need a sweep-and-mop, will not receive the body's care when the attention is outward most of the time. Without enough rest and inward focus during a cleanse, one can emerge feeling worse.

For those who do not feel strong, who are in a very active time of life (such as breastfeeding or raising young children), or who are contending with a disease diagnosis, cleansing may not be the right thing. A detoxification period can upset an established status quo. In cases where healthy habits have slipped, approach a home cleanse as a marker to get started on healthy habits that will stick around. Beware of pushing yourself through a rigorous cleanse and then collapsing into old habits.


## TIMING A CLEANSE

Ayurveda recommends a juncture between seasons as the ideal time for cleansing. Spring is the time to get rid of excess heavy, moist, dense, slow qualities that have accumulated during the winter. The longer your winter is, the more important spring cleansing may be. Fall is the time to get rid of excess hot, sharp, penetrating qualities that have accumulated during the summer. For hot body types, this can be very wise.

While you get more bang for your buck when you cleanse at a change of season, the best time for you is the time when you can relax. Having a sit-down with the calendar ahead of time is a good idea to make some space for an annual home cleanse. Once a rhythm begins to emerge, your annual cleanse time will start to feel natural.

Changes in temperature and moisture are a good place to start paying attention to signs of the seasons. Watch for signs in your body like dry skin or scalp, cold hands and feet, loss of appetite or a heavy stomach, and oily skin and hair; start to think of how these signs can tell you that your body is becoming dry, moist, or overheated. Have it in mind to balance these qualities during your home cleanse, so they don't get a foothold as the season deepens.

When possible, time your purification period during a waning moon and new moon, and rejuvenate during the waxing moon.

## THINGS TO CONSIDER WHEN PLANNING A CLEANSE

Before you begin, it is important to begin phasing out products in your home that may contain EDCs. (You will find a link to a consumer guide for EDCs in appendix C.) During a home cleanse, be sure to use only natural cleaners and body care products, and wear natural fibers as much as possible. Avoid using anything that contains "fragrance," which includes scented candles.

Ayurveda's approach to cleansing has some aspects that do not appear in Western philosophies. Purification involves the diet, the mind and senses, and relationships (to self and other). Doing a juice cleanse, which is common in some wellness circles, addresses only one of these aspects of life (diet) and neglects the greater context.

Detoxing your physical body works in the following order:
- Improving agni to burn impurities and digest well postcleanse
- Loosening toxins from the tissues and channels
- Processing toxins
- Rejuvenating

## CONTRAINDICATIONS

Cleansing is not recommended while breastfeeding or if you could be pregnant.

If you have health complications or any doubts whatsoever on how to go about a home cleanse, you will get better results by working with a practitioner to tailor something specific to your body at this time.

Those with any history of restrictive eating should proceed with caution and compassion on any food-based program.

# HOME CLEANSE PROGRAM

This simple, moderate program for home cleansing is an opportunity to slow down and take stock of your current food and dinacharya routines. Perhaps you've lost your rhythm, and this home cleanse isn't about food at all but a chance to get rhythms back on track. Keep a broad view of what cleansing means, and be in the moment to make the choice about what feels beneficial as you set your intentions for a three- to seven-day journey (or anywhere in between). I have provided two meal plans: one is a supersimple, one-pot meal you can make daily, and the other offers more comfort foods and variety. All the recipes in this book can be used, provided you follow the guidelines from the table on page 85, and if you have the time and space to go deep, simply use the Easy Meal Plan.

## WHAT TO EAT FOR DETOXIFICATION

During a cleanse, choose from food groups in the left column of the table. Favorable foods are easy to digest and nourish the body without creating any imbalances. The foods in the right column are OK to enjoy occasionally, but they are irritants, potential allergens, or difficult to digest and don't support a detoxification period. Choosing from the Foods to Favor list provides the conditions your body needs to detox.

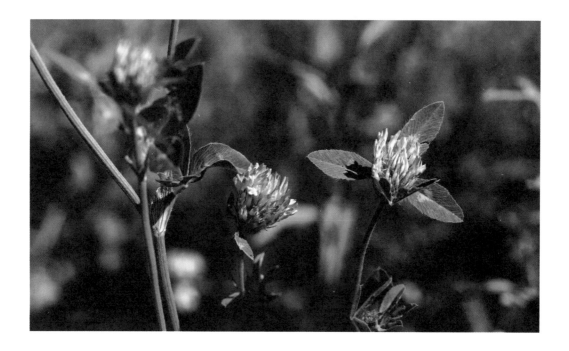

| FOODS TO FAVOR | FOODS TO AVOID |
|---|---|
| Herbal tea and spiced waters | Coffee and caffeinated tea |
| Date sugar, coconut sugar, raw honey, maple syrup, stevia (all only in ½ tsp portions) | White sugar |
| Mung beans, lentils (red, green, black), small amounts of grass-fed whey protein, rice protein, hemp protein, if needed | Animal products and isolated soy products, such as protein bars |
| Whole grains, especially basmati rice | Wheat products and all refined flours |
| Raw dairy, when available, if needed | Processed dairy |
| Sweet potatoes, steamed leafy greens | Members of the nightshade family: eggplant, tomato, white potato, bell peppers |
| Fruits and vegetables in season | Foods out of season |
| Natural fresh juices, especially pomegranate and vegetable juices | Alcohol, iced drinks |
| Seeds: sunflower, hemp, pumpkin, flax, chia | Nuts and nut butters |

Don't forget about *how* you eat during your detox. While you choose from the above table, favor a bigger lunch and smaller dinner, avoid mixing raw fruits with food, and take care to relax while you eat. All these choices support agni.

Consider the following meal plans according to whether you are trying to lighten up or preserve grounding qualities while cleansing. If you feel puffy, stagnant, and heavy, choose langhana. If you feel stressed, tire easily, or have little body fat, choose brmhana. If you aren't sure, take it one day at a time. Remember to work toward sit-down meals with no snacks; this may mean eating four meals a day.

**Easy Meal Plan**

If you don't want to think too much about planning and cooking, focus on New Moon Kichari (page 286); make a big pot and eat it for all your meals that day. Make a new pot the next day, and use different vegetables for variety. Between meals, sip Essential Spiced Water (page 231).

**Lightening Meal Plan**

    **Breakfast:** Strawberry Rose Smash (page 259) or Moringa Green Drink Three Ways (page 250)

    **Lunch:** New Moon Kichari (page 286) with Mixed Greens Chutney (page 297)

    **Dinner:** Red Rice Kanji (page 271) with Warm Arame and Kale Salad (page 292)

    **Between Meals:** Cleansing Herbal Infusion (page 222)

**Grounding Meal Plan**

    **Breakfast:** Best Medicinal PSL (page 244) and/or Creamy Coconut Breakfast Kichari (page 264)

    **Lunch:** New Moon Kichari (page 286) with Pumpkin Seed Cilantro Pâté (page 293)

    **Dinner:** Every Body Dal (page 280) with Warm Arame and Kale Salad (page 292)

    **Between Meals:** Essential Mineral Vegetable Broth (page 272) or Nourishing Herbal Infusion (page 218)

Choose one of the therapies from the following lists to practice during your cleanse.

Lightening Therapies
- Exercising, especially outdoors
- Sweating, via working out or a dry sauna
- Dry brushing
- Drinking Triphala Tea (page 224) or gargling with saltwater

Grounding Therapies
- Making time for relaxation—less moving around and more lying around
- Oiling the ears and feet at night
- Doing a sesame oil massage and/or a coconut oil head massage

## POSTCLEANSE REJUVENATION

Follow a cleanse with a period of rejuvenation. Imagine your tissues soaking up all the prana, minerals, and building qualities of natural foods after a light diet. Optimize your rebuild by taking a spoonful of Chyawanprash Herbal Jam (recipe on page 256, or purchase it from a supplier in appendix C) daily for about a month. The tonics from chapter 22 are also an excellent follow-up. Find more about rejuvenation therapies in chapter 18; you can benefit from them at any age. You can also find specific information about rejuvenation before conception in chapter 13.

# 9

# Lunar Rhythms for Health and Evolution

Essential to nature is an ebb and flow, regulated shifts between mobility and stability. This flow is present in the solar rhythms of a day—sunrise and sunset—and in annual seasons of growth, change, and decay. In Ayurveda practices, women can connect to a lunar rhythm that operates on a monthly cycle for stabilizing the generative system, as well as the mind and moods. A solar-leaning hormonal imbalance causes a lot of women's health issues (see chapter 1). The body of the moon itself is a direct line to soma. Balancing solar and lunar energies can lead to physiological healing: smoother menstrual and menopausal transitions, enhanced fertility, and a balanced mind. Cultivating a healthier hormone matrix throughout life has profound effects on the hormonal axis of our bodies and all the systems governed by it.

Throughout life, we react to desires, we plant seeds, we cultivate and establish. Then we cleanse, harvest, and let go of things we no longer desire or no longer benefit from. There are times we crave stillness and times we crave activity. It seems that too often we don't find the opportunity to reflect on the desires and actions that drive us. In a culture of "go," we end up operating through solar channels and rejecting the pause, the times between the tides when the wall of water is swollen with potential movement but momentarily still. It is in these moments of inaction when deeper awareness and meaning arise: the sacred pause.

Within the lunar rhythm framework, there is a possibility for spiritual healing too. Aligning with lunar energies attunes us to deeper aspects of nature and its pull, of our own cosmic nature, and the nature of Life itself.

## THE WAXING AND WANING MOON PHASES

The moon becomes "new" each month and waxes (builds) for two weeks. The waxing moon grows from a sliver to a circle, becoming brighter each night, and culminating with the full moon. During the waxing moon, the nourishing, soft, and cool qualities of the moon are on the rise. Approaching the full moon, the water element rises in the body, as when the ocean's tide shifts from low to high. The water element is most prevalent in rasa dhatu, our milk-like, juicy plasma.

Just as the tides swell with the full moon, rasa dhatu and its water element become expansive and full of building qualities. In women at the childbearing stage of life, this "juiciness," or shukra, provides the egg, the fertility component, with strong, energetic fullness. For women in later stages of life, these qualities also give generative energy and can be harnessed and directed into the deep tissues for nourishment, as well as toward creative endeavors. The time of the waxing moon is like springtime for the body and supports life-giving energies and higher activity levels.

The waning moon is also a two-week phase, beginning after the full moon and culminating with the new moon. Each night the moon grows darker, shrinking to a sliver, and on the fourteenth day, no moon is visible. The waning and new moon are the "dark" time. Energies naturally recede from external engagement and increasingly turn inward. The social and creative energy of the waxing moon is balanced by the quieter, contemplative waning moon.

Slowing down and turning in calms the wind and space elements. For women in the childbearing stage, rakta dhatu contributes to building the uterine lining, and fiery qualities of rakta may predominate, making this phase hotter and more irritable and a great time for cooling and calming practices. In any stage of life, the contemplative, dark time can be a window of personal and cosmic revelation and promotes deep wisdom building. Creating space for self-reflection during this time optimizes nature's potential for the mind and body. The time of the waning moon is like autumn and supports mental and physical purification.

Ayurveda texts divide a woman's monthly cycle into three parts, in which each of the doshas is physiologically more active. Most of the information in the classic texts is concerned with fertility and gestation. The texts do not provide much on the stage of life we call menopause. Therefore, texts relate the phases of the month to the activities of menstruating women and the corresponding cyclic dosha changes. (For those who menstruate, information on the three phases of the monthly cycle is given in chapter 11.)

A woman menstruates for about half her life, and as we live longer, information about living well postperiods is important. Let's explore the two cycles of the moon, waxing and waning, to consider how working with this flow fosters an essential balance at any age.

## LUNAR RHYTHM CONSIDERATIONS

Before we begin, take care not to adopt an all-or-nothing or too literal approach with the lunar rhythms in this chapter. This is not about following a protocol, but more about developing a perspective on how our energy moves between solar and lunar channels during a moon cycle. What resonates most with you? If you attune to this cycle, there will be an obvious element of your energy, sleep, periods, doshas, or moods that wants your attention. Just start integrating some awareness during the month, and try to establish a practice rhythm around it.

For example, if you are always tired, note when the new moon is and try to go to bed earlier for a few days during the dark time. Do this for a few months and see how you feel. When you establish one rhythm, it becomes the touchstone for a monthly awareness of flow.

These guidelines about rest and activity, and the shifting focus of inward to outward and back again, are good for most people most of the time. But remember that you are the one in your body, and if a practice doesn't feel beneficial, skip it and focus on something else.

# A Lunar Cycle

Over the course of a month, we move from a release of the previous month's energies to cultivating new energy and intentions, celebrating and manifesting, and looking inward for regeneration.

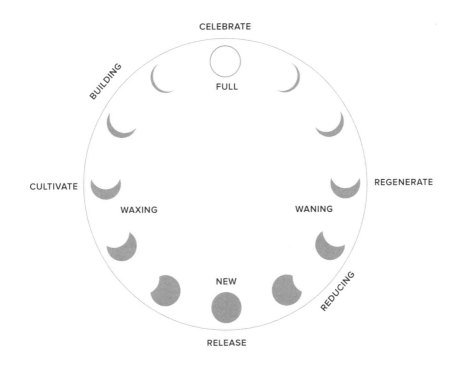

# NEW MOON: RELEASE

The new or "dark" moon is a time for dwelling with shadow, for promoting introspection, for getting rid of the old and making space for new growth. During the dark moon, activity reduces, tides are gentler, animals and hunters rest because they cannot see their prey. In a woman's cycle, this phase has the energy of winter, an inward-dwelling, restful, and quiet time. It is the time of release. What are you holding on to? The following new moon guidelines help the natural flow of energy turn down into your core by reducing stimulation, calming vata, and opening the channels.

**Make time to slow down.** Have a sense of when the new moon is going to be, and schedule fewer activities at that time.

**Fast (from food and stimulation).** On the new moon day, clear your mind by practicing silence, or observe a day of social media fasting. If you are no longer menstruating, a one-day kichari fast on the new moon is an excellent ongoing detox regimen. A one-day cleanse can take many forms—a monodiet of anything easy to digest, for example. In cold weather, it may be oats; in warmer weather, quinoa. Kapha types or overnourished folks can fast on hot water, Cleansing Herbal Infusion (page 222) or Essential Spiced Water (see page 231).

**Quiet the senses.** The ever-attentive sense organs pull prana out of the body. Taking care to reduce stimulation for a sense cleanse on a monthly rhythm not only preserves and rejuvenates the sense organs but also calms vata, restores apana, and reduces stress levels.

**Nest.** Socializing is great and community is nourishing, but if you find you are busy all the time, consider a new moon stay-home routine. Use the opportunity to organize an aspect of your space (not everything at once!), get rid of clutter, and/or do a creative home-improvement project. Put energy into your nest.

**Practice introspection.** Do some free-form writing, music making, or whatever helps you reflect, take stock, and release nonbeneficial thoughts.

**Ground yourself (literally).** Send energy down by connecting your bare feet to the earth. If it's cold, go outdoors and visualize the connection. Breathe down through your feet and into the earth.

**Bathe ritualistically.** Do an abhyanga (see page 323) or warm the room, dim the lighting, and settle into an Epsom salts bath, adding relaxing nervine plants such as lavender and rose.

**Work with herbs.** Incorporate herbs that support downward flow and pacify vata into your routine during the new moon; try Nourishing Herbal Infusion (page 218). If you are not menstruating during the new moon and looking for purification, drink Cleansing Herbal Infusion (page 222). Triphala Tea (page 224) also assists detoxification and downward flow, but do not use it while menstruating.

## WAXING MOON: CULTIVATE SHUKRA

The "bright fortnight" is the fourteen days after the new moon when the moon grows brighter each day until the full moon. In nature, activity begins to bustle and increase as the moon gets brighter. Tides rise even higher. The milky moonlight brings qualities of kapha, cool and moist, to the cosmos, and energy builds. The moon governs soma, the essential juice of substances and bodies. Soma is at its highest during the waxing and full moon. Any food taken during this period will yield the best nourishment. In farming practices, anything planted during a waxing moon will be stronger and produce the best seed. This also applies to creative projects and intentions.

As in springtime, the body directs resources toward creation during the waxing moon. It is a time of renewal after the dark phase. Some women, especially those who menstruate, may feel hungry for ojas-building foods during this phase. The fires of transformation are at work, and digestion and elimination tend to be easier. This is the time to build up your stores of physical, mental, and spiritual energy that culminate in manifestation on the day of the full moon. Water the seeds of your intentions.

We can assist nature's building energies with the following guidelines for food intake, daily living, balancing practices, and herbal support.

**Nourish.** The bright moon is a time of month for living at full power. Fuel up with sweet tastes from whole grains; meats and dairy (if you eat them); dense fruits like dates and figs; sweet and sour citrus; and root vegetables, especially yams and sweet potatoes. Balance all this with smaller amounts of bitter and astringent fruits, vegetables, and herbs.

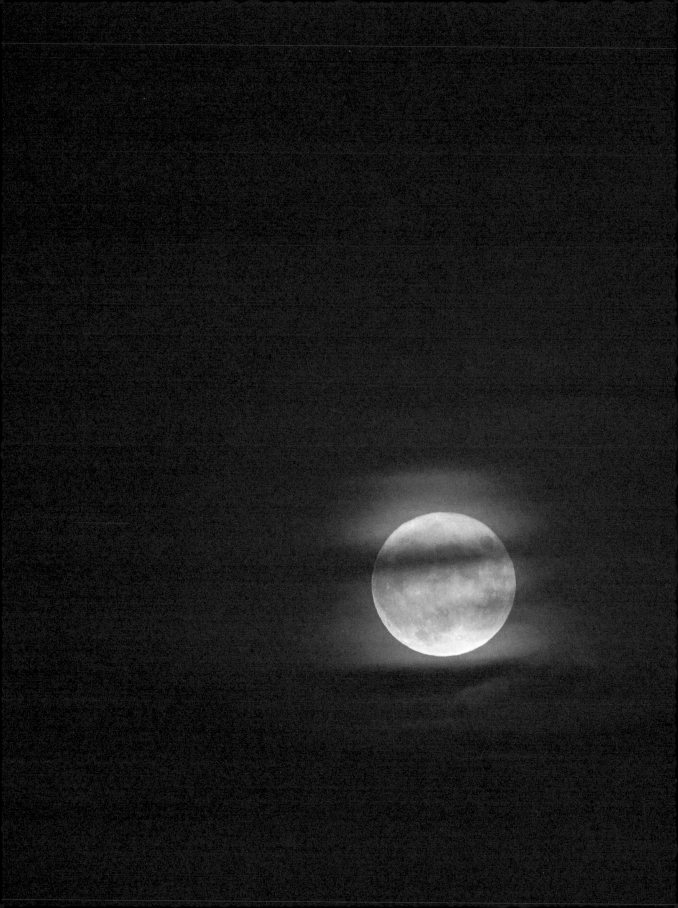

**Avoid poor-quality, heavy, sticky foods.** The body is integrating building qualities at this time, so foods that are heavy, sticky, oily, and denatured are not what you want. Watch out for processed oils, conventional meats, pastries, conventional dairy, excessively salty and sour foods, and white sugar.

**Support ojas.** Concentrate on life-giving substances, such as local milk, ghee, and produce; Nourishing Herbal Infusion (page 218); Essential Mineral Vegetable Broth (page 272); and meat-based soup. Remember that during this moon phase the body most effectively extracts the essence of foods into rasa dhatu. Ojas is preserved by lifestyle factors like moderation, getting enough nourishment and enough rest, and practicing wholesome behaviors not limited to diet.

**Moonbathe.** Soak up soma by walking or relaxing in the moonlight.

**Move more.** It is natural to want to be more active during the waxing moon. You may feel like jogging a little farther or choosing more active pursuits outside. Go for it now, as you may feel more tired as the cycle shifts.

**Be clear.** It's easy to get high on the energy ride as the moon grows and charges up the mental field. The potency of this time for deep nourishment and manifestation of intentions lies in extracting shukra from food and activities. It is good to have a daily check-in to be sure your actions are aligned with your true desires and you aren't just being knocked around like a tetherball.

## FULL MOON: CELEBRATE

In traditional agriculture, seedlings planted during the bright moon are said to absorb more water, which results in better germination and stronger plants later in the season. The full moon pulls moisture to the surface of the soil, in the same way it affects high tides. In women's bodies, this pull results in ultimate juiciness, fertility, and creativity. Take advantage of this magical window in a monthly cycle to nourish, manifest, and celebrate.

The full moon is a twenty-four-hour period when the light of the moon is brightest. Nature hustles and bustles, plants grow faster, as do your hair and nails. The energy of the full moon is akin to the juiciness of kapha. Vaginal juices are plentiful and the heart and mind are likely to be more active. It is common to sleep less and socialize more on the full moon.

The full moon is the time for an outward flow of activity and attention, and it is an ideal time for calling in abundance, whether it's money, opportunity, or fertility—bring it on! Take advantage of the cosmic support to start new projects and foster relationships. Harness full moon energy with the following guidelines.

**Share treats.** Celebratory milk- and ghee-based sweets, such as Almond Cardamom Diamonds (page 306), are often offered on the full moon. Baking or making treats is an excellent full moon ritual. Offer this abundance to loved ones by gifting or hosting and feeding others.

**Make ghee.** Ghee made during the full moon has maximum benefits both for generative tissues and for brain and nerve health. Some believe that the habit of making ghee on the full moon day each month makes a magical cooking oil. Moon Milk (page 247) also builds shukra on the full moon.

**Grow sprouts.** The explosive energy of the full moon is like that of a sprout bursting from a dormant seed. Bring this energy into your days by eating sprouts, which manifest change and growth with the transformative energy of pitta. Green mung beans are very easy to sprout at home and can be used in kichari instead of the split variety. Other common homemade sprouts are alfalfa, radish, and sunflower.

## Full Moon Sprouted Almonds

Four days before the full moon, soak ⅔ cup raw almonds in water overnight, then drain and rinse them. Place them in a dish, covered with a towel, for three more days. Rinse and drain them well each day until the sprouts begin to emerge. Once they sprout, they need to be refrigerated until you use them. Remove the skins, and use the almonds to make a quart of ultra-potent Basic Almond Milk (page 240) on the full moon.

# Gathering as Women

There is power in numbers. When getting women together to call in divine energy —whether it's through sharing stories or food or doing creative activities like in sewing circles—make your gatherings intentional. Consider holding a full moon gathering where your participants are invited to share an intention for the coming month. You may choose to hold these monthly or seasonally, to check in on the intentions shared and support each other's changes and challenges.

Gathering with intention can be as simple as taking a few moments of gratitude before eating. Sometimes we may feel awkward or like we are imposing on our guests by asking them to focus, but in truth, we need more conscious gatherings in the world.

# See Soma in Your Eyes

Moisture changes are visible in the eyes during the lunar cycle. When shukra is building, you may notice that your eyes appear larger and more lustrous. In the same way that you can track digestion by scraping your tongue, daily inspection of your eyes will show changes. Stress and exhaustion reduce luster, whereas juiciness increases it. Look for the luster to build, especially during the bright moon.

**Boost libido.** The full moon supports the highest sex drive in a lunar cycle and boosts fertility. You can stimulate your libido, if needed, by eating onions and garlic. Keep in mind that these alliums are quite heating and may aggravate an acidic stomach. Their powers are considered so potent that, traditionally, people practicing celibacy avoid eating them.

**Manifest.** After clearing the cobwebs and reflecting on motivating factors during the new moon, then watering the seeds of your heart's desire over the waxing moon phase, the full moon is the moment to manifest. Bring the confidence of the previous two weeks' cultivation to a rite to call in what you crave. Choose a ritual that can be done ceremoniously: making ghee or Moon Milk (page 247), for example, or lighting a candle and saying a prayer.

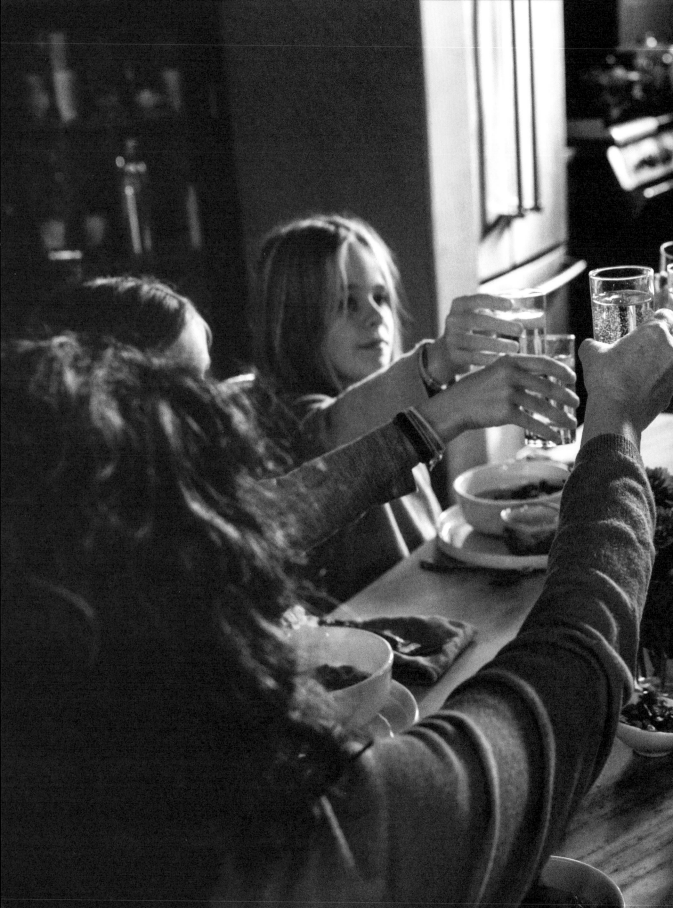

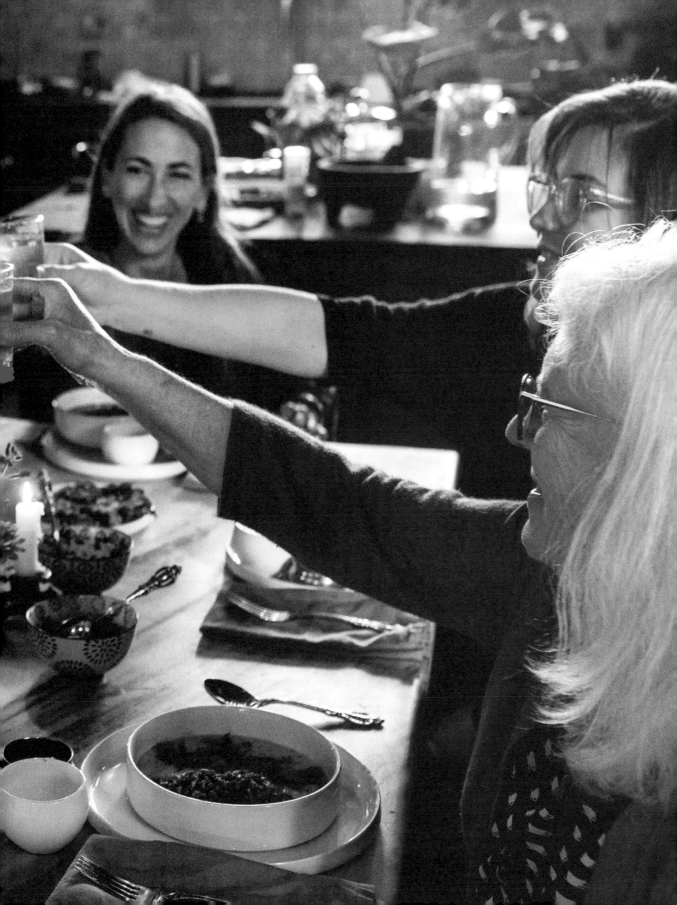

# WANING MOON: REGENERATE

Like autumn, the waning moon is a gradual shift from outward energy and awareness to spending more time with inner work. Regenerate your intentions and investigate how actions during this period do or do not support your deepest desires. Take time in this two-week period to dial down spicy, hot, sour foods and alcohol that could start to aggravate your system as the dark moon approaches. Work in a cycle of regeneration with restful and contemplative self-care rituals for at least the week or so before the new moon. The following practices support the inward flow.

**Taper down.** The week before the new moon is the most potent time to reduce spicy, sour, salty foods and alcohol, especially for those experiencing hot flashes or pitta in the menstrual cycle. This reduction in itself can sometimes alleviate perimenopausal and menstrual symptoms.

**Exercise less.** Work with your energy levels, but don't be surprised if you don't have the same oomph as the moon wanes. Connective tissues may not feel as stretchy and springy without the shukra of a big moon, especially as we get older. Be careful about injuries during the dark moon, as they may take longer to heal.

**Be in bed by ten.** As the moon wanes, sleep comes to the forefront, and it's easier to get back to that early bedtime. Support natural detox by being asleep between 10 P.M. and 2 A.M. Eat dinner earlier too.

**Practice calm.** For many, the natural shift of attention inward can feel uncomfortable. It takes time and practice to slow down if you are used to moving fast. While you might not notice a desire for reflection when the moon is bright, if you pay attention to your energy and consciousness for a few months, you may start to notice an inward mental flow arising. Induce calm in this moon phase by experimenting with a weekly herbal bath or home facial (see appendix A). It's often easier to slow down when you are doing something nurturing.

If you are fairly new to Ayurveda and working in some simple daily routines, you might just allow these ideas about lunar cycles to sit in your consciousness and not act to integrate them now. When the time is right, these concepts will emerge to bring a deeper sense of agency to your movements and a true feeling of cosmic interconnection and living the life you are meant to live. There's no rush.

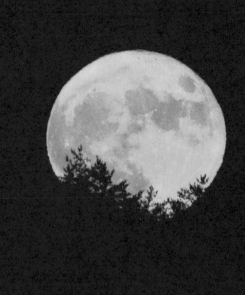

# PART THREE

# FINDING BALANCE THROUGH *the* SEASONS *of* LIFE

Womens' bodies undergo marked changes with menarche, childbirth, and menopause. While the body's transformational processes may not always be as temperate as we would like, understanding the qualities of life's stages and how the doshas manifest gives us big clues about how to manage our transitions smoothly. The lifestyle and diet practices in part two provide tools to set you up for success. In part three, we look closely at the challenges that may be present as women move through different life stages, from fertility to pregnancy to menopause and beyond. The tools in this book empower you to embrace natural changes, recognize signs of imbalance that may arise, and manage the doshas for optimal health.

# 10
# Navigating Principles

## MONEY, FAMILY, DESIRE, AND DHARMA

Persons desirous of (long) life which is the means for achieving dharma (righteousness),
artha (wealth), sukha (happiness; good space)
should repose utmost faith in the teachings of Ayurveda.

—*ASHTANGA HRYDAYAM*, SUTRASTHANA I:2

Front and center in the first section of the Ayurveda texts, Sutrasthana, is an introduction to the *purusarthas* (objectives of life). As you can see in the quotation above, Ayurveda is an important study for those who wish, not only to live a long life, but also to apply their life energy toward spiritual growth. The Vedic underpinnings point to the *meaning* of life, not simply its preservation. In this context, the maintenance of health becomes a philosophical undertaking, as the point of a long, healthy life is to devote plenty of time and energy to living fully and satisfying the aims of a human birth. Weaving the purusarthas into our understanding of the *ashramas* (four stages of life) gives us an even deeper perspective on what life's about and how to do and experience life in the most fulfilling ways.

Through my work with women, I see how helpful this perspective is in illuminating transitional periods. These ideas are a road map for life. Not that we should cleave to a preordained route and follow its course, but we can use this map as a navigational tool: "you are here." While Ayurveda clearly teaches that parinama (change) is the only constant, we find ourselves flabbergasted when that glass of wine begins to yield a hangover. We think, "Wine never had that effect on me before. What the . . . ?" Turns out that bodies, and how they are affected by the environment, are always changing.

Due to these physiological changes of growth and aging, the body's qualities reflect the doshas' qualities in different stages of life. Childhood is the kapha time of life, pitta lasts from puberty to menopause, and vata comprises menopause until the end of life. It will support your health to introduce balancing qualities to manage these changes during the corresponding stage of life. Changes in the body's qualities are unavoidable, but they don't have to bring on imbalances, especially if you understand what's next and are reasonably proactive.

Part three shows us how to look for the changes that are happening and what actions need to occur to support flow. Everything around us is undergoing transformation, as are we—in our bodies, our perspectives, and our objectives. The things we want in life may change, our values may shift, and we may draw satisfaction and pleasure from different activities and pursuits. (When did a "staycation" become so alluring? Why don't I like to travel like I did when I was in my twenties?) This ever-evolving process of *becoming* is the heart. We draw on our knowledge of life stages and aims to get a fresh look, find our "you are here" marker, and reorient with a renewed sense of purpose.

## PURUSARTHAS: THE FOUR AIMS OF LIFE

Imagine the impulses of a baby to discover; to touch, taste, and see everything; and to gain information. Imagine the driving karma to make a family or climb the career ladder in the active stage of life. Imagine this drive, decades later, giving way to a call to seek deeper meaning in this life, contemplate the nature of our desires, and take responsibility for how our desires propel us. Later, this culminates in an impulse to detach, let go of this "self," and merge into Nature. In the first half of life, we move toward possessions and experiences, and in the second half, we move away from them.

*Purusartha* can be translated as "object of human pursuit." The four aims of life are dharma, *artha*, *kama*, and *moksha*. As philosophical ideals, they are the pillars of a human life. The Sanskrit words that describe these objectives are complex, and it's beyond the scope of this book to consider all their meanings. For our purposes, I have listed them briefly and applied the meanings that feel most potent within our context.

Dharma: Righteousness, ethical living

Artha: Wealth, material goods, security

Kama: Desire, gratification

Moksha: Emancipation, spiritual freedom

Women are often at the mercy of so many demands on their time, energy, and attention. Personal goals, career goals, pregnancy, and family are a lot to balance. It's common to feel conflicted between personal and spiritual goals and what family and culture demand of us. How can the purusarthas support that "you are here" feeling on the cosmic road map and help you integrate the specifics of your life? Looking forward to, or back on, these changes through the lens of these four objectives provides a big-picture sense of change and reveals one's driving influence at different stages.

## STAGES OF LIFE, AIMS OF LIFE, AND THE DOSHAS

This chart is a reference for drawing parallels between your stage of life, aim of life, and the doshas. Of course, life can take different courses, but this is useful as a point of reference.

| ASHRAMA: STAGE OF LIFE | PURUSARTHA: AIM OF LIFE | PREVALENT DOSHA |
|---|---|---|
| *Brahmacharya* (student) | Dharma: righteousness | Kapha |
| *Grihastha* (householder) | Artha: wealth, security | Pitta |
| *Vanaprastha* (forest dweller) | Kama: desire, gratification | Vata |
| *Sannyasa* (renunciation) | Moksha: liberation | Vata |

These philosophies on life are food for thought, not dogma. You may cultivate a spiritual anchor in the language of another tradition or in your personal worldview and still navigate the stages and aims of life with intention. A cosmic road map for life's changes can help you stay on the path and live with a feeling that your times of transition are natural—and beneficial! Everything is moving in the right direction.

## WHY KNOWING WHAT'S NEXT MATTERS

The life span of a person is one hundred years. Dividing that time,
he should attend to three aims of life in such a way that they support,
rather than hinder each other. In his youth he should attend to profitable aims (artha)
such as learning, in his prime to pleasure (kama), and in his old age to dharma and moksha.

—KAMA SUTRA 1.2.1–4

At age twenty-four, I had been studying yoga intensively for five years, and I was sick of cleaning houses for a living. I felt that after those years of diligent practice, I should be making a living teaching yoga. On my next visit to my teacher in India, I approached him one afternoon to express my goal.

"I have been a house cleaner for four years on Maui, and I am tired of cleaning. I am thinking of going to Boston where a group needs an instructor. What do you think, Teacher? Should I go?"

"Boston?" he said, shaking his head and looking confused. "You go to Maui. Maaaaany houses are there. Pleeeenty of work." He broke into a bright, assuring smile. "You come here and study yoga three more years, then you take teaching."

Easy for him to say with that big smile. I was crestfallen. But he put into context for me that my present situation, with which I was impatient, was part of a larger plan that would, when it was ripe, yield the best fruit. To start teaching yoga to others too soon can arrest the process of learning and embodying. A priceless lesson! This was one of several pivotal moments in my twenties when a mentor suggested that I keep my day job, study well, and look forward to being of service at a later time. The argument seems obvious to me in hindsight, but back then the discipline of patience was something I had to be taught.

Throughout the stages of life (ashramas), skills can be cultivated in preparation for what comes next, supportive as well as preventive measures to ensure that we are equipped to make the most of the strengths of each stage and are protected through its weaknesses. Our actions in one stage of life can manifest in the next. Learning patience as a student makes for a patient teacher, while learning how to relax during the active years makes for a smoother transition into the later years.

The Vedic view of life clearly describes four stages of evolution, which dovetail with the four aims of life and the doshas. Life begins with a building of the physical body, then a sharpening of the intellect. The active years naturally give way to a slow reduction of stimulation, more peace and quiet. As we age, we can devote more time and energy to spirituality and the life of the soul.

Life stages and aims can happen in a different order, there may be some backtracking or a natural focus on one lifelong aspect. This model may appear linear, but life may move in a zigzag or a spiral. Take care not to impose ideas on yourself. Considered in tandem, the concepts of ashramas and life aims provide a rich garden that, when watered nicely, provides fruits for living well.

# Opening the Channels for Change

Life energy coalesces around intention. Prana follows the mind because both are composed of air and space. It's not only the physical—doshas, hormones, metabolic fires, and such—that changes; it is also our perspective on and orientations in life, our very desires, that are shifting. Ayurveda teaches that bringing awareness to and supporting these inner shifts opens the channels for the physiology to flow smoothly. As we try to manage underlying tectonics with superficial structures, the inner world roils. Looking within, softening, and welcoming deep changes opens the subtle channels for change.

## BRAHMACHARYA: THE STUDENT STAGE

During childhood, the building qualities of kapha support the growing body, strengthen the immune system, and prepare a pliant mind to collect experiences and memories. Earth and water elements make up more of the diet, while physical activity is key to avoiding the stagnation that comes with a lot of kapha qualities.

The essence of brahmacharya is learning about what is right and wrong for us as individuals and as members of a community. Do you remember, when you were a child, someone saying to you, "One cookie is enough," or "You're overtired; it's bedtime"? As kids, we don't know that eating the whole box of cookies is going to cause digestive problems or that we will go crazy due to lack of sleep. We learn that certain things are "not right," while others are—concepts like nonviolence, cleanliness, and truthfulness.

The word *brahmacharya* is from *brahma* ("the divine") and *charya* ("movement"): to move in a way that is harmonious with the divine. (We also see *charya* in *dinacharya*, which means moving in a way that is harmonious with daily rhythms.) Learning how to live in the world is as practical as it is spiritual, and while we learn morality as children, it is also ideal to learn healthy daily rhythms. Girls' bodies will begin to sync with the moon at puberty, and attuning young girls to lunar rhythms is one way of helping them understand the world and their bodies that will serve them throughout their lives.

The first twenty-five years or so of life are a time of learning. It is important to support girls in gaining perspective on the world and finding meaning in it. Brahmacharya is about the *how* of life, not the *what*. The development of a sound moral and spiritual compass, an understanding that life requires nourishment and attention both internally and externally, is the best-case

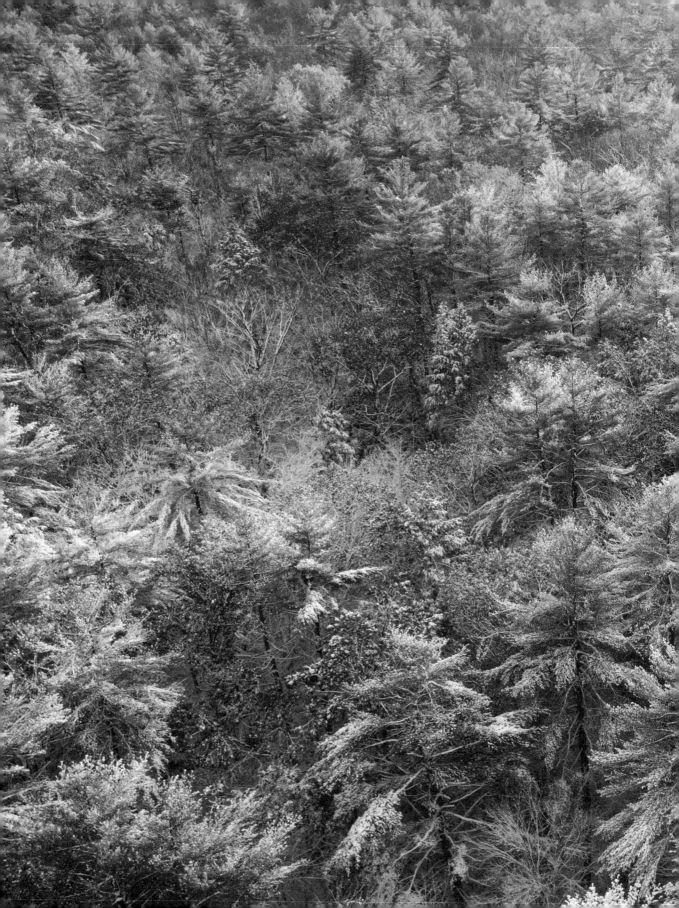

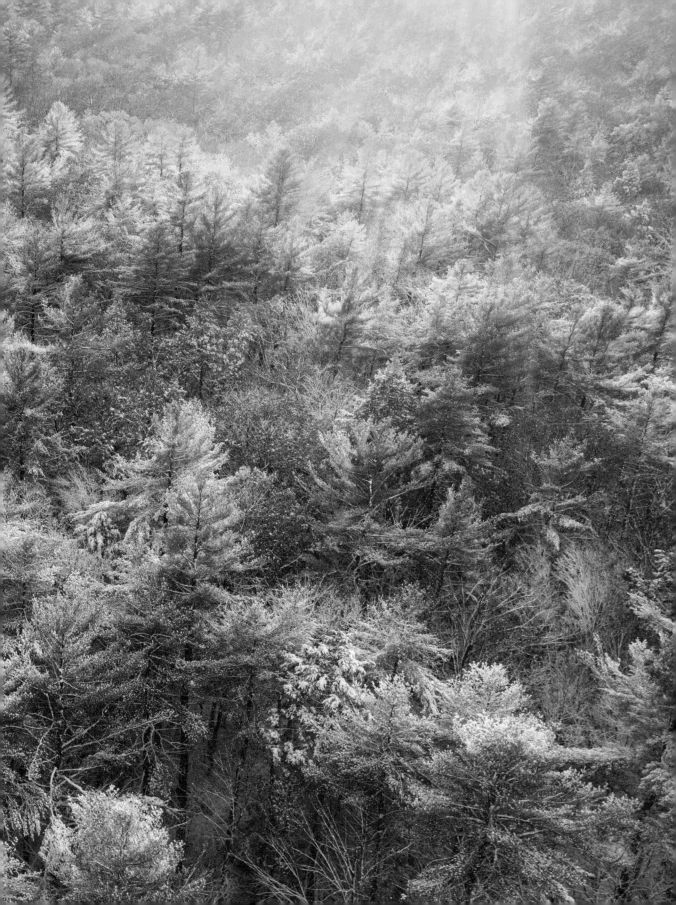

scenario for these younger years. If during this stage of life a girl is taught that only material success matters, she may be set up to work in that direction in the second stage of life and end up wondering what really matters when that stage shifts.

## DHARMA: HOW TO LIVE RIGHTEOUSLY

Many women at some point have to consider whether they intend to have children, which was at other times in history considered to be the pinnacle of the female experience. These days, the choice to be a mother is likely to be weighed against desires for other pursuits. While trying to "have it all" may end up creating imbalances for many women, an alternative goal of establishing *sukha*, with whatever we've chosen or been given, is the pinnacle of dharmic living.

The word *dharma* is often misused and confused. A simple way to clear this up: dharma isn't about the *what*, it's the *how*. "Am I living my dharma?" doesn't mean "Am I supposed to have kids? Am I in the career I am supposed to be in? Am I living my life's purpose?" It means "Am I manifesting in the universe in the way that is most beneficial for all beings?" This good space, called *sukha* (which also means "happiness") is, according to Ayurveda, the highest purpose of life.

*Dharma* means "to hold or support," and one can think of the cosmic laws of dharma, laid out in the ancient Dharmashastra texts, as that which holds and supports moral living instead of chaos. A best-case scenario is that a person learns and begins to adopt tenets of compassionate living when they are young, and dharma becomes their moral compass, a root of happiness and satisfaction throughout their life. Imagine making decisions from a place of compassion, moderation, and contentment instead of one that is rash, uninformed, and selfish. Seeds sown from a thoughtful place are likely to land us in better growing conditions.

For young women, learning healthy perspectives on menstruation, fertility, and birth control and finding role models who demonstrate different pathways for creating good space in the world are the ideal. Routines for good living frame all the choices and interactions to come and become a navigation tool. Nature's rhythms are a dharma of sorts, a support structure for the body, mind, and spirit as we move through the world. If healthy habits are not instilled in youth, or one has drifted away from them, it is never too late to adopt those habits one day at a time.

# GRIHASTHA: THE HOUSEHOLDER STAGE

"Householding" means taking care of the business of daily life. In this second stage of life (approximately age twenty-five to fifty), the focus is on engaging with the external world, being part of a community or society, working, making money, having a family, acquiring material goods. Women may bear and raise children or manifest creation and caretaking in other ways. One is no longer a child and needs to stand on one's own, find security and sustenance, and perhaps provide for others as well. This is a time of action and responsibility. The moral compass established in the first stage of life governs the activities of this second stage. Holding down the responsibilities of an employee, a parent, or a community leader may take up most of someone's time. The pursuit of self-knowledge can easily fall by the wayside and is often not a priority. While these years are intensely busy for many, setting aside time for routines that keep one grounded and healthy will ease the transition into the next stage, fortify the body, and keep imbalances at bay.

The activity of the grihastha stage will remind you of the hot, sharp, intense nature of pitta, and indeed this is the pitta time of life. An awareness of balancing pitta dosha with relaxation time, nature, and play—in addition to keeping stimulants, recreational drugs, and alcohol under control—will help maintain balance despite what may be a very busy time.

## ARTHA: THE MEANING OF MATERIAL GOODS

Considerations about money and abundance are at the forefront during this time. *Artha*, usually translated as "wealth," is a word that takes a little finessing to define. In the grihastha stage, one moves from being a dependent to being depended upon, such as in the case of being responsible for a family or business. Although you may not have been too concerned with possessions before, it gets real when you need to procure your own home, bed, and food. To take care of family and live comfortably becomes a priority. Building financial security manifests as "making a living."

Making a living is having an active and engaged relationship with community and culture. Brahmacharya sets us up to do so with a sound moral compass. Grihastha is a time for building, not letting go. What artha says in this context is, turn your attention to security and prosperity. Build a home, perhaps a family, and provide a product or service to humanity.

Amassing money and "stuff" becomes a problem when we lose sight of why we are doing so. A belief that happiness comes from material goods and that amassing wealth is our purpose will cause a rude awakening in later life, or at the doors of death, when we realize none of it goes with us. Placing the pursuit of wealth in the context of a larger life story keeps it in perspective. Artha calls us to consider what we value in life, what *feels* like wealth.

# A Woman's Story:
# Balancing Work and Pregnancy

So many women struggle to keep up with the demands of procreating while still maintaining a career. Most women have to keep working, and many wish to be mothers as well as to feed other parts of the self. This story is contributed by Emily Murphy Kaur, the owner of a retreat center in Vermont. I observed her building a small business from scratch, as well as becoming pregnant just a year after opening the center. I invited her to share a story about finding balance.

For many women, finding a balanced way to grow both professionally and personally is important to feeling fulfilled. As the owners of Sētu Vermont, a retreat center focused on Ayurveda living, my husband and I worked long hours, leaving no time idle. A year after opening, I became pregnant with our daughter, an experience that required many of the same qualities I had cultivated growing the business: adaptability to the unknown, focused effort, and clarity of purpose. And, like owning a business, there was no training manual that would guide me.

Owning a business required a lot of pitta and vata energy: pitta to transform and create systems, and vata to adapt and move. Pregnancy on the other hand, required that I pacify pitta and protect myself from vata, promoting the qualities of kapha, warm, nourishing, calm, and stable.

How did I strike a balance? I altered my diet to promote the qualities of kapha, integrating foods like yams, beets, and nourishing soups. I reduced activities that encouraged vata's mobility like strong vinyasa yoga, favoring a gentler practice, long walks, and being in nature. I was conscious of the imagery and sounds I took in through my senses, working to promote happiness by chanting and singing uplifting songs. Following the wisdom of Ayurveda promoted subtle experiences that I trust helped to shape my daughter's body and mind in the womb and will provide strength as she grows and flourishes for years to come.

# VANAPRASTHA: THE FOREST DWELLER STAGE

The shift into vanaprastha begins the vata time of life, which corresponds to menopause. Pregnancy, birthing, and rearing are behind you now. The growth governed by kapha and the hormonal activity of pitta both recede, and the body becomes subtler, more attuned to cosmic factors. It is time to focus on managing the qualities of vata dosha (dry, cold, light, and so on) through practicing Ayurveda's longevity techniques—such as eating warm, moist foods and practicing oil massage—and devoting more time to spirituality.

At this stage, roughly ages fifty to seventy-five, more than half of your life is behind you. The idea of "forest dwelling" is a retreat of sorts, taking a step back, but not all the way into a cave. Imagine a figurative retreat from the city into the quietude of forest living. As the responsibilities of the active years wane, it is time to shift your attention toward your inner life. This doesn't require moving into the actual forest (though nature inspires contemplation), but it does require making space for a sense of self that is not dependent on a job or family. It is at this time that it becomes clear, if you've lost track, that you are not your responsibilities or your achievements. You were ensnared by a role—you are a luminous heart!

Vanaprastha can be a challenging time for those who aren't used to resting or dwelling on the inward aspects of being alive. In a culture where productivity is often at the top of the ladder, a shift toward doing less can bring on a midlife crisis. I, for one, am grateful for this aspect of my Ayurveda studies, which has helped me enrich grihastha with simple daily practices that keep me grounded in my Self, while keeping an eye on my tendency to rely on outward success for meaning in life.

## KAMA: THE NATURE OF DESIRE

Once artha meets our basic needs in "retirement," we may enjoy the freedom to consider what desires we have, aside from security. In my observations, I've seen women naturally shift into contemplation with menopause, desires flowing in new directions. *Kama* literally means "desire, pleasure," but not necessarily related to sex. Kama's reputation came from its association with the Kama Sutra, an ancient text on the nature of love and pleasure, which covers family life and sex. The highest kama is actually for union with the divine. Traditionally, the progression from taking care of a family and providing for self and others gives way to a retirement age where one begins to contemplate the absolute (now that there's plenty of time). Spirituality can take center stage. One idea with kama in the third stage of life is to work out desires of the senses, not by fulfilling them, but by tempering them and discovering true satisfaction. Which leads us toward the next, and final, aim of life: moksha (liberation).

If *artha* can mean both "wealth" and "meaning," maybe we need to be manifesting both of these things throughout the grihastha stage. The importance of keeping some time for self-care and spirit, even in the busy years, keeps the pilot light on for dharma.

In a worldview in which leaving the earth better than you found it is the highest dharma, having later years to do good works, purify the self, and offer wise counsel to others is dharma indeed.

## SANNYASA: THE RENUNCIATION STAGE

Moving deeper into the vata time of life, the word *sannyasa* suggests a wandering ascetic, a practitioner of subtle arts. This brings to mind the image of the crone, a wise, supernatural, master of earth magic. She is not a wanderer but rooted, possibly at one with the natural rhythms and medicines that have surrounded her for decades and supported her through life. As the body becomes more and more subtle, communications with the mystic aspects of reality supercede the physical.

The "wandering" ascetic is symbolic of a withdrawal from the likes and dislikes, the doing and desiring, that have characterized life thus far. Beginning to disengage from the objects of this world before death will make dying a lot smoother. In this final stage of life, around age seventy-five to one hundred, we prepare to pass on with a sense of satisfaction and find the prospect of death much less intimidating. This final stage is a time of simplification, connecting deeply to the spiritual aspects of life without much distraction. Now that's something to look forward to.

## MOKSHA—SIMPLIFY, SIMPLIFY

The wandering ascetic is seeking moksha, liberation from an endless cycle of desire and gratification. Contemplating the nature of satisfaction, as in kama, is a practice of liberation. Many humans tend to attach to an object of the senses to gratify their desires. Such an object might be money, power, sex, or food, to name a few. Desire is a spark in humans that propels us forward into action, that keeps the wheel of this life going around. Moksha, spiritual liberation, is described as a release from this cycle, when a person learns to live in satisfaction as a state of mind.

Old age, in this model, is about learning to do nothing. Liberation requires a purification of sensory desires and the cultivation of the skill of contentment (*santosha*). I've been studying and contemplating these ideas since I was a teenager, and aging and death talk still makes me feel a little sad. It's natural to feel attached. Hence, the need to devote one's final years to the purification of attachments in life. A conscious and fulfilling death process is a lucky thing, if you have the security in old age to mature in this way.

The concept of liberation in old age (or at any stage of life, should it arise) is the cream of life in the Vedic model. In a culture where aging can be viewed as becoming irrelevant, even invisible, I find comfort in this model of spiritual work as an elder.

This description of the stages of life is a guideline, not an absolute timeline. Stages can overlap, or a person might engage mostly with one of these paradigms for their whole life. Maybe a lot of stages are already behind you, or maybe you are backtracking, but holding a view of the overall context is meaningful.

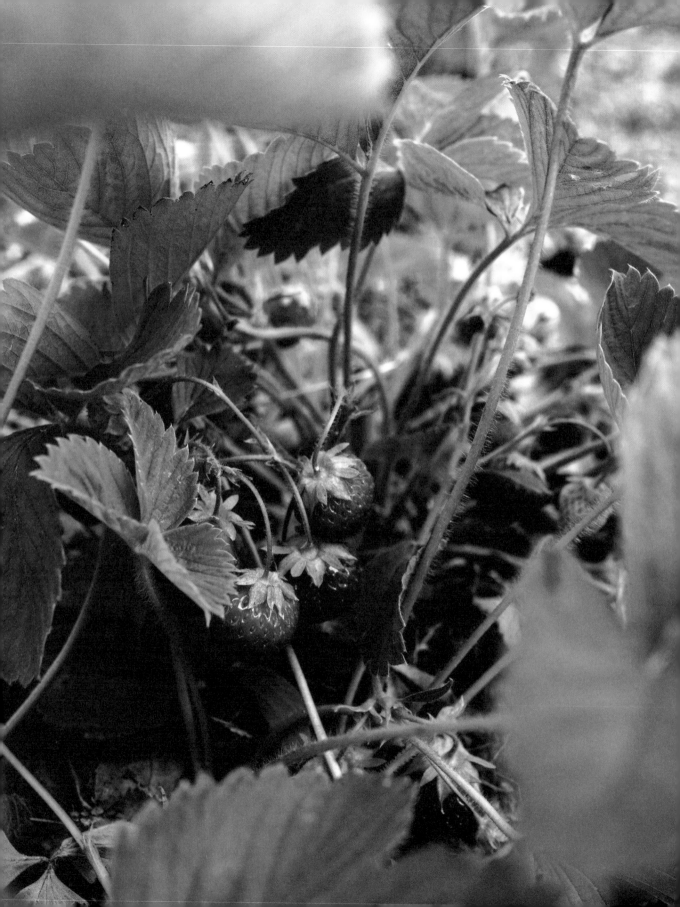

# 11

# Healthy Menstruation

The monthly regeneration of the generative system and the mobilization of rasa, rakta, and *apana vata* to build, cleanse, and build again is a wonder of nature—and a centralizing force in a female body. The yoni, a symbol of *shakti* (cosmic generative energy), is an aspect of universal creative power unlike any other. The womb is the seat of a woman's power, not because of its ability to gestate, but because of its essential relationship to shakti. Womb health equals shakti. Shakti is the principle behind all creativity, energy, and movement in the universe, and each woman's body is a piece of this manifestation. Caring for menstrual blood during the second stage of life is an act of love for all beings.

In Ayurveda, the care of artava (generative tissues) during a menstrual cycle involves protecting agni, promoting downward flow, and nourishing the blood. While each of the doshas has its peak during a part of the menstrual cycle, vata dominates the movement of the blood. Making space for downward flow and nourishing the body well to support regeneration are the most important factors in menstrual health.

## WHAT IS A HEALTHY PERIOD?

A healthy period is generally regular in timing, amount of blood, and color of blood. These aspects give us information about a woman's overall health, as well as hormonal health and the health of the generative organs. Kind of like the perfect poop, a comfortable, easy period can be elusive and doesn't mean that something is wrong. Getting a sense of what's healthy for you is the key to recognizing unhealthy changes.

Here are general characteristics of a "healthy" period, according to traditional Ayurveda and to Western medicine.

Ayurveda Texts
- The period occurs about every twenty-eight days.
- It lasts three to five days.

- It comprises bright red blood.
- It arrives on the new moon.
- It has a honey-like smell.
- It comprises about four *anjali* (handfuls) of blood

Notice how the amount of menstrual blood is not expected to be the same for everyone but is relative to one's body size. A smaller frame likely has a smaller hand and less blood in general; therefore, the amount of flow is individual to the person.

Western Medicine
- The cycle length is between twenty-four and thirty-eight days. (The average is twenty-nine, and teens are more likely to have longer cycles.)
- Variations in the cycle length (within six days) are considered normal from month to month.
- The period lasts three to seven days.
- It comprises about 30 to 80 milliliters (around 2 ounces or 1/4 cup) of blood.
- There is no cramping.
- One may experience mild shifts in mood that do not disrupt daily activity.

## AYURVEDA'S ANATOMY OF THE MENSTRUAL CYCLE

According to Ayurveda texts, a woman's roughly twenty-eight-day moon cycle has three parts, give or take a few days:

**Days 1-5** (*rajahkala*): The uterine lining sheds, menstrual blood flows, and vata predominates through *dhamanee* (tiny channels, blood vessels). The queen of movement and flow is vata's downward-moving current, apana vayu.

**Days 5-16** (*rutukala*): Kapha increases through nutritive juices, building rasa dhatu and providing building qualities for the fertility component.

**Days 16-28** (*rutavateetakala*): Pitta increases through rakta dhatu, and the uterine lining matures.

These phases of a woman's cycle correspond to the moon phases. They may not literally overlap, but the energy that governs each phase can guide us on how to integrate this wonderful bit of intuition. Even as a metaphor, the lunar cycle can be instrumental in embodying the wisdom of the menstrual cycle.

First, rajahkala and letting go—prioritizing inward and downward movement, releasing menstrual blood—is natural at the new or dark moon. It is natural to be a homebody, to crave a bit of solitude, to cleanse and reflect.

Then, rutakala mirrors the growth of building and nourishing qualities as the waxing moon grows to the full moon and the ovaries release an egg. This is the time of full power, and the body naturally craves more activity, more interaction, and more food.

From the waning moon to the new moon, as during rutavateetakala, pitta and the qualities of transformation dominate, simmering the pot full of the previous cycle's activity and maturing the uterine lining. This is like late summer and early fall: with growth going to seed, the bustling energy of the full moon settles into a time for storing seeds, resting more, and cultivating intuition and self-expression.

## WESTERN DEFINITION OF THE MENSTRUAL CYCLE

In the Western model, a roughly twenty-eight-day cycle is broken down into four parts:

**Days 1-6 (menstruation):** The uterine lining sheds, and sex hormones are at their lowest.

**Days 1-13 (follicular phase):** Estrogen rises, building the uterine lining, and the ovary is ripening for the release of an egg.

**Days 14-18 (ovulation):** An egg is released from the ovary, and estrogen peaks. This is the fertile phase of the cycle, when the ovum is available for fertilization.

**Days 14-28 (luteal phase):** The body prepares for pregnancy or menstruation. Progesterone increases, allowing the uterine lining to mature. In the second half of this phase, estrogen and progesterone both decrease if fertilization does not occur, signaling the uterine lining to shed. Body temperature is slightly higher during this phase.

# Menstrual Cycle and Doshas

**Vata time** is associated with the **new moon** and menstruation, and it is a time for rest, inward reflection, and new beginnings.

**Kapha time**, the growing and building stage of egg and endometrium, is like the **waxing moon**, and it is a time for brmhana qualities to support new growth. Women will generally feel most energetic and fresher during this time.

The **kapha peak**, ovulation, is associated with the **full moon**, and this is a time of fertility, increased libido, outward focus, and interconnection.

The third stage, **pitta time**, has a langhana energy of slowing down endometrial tissue growth to allow for maturation and potential implantation of a fertilized egg. Body temperature rises in the latter half of this phase, associated with the **waning moon**. Women may feel energy and libido waning in the latter half of this stage and crave more quiet time.

(For more information on moon cycles, see chapter 9.)

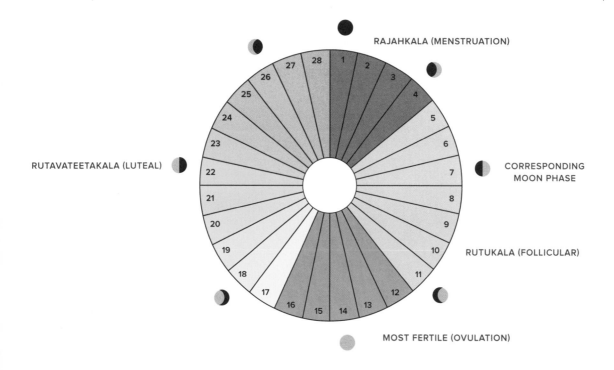

## SYNCING WITH THE MOON

Not everyone will naturally menstruate at the new moon, though the internal energy of the dark moon is most similar to bleeding time. As long as the cycle is reasonably consistent, there is no need to be concerned about when your period falls in a lunar cycle. You may notice that some factors, such as the amount of blood or intervals between periods, shift seasonally.

When working with lunar rhythms over time, your cycles may begin to align with nature. Life loves rhythm and patterns. A life that can sometimes feel chaotic becomes organized. The nature of a meaningful life may not lie in what we do each day, but how we do it. Our periods are an opportunity to connect with the cosmos.

In many indigenous societies, menstruation on the new moon was considered ideal for fertility. In modern times and urban lifestyles, especially due to artificial light at night, periods align with the moon much less often. Some women tend to menstruate around the new moon and others around the full moon. Some conjecture that women in hunter-gatherer groups bleed on the full moon during summer, when men go out hunting to take advantage of the light. This way ovulation would coincide with men being home on the dark moon. (Women's cycles may shift from menses at the new moon to the full moon seasonally.)

While getting your period on or near to a moon day is a sign of superb health, it doesn't mean something is wrong if you don't. Many factors can influence the timing of your cycle. Travel, especially changing time zones or climate, is most likely to cause irregularities, as are stress, undernourishment, and overexercise. Women with regular daily routines, or those who live in rural areas or spend a lot of time outdoors, are more likely to notice their periods aligning with the moon.

Consistent biorhythms, reduced artificial light at night, getting more exposure to the sun and moonlight, as well as shifting your energy focus as moon phases change, are likely to move your period in the direction of a full or new moon expression. The health benefits of moving with the energy generated by the ebb and flow of the moon increase soma (the nectar of life).

I offer these lunar rhythms not to create self-consciousness about when you bleed, but as a practice to link us to natural energy tides and allow us to harness the power and intelligence of these cosmic forces. These forces are at work in all bodies, regardless of sex or stage of life. Practice begins with simply being aware of the moon cycle. Add the full and new moon days to your calendar. Tune in to when it is waxing or waning. Look for the moon in the sky at night, and go outside to view it. This practice itself creates connection.

When you feel ready, start to look for patterns in your energy, your sleep, and your libido throughout your cycle. Track these patterns in a journal, if you like. I give you journal prompts for period tracking in chapter 12.

To sync your energy with lunar phases, apply these essential practices:

- Do not do vigorous exercise on the new moon or the day before or after the new moon. Instead, practice oil massage, take a floral bath, practice yoga that promotes apana vayu, or take gentle walks. Sleep more if you can.
- Spend time outdoors in the moonlight. Allow moonlight to reach your eyes, your skin, and the crown of your head as often as possible.
- Do not use screens after dark, and wear blue light blocking glasses if you need to use screens after sunset. At the very least, do not use screens for a *minimum* of one hour before bedtime. Keep smartphones out of the bedroom!
- Eat more nourishing foods around the full moon, especially good fats from almonds, seeds, ghee, and coconut. Try the Moon Milk recipe on page 247.

## The Light Factor

Light is the biggest factor in how the moon affects women's reproductive rhythms. Exposing the skin to natural moonlight, known as moonbathing, is the single best way to sync an irregular cycle with the energy of the moon. Reducing artificial light at night, especially during the waning and new moon phases, is also essential in promoting good sleep and healthy hormones.

## SELF-CARE DURING YOUR PERIOD

Ayurveda recommends general diet and lifestyle principles to prioritize menstrual health, some of which make more sense than others in modern times. Some of the traditional practices had to do with cleanliness. Others seem to be geared toward prioritizing fertility and providing complete rest.

The key is to emphasize apana and agni during menstruation. Anything that overwhelms agni (like heavy meals), aggravates vata (cold, travel, excessive exercise), or impedes apana (restrictive clothing, overuse of the senses) is suspect. Learning to prioritize downward flow and allowing prana to turn inward during the period is the most important lesson.

Deepen your understanding of apana vata by reviewing chapter 3.

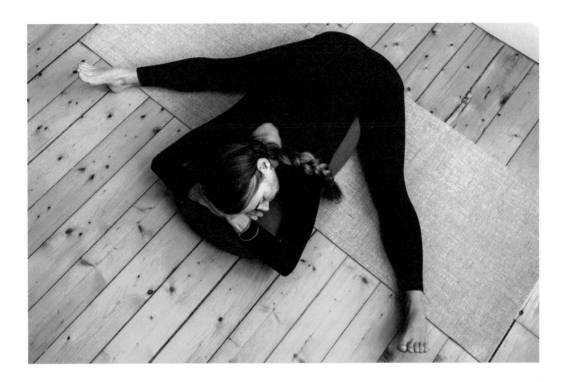

## Free Flow and Menstrual Collection Methods

Ayurveda believes that internal methods of collecting period blood cause a disturbance to the downward flow. It is subtle, but the vaginal canal, while trying to expel something, senses a block there. A free flow is the ideal. This can be achieved with period panties or washable cotton menstrual pads without creating a lot of trash. According to the Ayurveda view, tampons and menstrual cups disturb apana.

## BEST EXERCISE DURING YOUR PERIOD

From your body's point of view, having a period *is* exercise. The job of shedding the endometrial lining and prepping the ovary to release an egg is a task to be respected, supported, and even revered. In a culture where vigorous exercise is promoted, the physiological demands on a body can be seen as a disruption to one's workout. To take rest and allow energy to move down and into the uterus, the ovaries, and the blood—not the biceps, the quads, or the mind—takes courage. Resting during one's period was traditional wisdom that in today's world is countercultural. I dare you to rest during your period!

That being said, some women find the body needs a little help in shedding the uterine lining. Gentle walks can be sufficient movement to open the channels and instigate the flow. The lower abdomen is swollen during the menstrual cycle, and movements that compress the region, like crunches or deep twists, aren't helpful during your period and can lead to cramping. Less of anything that causes contraction in the abdomen, whether tight clothing or emotional stress, is best.

## BALANCE VATA WITH REDUCED SENSE ACTIVITY

During your period, allow apana vata to receive all the resources it needs. Too much activity, of any kind, pulls prana away from the downward wind. Too much talking, overstimulating the senses (loud noise, too much screen time, or stimulants like caffeine and white sugar) are also best moderated for a healthy period. To intuit why this is recommended, visualize how any of these activities instigate an outward flow of energy from the body's center. While you may be able to get away with a bit of vata provocation, imbalances that are fed too often over time lead to irregularities in your period.

## PLAN LESS, STRESS LESS, AND REST MORE

Do you push against your period to keep up productivity or activity? In the long run, this will cause imbalances. Make fewer plans. Stay home, wear your loungewear, and give your breasts and pelvis a break from restrictive clothing. If you have the energy, do some nesting activities, such as decluttering or organizing, or creative projects. Relaxing completely is ideal! Of course, it is not always possible to reduce stressors during your period, but avoiding opportunities for being stressed or overwhelmed is a good move. Do less and plan to be less productive during your period.

Observing the moon phases, and scheduling activity and rest accordingly, is likely to bring about a natural, more lunar rhythm in your periods.

## PAUSE THE ABHYANGA

The application of heavy oils during your period, including abhyanga, is not recommended on heavy flow days as this taxes the agni. A light application of oil for dry skin is fine, but lots of oil followed by heat, such as a hot shower or bath, will disturb the flow of apana. Texts also recommend abstaining from fragrance and cosmetics during your period. During this time of cleansing, keep what comes in contact with your body natural to encourage purification. Tongue scraping and other care of the senses are excellent routines to practice during your period.

## CURB AGGRAVATORS

Coffee and alcohol, both pitta-aggravating, increase the hot and damp qualities in the breasts. You will find relief from PMS swelling and pain if you reduce these substances, especially in the week or two before your period.

## PRACTICE GRATITUDE

Throughout the days of bleeding, remind your body of how great it is, and how grateful you are for all the hard work. Reflect on the presence of shakti and invite her power into your life.

### Elimination and Menstruation

In working with women's health, I have observed clear links between comfortable digestion and comfortable menstruation. The channels of elimination of poop, urine, and menstrual blood are all in close proximity, and stagnation in one can affect the others. Women who experience constipation are likely to have low back pain before menses and possibly cramping on the first day or two. Constipation, compounded by the natural swelling of the uterus before menstruation, blocks the free flow of all apana functions. If the colon is full of stool or wind, you will feel uncomfortable during your period. If shifting to warm, moist foods doesn't get the stool moving, consider using Triphala Tea (recipe on page 224) for a few months.

Loose stools in conjunction with the period are likely for many women, as pitta increases and apana kicks into gear. Do not suppress the urge to release. Eat simply, and reduce raw food, alcohol, spice, and sour foods to calm loose stools during your period.

## WHAT TO EAT DURING THE MENSTRUAL CYCLE

The most important thing about diet during the menstrual period is to keep your foods easy to digest. Vata-pacifying foods—warm, cooked, and moist—will reduce the likelihood of gas and bloating, which can disturb the downward flow. Sitting down while eating is of supreme importance at this time to respect apana vayu.

You may notice fluctuations in your appetite during your period. It is common to feel less hungry on heavy days as the wind that stokes agni is working on the downward flow, and the body is more about *out* than *in* at this time. Eating simple, warm, moist foods during your period keeps a smooth flow in the bowels. Eating according to appetite is key; a low appetite will give way to more hunger soon.

Keeping the diet light, lower in fats, and free of heavy, hard-to-digest foods like cheese and meat allows the body to bring more of its energy to the task of cleansing the uterine lining. If nourishment is balanced throughout the month, eating light foods during your cycle will feel natural. Some women report cravings for blood-building foods like red meat just before or just after bleeding. Listen to those cravings: it is more beneficial to eat building foods before or after than during.

Think of your period time as a monthly cleanse. The loss of menstrual blood stimulates building a fresh uterine lining. Rakta dhatu is refreshed by bleeding. Allow for your body's natural inclination to detox at this time by simplifying your diet. Include only easy-to-digest foods such as kichari, cooked vegetables, and fruit compotes. Focus on warming and sweet spices like cinnamon, cardamom, and nutmeg and carminatives like fennel and *ajwain*, especially if you feel bloated. Avoid excessively spicy, sour, and salty foods. These tastes predominate in restaurant food, and it's healthier to cook at home when possible. Raw juices and fruits or light salads can disturb the downward flow. Too much bitter and astringent tastes cause constriction.

## Foods to Favor for Healthy Periods

**Foods that support downward flow.** Focus on foods and spices that assist in downward flow, such as fennel, hing, and eggplant in moderation. Drink only warm liquids, nothing cold. *Sit down anytime you are eating* or the food will not move down well.

**Blood-building foods.** If you have heavy cycles, or are low in iron or other minerals, it may feel important to keep up your strength. Eat cleansing foods for two of your heaviest flow days, then add in blood-building foods like broths, meat-based soup, nuts and seeds, sea vegetables, and red and blue fruits. Consider drinking Raisin Mantha (page 261) if needed between meals to keep your energy up without taxing the agni while you are bleeding.

### Support Healthy Periods by Eating More of These

Ajwain

Asparagus, celery, dandelion, burdock, and daikon

Barley water

Bone broth

Cooked vegetables, especially winter squashes, sweet potatoes, lotus, and dark greens

Kichari

Meat soup

Mung beans

Red and blue fruits, including raisins, prunes, blackberries, blueberries, pomegranates, and cherries

Rice, especially red

Sea vegetables

Seeds, especially pâtés and butters

### Favor These Recipes during Your Period

Creamy Coconut Breakfast Kichari (page 264)

New Moon Kichari (page 286)

Red Rice Kanji (page 271)

Beets and Barley Stew (page 284)

Black Sesame Balls (page 303)

## HERBAL SUPPORT DURING YOUR PERIOD

Herbs that support downward flow and pacify vata, such as those in Nourishing Herbal Infusion, on page 218, are supportive at this time. Raspberry Leaf and Nettle Brew (page 223) is a classic formula for balanced artava as an infusion.

In general, Ayurveda recommends holding off on using concentrated herbal *churnas* (fine powders), tablets, and vitamins during the heavy days of your period as they tax the agni. For bloating or abdominal cramps, sip warm Ajwain Water (page 232).

# PRACTICES FOR YOUR MENSTRUAL CYCLE

A little cycle awareness goes a long way. The chart below is a reference for seeing the bigger picture of your monthly flow. You can eat simple, vata-pacifying foods during the vata phase and mellow your exercise. Shift to more nourishing foods during the follicular phase, and enjoy feeling full power this week; harness creative energies. During ovulation, prioritize your generative factor, favor juicy foods, and feed your cravings. As the moon wanes, avoid burning out by slowing down a bit, and reduce foods that aggravate pitta. Keep the channels open by encouraging a downward flow.

| DOSHA / CYCLE PHASE | MOON PHASE | ACTIVITIES TO FAVOR | FOODS TO FAVOR | FOCUS PRACTICE |
|---|---|---|---|---|
| VATA / MENSTRUATION | New moon | Rest and reflection, bathing, sleep, journaling, cleansing | Light, soupy cooked foods that are easy to digest | Support downward flow |
| KAPHA / FOLLICULAR | Waxing moon | Exercise, building | Building foods, especially good fats | Moonbathe |
| KAPHA / OVULATION | Full moon | Connecting, enjoying, full-power | Building foods | Promote shukra |
| PITTA / LUTEAL | Waning moon | Slowing down a bit; resting if tired | Cooling and calming foods; high-mineral foods; less alcohol, coffee, and spicy food | Pitta-balancing |

Her period is a woman's top tool for assessing overall health on a regular basis. It is also integral to the health of the seat of cosmic creative power. Maintaining balanced routines throughout a month that support a robust menstrual flow is one of the most important rituals for health and fostering inner strength from the core to take you anywhere you want to go.

# 12

# Managing PMS and Menstrual Imbalances

*The balanced state of the three doshas causes a normal menstrual cycle while any sort of imbalance causes abnormality.*[6]

—NIRMALA JOSHI, *AYURVEDIC CONCEPTS IN GYNAECOLOGY*

The body and the doshas undergo natural changes throughout the month, just as they do during a daily cycle. Getting in rhythm with this flow supports hormonal balance and healthy periods. When the body is working smoothly, the ebbs and flows of the doshas ensure a balance. When doshas become out of balance, any aspect of the monthly cycle can be affected, leading to undesirable changes in ovulation, menstruation, or hormonal activity.

Living harmoniously with the rhythms around us is the best medicine for the doshas, as we saw in part two, but what do we do when things get wacky? Having a sense of what is normal and not normal for you, and how to read the signs your period is giving you, is step one of learning to manage any effects the doshas may be having on your cycle. Read on for how to determine what your healthy cycle looks like and what to do when it doesn't feel right.

## DOSHAS' ROLE IN MENSTRUATION

From the Ayurveda perspective, variations from a healthy period are likely to lean in the direction of one's constitution. For example, vata is dry, light, and prone to change. Vata cycles are generally lighter, may have longer intervals between periods, and may tend toward irregularity. Pitta types are likely to have shorter intervals (especially in hot weather), comprise robust blood sometimes associated with heat, and be very regular. Kapha types are likely to have longer or heavier periods, sometimes associated with dull pain, and are very regular.

These variations can become more noticeable when a dosha is out of balance and become mild or obsolete when doshas are in balance. The qualities of a prominent dosha are likely to show up in your period, and this makes your period an excellent barometer for general states of balance and imbalance.

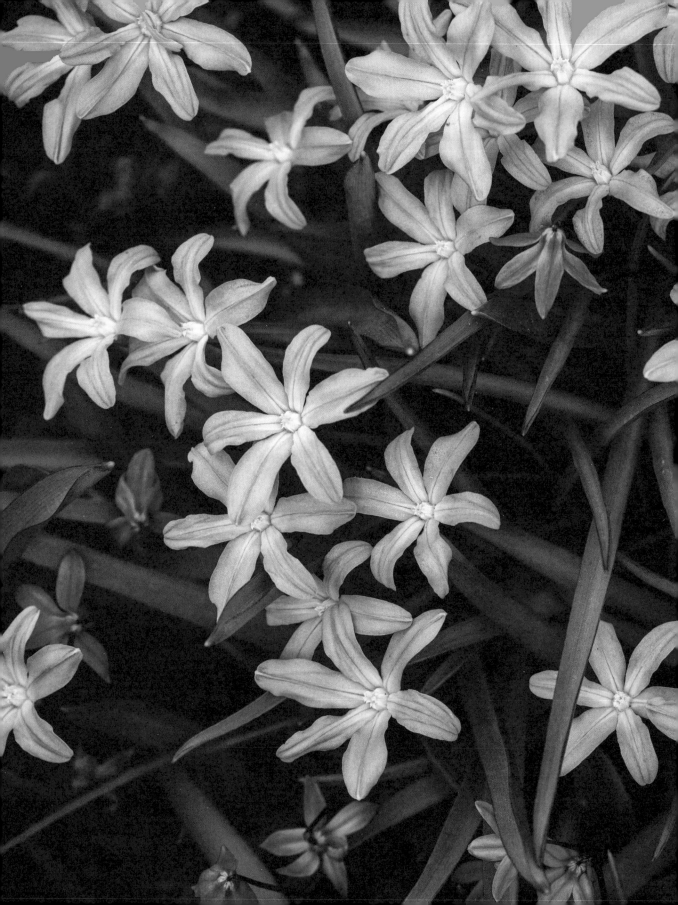

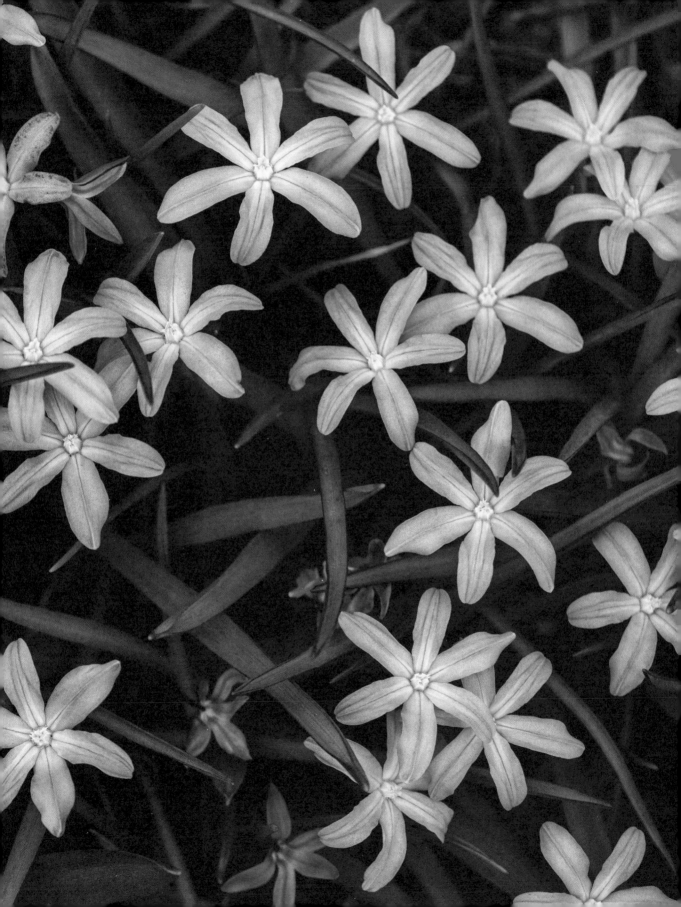

Period health is an indicator of health in general. Knowledge of your own period and how to keep it healthy is an empowering path toward self-reliant health. Track your cycle over time, keep a period journal, or use an app if that works for you, though the less time spent on phones the better. A little book by your bed for jotting down and looking back is a perfect tool. Give it about six months to notice patterns, and once you do, this information is gold.

## WHAT YOUR PMS IS TELLING YOU

From the Ayurveda viewpoint, many of the symptoms known as PMS—mood swings, swelling, food cravings, fatigue, and tender breasts—are signs of aggravated doshas. In other words, a healthy cycle is not associated with any of these symptoms. PMS symptoms do not mean you are unhealthy; they may be early signs of imbalance but not disease. Points to keep in mind are (1) discomforts associated with your cycle can be alleviated, and (2) you are not "sick" or "doing something wrong" if you do not have an easy period all the time. Your period may arrive as a surprise, unheralded by any discomforts, and be a nonevent. But the majority of women have some PMS, some of the time. Targeted regular self-care, based on the knowledge of what your symptoms are telling you, will steadily reduce your PMS.

Knowing the signs of vata, pitta, and kapha qualities in your cycle can help you keep things in balance well before more serious disorders get any real estate in your generative system. All women's concerns about fertility, uterine and ovarian health, and hormone balance are coded into the Ayurveda model, the general principle of observing imbalance in qualities early on, and introducing opposite qualities to foster balance. Read on to apply the knowledge of what your PMS is telling you and be an agent in your own reproductive health.

**Note:** You will find general principles for self-care during your menstrual cycle in chapter 11, with everyday considerations for maintaining healthy states. Here, we go into abnormalities of the menstrual cycle caused by the doshas. You can find specific diet and lifestyle guidelines for the effects of doshas on your cycle in this section, as well as how to modify your self-care routines when doshas are making mischief in your cycle. Recognizing many signs of a certain dosha in your cycle does not mean you are on the road to disease. These early signs are manageable with the correct application of knowledge. At the end of this section, we will discuss more serious menstrual disorders, what to look for, and when to see a medical professional.

# Period Tracking

If you choose to track your periods, the following are all helpful aspects of the cycle to focus on. Consider this a data-gathering journal project: without judgment and without trying to "fix" anything.

## Timing

- How many days is your cycle? The first day of bleeding is day 1; the last day is the day before bleeding starts again.

- Is there spotting for any number of days before the blood begins to "flow"?

## Blood Color and Texture

- Does it start out brown and turn to dark or bright red? Is it bright red and flowing from the start?

- Are there clots, which are normal, up to about the size of a quarter?

- Is it pale? (A light pink color can mean anemia.)

- Is there mucus?

- How many days do you have a heavy bleed, and how many days do you have a light flow or spotting?

- How much blood is there? You can gauge this by observing your blood through whatever method you use to collect it. Over time, you will have a sense of your "normal," although you may not be able to measure the actual volume of blood.

## Pain

- Do you have cramping? On which days?

- Do you have low back pain or pelvic pain?

## Premenstrual Signs

Do you experience any of the following?

- Water retention
- Breast swelling and/or tenderness
- Constipation or diarrhea
- Headaches
- Food cravings
- Mood changes: sadness, fear, or irritation (in addition to your usual ups and downs)

# HOW DO MENSTRUAL CYCLES BECOME IRREGULAR?

> Without the aggravation of vata, the vagina/uterus does not get disordered in women;
> hence that should be won over (mitigated) first, and the others treated next.
> —*ASHTANGA HRDAYAM*, UTTARASTHANA, 34:23

As we know, doshas are that which cause trouble in the body. It would follow that their trouble-making extends to the menstrual cycle. The beauty is that doshic imbalance in the body is likely to manifest in your cycle (if you pay attention), and healing your cycle brings this dosha into balance. Listening to what your cycle is telling you and adjusting your routines accordingly is a reliable tool for maintaining good health.

Vata dosha and its qualities dominate below the navel, so the activities of the reproductive organs fall under its domain. For this reason, keeping vata smooth and rhythmic is the first consideration in addressing irregularities in the menstrual cycle. This being said, pitta and kapha, in states of aggravation, can also promote deviations from a normal cycle.

## VATA IMBALANCES OF THE MENSTRUAL CYCLE

When the channels are open and the downward flow of energy is smooth, the menstrual cycle comes on without pain, spotting, or mental or digestive disturbance. Apana, the aspect of vata that flows downward, is the most likely instigator of menstrual problems. This direction of energy can be challenging for those with more air and space (both upward moving) in their constitution. However, everyone is at risk of apana problems from being too busy, staying too outwardly focused, and recruiting too much energy above the neck to the activities of the mind and sense organs.

Additionally, the tendency to suppress urine, gas, and poop disturbs downward flow. Over time, suppressing these urges results in a "redirect" of the downward flow upward. When the monthly cycle approaches and the downward flow is unfamiliar, or redirected, there will be pain in the abdomen and low back, a tendency toward constipation, and possible headaches. This same redirect can be the cause of menstrual cramping in the first day or two of the period.

Stress can contribute to the hard and constricting qualities of vata, especially in muscular contraction in the abdomen. This tightening of the apana region can result in cramping during the period.

With vata's dry and light qualities, one is likely to see a shorter or lighter cycle, or a day of spotting where it feels like the flow just can't find its way down. Vata's mobile quality will be aggravated by travel, which throws off the cycle's rhythm. The expanding nature of air may cause bloating, and the space element is cramped by uterine swelling before the flow starts, which contributes to abdominal and low back pain, constipation, gas trapped in the large intestine, and perhaps an insistent bladder. When vata flows downward excessively, it can result in overactivity of the bladder and bowels, frequent urination, and loose stools.

Vata is also sensitive to nutritional deficiencies. Artava is the last in the nutritional hierarchy. This means the reproductive tissues are the first to show signs of depletion. Depletion looks like a short or light cycle; spotting instead of true bleeding; dark red, brown, or blackish blood; exhaustion; and cravings for sweet, sour, and salty foods before or during the cycle.

## Signs of Vata in the Cycle

Intervals between periods becoming longer

Cycle becoming irregular due to travel

Period becoming light due to vigorous exercise

Scanty bleeding

Low back pain

Restless or aching legs

Constipation associated with the period

Spotting on the first day of the cycle

Bleeding stopping and starting during the period, instead of having a smooth flow

Dark blood, dry blood

Mood swings

Anxiety, fear, feeling overwhelmed

Cravings for dry, crunchy foods or iced drinks

## BALANCING VATA IN ARTAVA

Doing your best to establish routines around sleep, food, and activity (outlined in part two) all keep vata regular. Introduce warm, soft, and moist qualities through your food and drink, your clothing, your attitude, and your environment whenever possible. Choose one or two of these rhythms and practice diligently a few days before and during your period.

### Food

- Reduce or avoid dry foods like crackers, chips, and popcorn.
- Reduce dehydrating beverages like coffee and alcohol.
- Avoid heavily refined foods like white flour and sugar.
- Reduce cold and raw foods, such as salads and frozen desserts.
- Reduce gas-forming foods like kidney beans, bubbly water, and cruciferous vegetables.

- Drink warm water.
- Increase good fats in the diet from nuts, dairy, and good oils.
- If you crave meats, eat meat soup.
- Drink 1 quart of Nourishing Herbal Infusion (page 218) daily.
- During your period, eat only warm, moist, grounding foods—nothing cold.
- Eat meals, not snacks.
- Sit down or squat when eating or drinking.

### Rhythms

- Go to bed early.
- Shut all screens off one hour before bed.
- Reduce food intake at night, and enjoy more at midday.
- Practice sense care (see the discussion of dinacharya in chapter 5).

- Wear loose clothing.
- Practice relaxing your abdomen.
- Do not suppress the urge to pee, pass wind, or poop.
- Keep warm.

### Activity

- Wind down your exercise during the week leading up to your period.
- Rest on the first two or three days of bleeding. If your period is irregular or absent, rest as though you have your period for two or three days at the new moon. Enjoy a bath, a walk, read, and take time to daydream.

- Schedule downtime and sedentary activities.
- Apply Castor Oil Packs (page 318) to the body where you're feeling constriction/stagnation.
- Yoni Steaming (page 318) can soften constriction before your period and open the channels.

The more often you adopt these foods, rhythms, and activity levels, the more you can expect to see the signs of vata affecting your cycle decrease over a few months' time. Balance doesn't require following all of these routines; take one change at a time and notice how it affects you.

# PITTA IMBALANCES OF THE MENSTRUAL CYCLE

While we have established the significant role vata plays in menstruation, pitta is a likely instigator because rakta dhatu (red blood) is a place where the pitta qualities of hot, sharp, and spreading predominate. This tissue is also a major contributor to menstrual bleeding, and its qualities influence how your period manifests. Healthy pitta opens the channels with the warmth of the fire element, while the water element supports viscosity and flow. Pitta's subtle governance of transformation keeps the monthly hormone cycle moving smoothly. Healthy blood flows easily without pain and has a faint (not strong) smell, and periods feel calming and refreshing to pitta types. Increased hot, sharp, oily qualities in the blood can make cycles "angry," manifesting as heat or burning sensations, acne before your period, and a stronger, acrid smell to the blood. An increase in the quantity of blood and the hot, sharp, oily, spreading qualities of pitta can be at the bottom of a host of angry, hot premenstrual symptoms and heavy periods.

Pitta tends to aggravate during the luteal phase, after ovulation and before menstruation, as progesterone (hot) rises and estrogen (cool) drops. While a gentle increase in heat is normal, intensity increases for those who have more fire in the constitution or those who, due to stress or diet, have accumulated pitta qualities. Aggravated pitta causes cravings for spicy, sour, or salty foods before the period, while balanced pitta craves natural sweet tastes, such as fresh fruits, to cool the heat.

The hot quality of pitta is responsible for night sweats and feeling hot in general just before or during the period. Hot, oily, and spreading qualities liquefy the stool and cause the infamous "period poop," an urgent, hot, stinky, loose bowel movement that can occur several times daily during heavy days and may show signs of undigested food. This phenomenon is supported by indulging in too much spicy and sour food and drink.

The red blood has all the qualities of pitta, and if it becomes hotter, sharper, and faster—or increases in quantity—periods can become heavy and intense. Blood will come fast and generally in greater quantity when pitta is accumulated. Time between periods can decrease as the body craves the cooling effects of releasing these qualities via the menstrual flow.

Hot and sharp qualities also feed the emotions with irritability and anger. For some women, these emotions may be familiar but harder to manage around their period. Overscheduling and lack of personal space during or before the period aggravate emotions further.

# Signs of Pitta in the Cycle

Intervals between periods becoming shorter

Heavy bleeding associated with heat or burning sensations

Loose stools with the period

Acne before the period

Fleshy smelling blood

Hot, swollen breasts

Anger, irritability

Cravings for spicy, sour, or salty food

## BALANCING PITTA IN ARTAVA

Reducing foods that are heating, oily, and sharp during the second phase of your cycle, and especially the week before bleeding, makes a big difference in alleviating symptoms. The body is good at transforming and balancing; it just needs a reduction in the pitta qualities going in. Paying attention to food and drink during the days when things are heating up naturally will help the body manage it. I have seen women relieved of migraines by omitting red wine for two weeks before their period, without giving it up altogether. Moderate changes often work!

Introduce cooling, calming, and refreshing qualities in your food and drink, your work/relaxation balance, and in your approach to projects and deadlines.

We know that stress increases heat in the body, and the stress factor affects the menstrual cycle in relation to pitta symptoms perhaps more than any other dosha. The trick is to slow down—when fire is high, it wants to keep burning, and it takes a gentle and steady effort to learn how to mellow out in the face of aggravated pitta.

### Food

- Reduce or avoid spicy, sour, and salty foods like chilis, ferments, and salted nuts.
- Reduce acidic beverages like orange juice, coffee, and alcohol (especially red wine).
- Reduce or avoid fried foods.

- Drink warm water and mint tea.
- Enjoy naturally sweet and juicy fruits, especially pomegranates, plums, and red grapes.
- Eat cooked greens to purify the blood.
- Increase soft, gently spiced, sweet foods like oatmeal and whole-grain breads.

- Drink 1 quart of Cooling Herbal Infusion (page 220) or Refreshing Phanta Infusion (page 221) daily.

- During your period, eat more cooked foods and fewer raw vegetables.
- Sit down to eat.

## Rhythms

- Sleep more if you can.
- Shut all screens off one hour before bed.
- Get to bed by 10 P.M.
- Reduce food intake at night, and enjoy more at midday.

- Practice sense care (see the discussion of dinacharya in chapter 5).
- Wear loose clothing.
- Practice relaxing your abdomen.

## Activity

- Rest on the first days of bleeding—the day before or after too, if you're tired.
- Enjoy unstructured, less productive time. Balance fire with space. Allow the bleeding to be your productivity.
- Schedule downtime and sedentary activities. Look ahead on the calendar and try

  to schedule less during the heavy days of your period.
- Reduce stress any way you can (see chapter 10).
- Practice Sitali Cooling Breath (page 323).

The more you embrace these foods and rhythms and shift your activity levels, the more you can expect to see the signs of pitta in your period decrease over a few months. **Warning:** If you "follow the rules" exactingly for one week but practice the opposite the rest of the time, mixed messages are likely to keep you in a place of imbalance. Try working a practice or two into your days at other times of the month (and don't try to be perfect, ever).

## KAPHA IMBALANCES OF THE MENSTRUAL CYCLE

Kapha is heavy, cool, moist, sticky, building, and slow—all the qualities a body needs for healthy ovulation. Among the three doshas, kapha is the nourisher, and a healthy kapha brings the nourishment needed to build blood and ova. Kapha body types will naturally have heavier periods and lose a larger volume of blood. When kapha gets too heavy, sticky, or slow, however, it can cause problems. The heavy quality can cause an accumulation of tissue leading to even heavier periods, while the slow quality of kapha may lead to stagnation. This presents as a dull pain in the lower abdomen or cramping pain during the period, and it may cause a slow start to the blood flow. It may feel like the womb is holding on to the blood instead of letting it go.

The increased water of accumulated kapha causes swelling of the breasts, legs, hands, and feet. If kapha is aggravated, these PMS symptoms are more likely. Water is also the emotional element, and out-of-balance kapha can make you feel sad, heavy, and sluggish. Emotional eating before or during your period, and cravings for heavy, oily, sweet foods during your period are signs of kapha imbalance.

## Signs of Kapha in the Cycle

Intervals between periods becoming longer

Period being slow to start and associated with pain or spotting

Dull pain in the low abdomen

Cramping

Premenstrual swelling

Mucus in the blood

Sadness, sluggishness

Emotional eating

Cravings for heavy, oily, or sweet foods

## BALANCING KAPHA IN ARTAVA

A kapha-provoking diet or sedentary lifestyle are the biggest factors causing imbalance, which will manifest in the cycle. Keeping kapha in balance requires regular physical movement, and finding a way of moving your body that you can easily fit into your schedule will be key. Digestion is also a big factor in kapha imbalance, when slow and sticky qualities may lend themselves to low agni and the production of ama, so taking special note of the general food guidelines in part two is sure to yield results. Processed foods, especially flours and oils, greatly contribute to the sticky quality.

Introduce warming, penetrating, and mobilizing qualities through your food and drink, your clothing (wear some bright colors!), and your activity levels.

### Food

- Reduce oily, sweet, and salty foods like takeout, oily meats, dairy, and pastries.
- Enjoy more astringent stone fruits and berries, cooked greens, and digestive spices.
- Eat Spiced Barley Soup (page 269).
- Drink ginger tea.
- Do not eat when you're not hungry.
- Favor cooked food over raw.
- Drink 1 quart of Cleansing Herbal Infusion (page 222) daily.

### Rhythms

- Avoid sleeping in the daytime, especially after meals.
- Avoid oversleeping, especially into the late morning hours.
- Eat a light dinner.
- Do not suppress the urge to pee, pass wind, or poop.
- Be sweet with yourself during your period, and notice if you give yourself a hard time about resting.

### Activity

- Rest or take gentle walks during the heavy days of your period if you crave it.
- Move (walk, dance, etc.) for 45 minutes or so five days per week.
- Use Castor Oil Packs on the lower abdomen (page 318).

# HOW DOSHAS AFFECT YOUR PERIOD

The following table will help you see the big picture and that there can be more at work in your cycle than just general tendencies. If one or more of these signs is chronic, get it checked out.

| SYMPTOM | DOSHA AT WORK |
| --- | --- |
| Increased length between periods | Vata and/or kapha |
| Occipital headaches | Vata and/or pitta |
| Scanty periods | Vata |
| Sharp pain | Vata |
| Dark blood (dark red, black, or brownish red) | Vata |
| Decreased length between periods | Pitta |
| Temporal headaches | Pitta |
| Burning pain | Pitta |
| Hot, swollen breasts | Pitta |
| Acne before period | Pitta |
| Heavy periods | Kapha |
| Increased mucus in the blood | Kapha |
| Swelling | Kapha |
| Dull pain | Kapha |

## WHAT DOES AYURVEDA SAY ABOUT PMS?

Although PMS is quite common today, it is not considered normal in Ayurveda, which sees such symptoms as signs of imbalance. The approach is not to address the symptom, such as hot tea for bloating (which does work but doesn't keep the PMS from recurring). Instead, one must address the dosha that is causing the problem. Most often, working with the lifestyle and diet factors in part two makes the shift, even without a specialized knowledge of doshas. That is great news for you, dear reader. The general principles of living with natural rhythms, optimizing digestion (and therefore immunity), and circulating prana most of the time alleviate a lot of discomforts.

Observing slow and steady improvements in your PMS symptoms after a few months of working with Ayurveda tells you, *Yes, this is improving.* Even better, you will become attuned to "flare-ups" when symptoms increase. Keeping track of your monthly routines can help you root out causes of imbalance. For example, things may get wacky after a month during which you traveled a lot. Maybe you don't have a choice about that travel right now, but you know that because of it, you need to incorporate more consistency in your food and sleep schedules when you are not on the road. (This is called vata management!) PMS symptoms are one of your best tools for understanding your doshas and your body's needs.

## WHAT'S NORMAL, WHAT'S NOT: WHAT TO LOOK FOR

Imbalances described in this section that do not respond to your therapeutic efforts may be warning you of something more serious that needs professional evaluation.

Disorders of the menstrual cycle can sometimes be due to deeper imbalances, and it is important to know what is "normal" and when to see a doctor. *Your* normal may not be exactly what is shown here, and that doesn't always mean something is wrong. With observation, knowing your normal makes you alert to your abnormal too. You may have five heavy days instead of the "normal" two to three, and if that's your normal, it doesn't mean something is wrong. But take note if the number of days of heavy bleeding suddenly starts to extend beyond your normal. Taking care to know as much as you can about your cycle, PMS symptoms, and ovulation is the number-one factor in taking charge of your generative health.

It is never a bad thing to rule out serious disorders or to look for a second opinion when something doesn't feel right. Taking time to write down and track notes about your symptoms will make it easier for you to communicate this information to your health care provider. Take your notes with you to your appointment and rely on them to be sure, in the moment, that you share everything you have been tracking and express any concerns freely.

As I age and things sometimes happen that aren't in my normal, I do consult with a doctor. I ask what I should be looking for and what the Western interventions are in the event of an imbalance or diagnosis. I see myself as a co-creator in my own health narrative. I have the information from two viewpoints, Ayurveda and Western medicine, and I have a direct line of prevention through my Ayurveda practices. I trust I am doing my best to take good care of myself. Ayurveda isn't about worrying about imbalances; it is about feeling agency in the process of maintaining health.

While I am not a medical doctor and this book is not meant to diagnose any menstrual problems, it felt important to mention a few red flags that may indicate something deeper is going wrong. The following lists of the most common generative organ diagnoses and signs to look for will help you understand what sorts of imbalances might signal a need for urgent attention.

- Uterine or ovarian cysts: fluid-filled sacs that grow in or on the ovaries, many of which dissolve on their own
- Uterine fibroids: tumors of the uterus that can shrink on their own
- Polycystic ovary syndrome: a hormonal imbalance rooted in the ovaries
- Endometriosis: endometrial-like cells growing outside the uterus
- Amenorrhea: absent periods
- Dysmenorrhea: severe cramps and pain during periods.

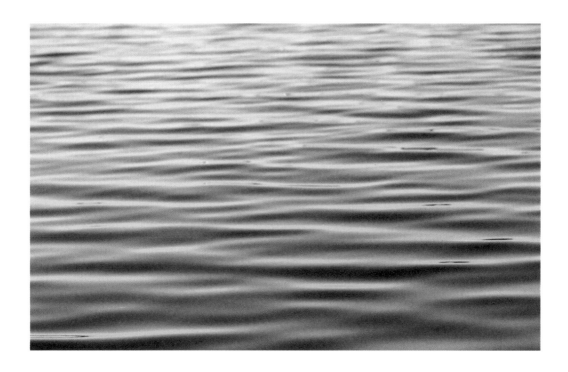

The following symptoms can be indicators of any of these disorders. Watch for unusual occurrences that deviate from your normal. Tracking your cycle and periods over time can help you establish a status quo and recognize changes.

- Heavy bleeding (soaking through a pad or filling a cup, period panty, or tampon in less than two hours)
- Bleeding that lasts more than seven days
- More than normal pain during your period
- New onset of pelvic or abdominal pain during your period
- Persistent bloating
- Fever-like symptoms or foul-smelling discharge (can be signs of bacterial infection)
- Dizziness or fainting (may be anemia due to heavy blood loss)
- Bleeding between periods
- Suicidal thoughts during periods
- Absent period for three months or more (unless you are breastfeeding, pregnant, or using a cycle-suppressing hormonal form of birth control)[7]

**Note:** It is normal for periods to be irregular during the first two years after menarche. Look for a new onset of irregularity, a variation from your normal, as a potential sign of a problem.

Ayurveda may be of help in these disorders, but if symptoms persist despite interventions, they should be evaluated further. Knowing your body's signs will help you get the care you need sooner.

Ayurveda's medicines are extremely effective in many cases, but they are always used in tandem with personalized dietary and lifestyle choices. All the general guidelines for health maintenance through regular self-care remain the substratum for healing, and these practices will provide the ideal circumstances for an Ayurveda specialist to build on.

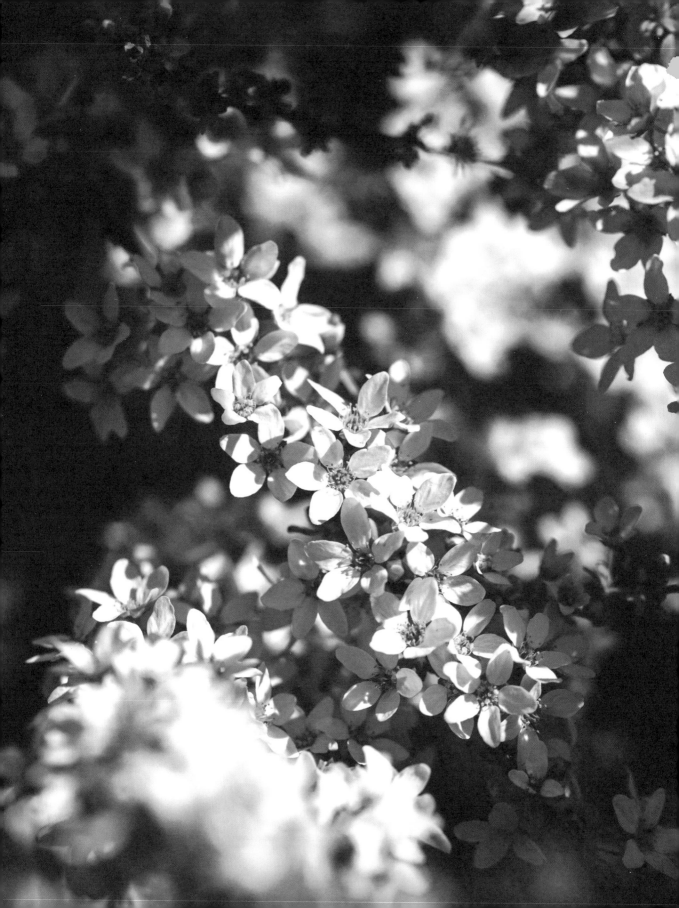

# 13

# Fertility Enhancement and Pregnancy Prevention

Knowing your body's ovulation cycles can help you avoid getting pregnant or help you get pregnant. Tracking your fertility is tracking your full-moon energy and being aware of when shukra's potency is highest. Whether you choose to channel that juiciness toward sexiness, fertility, or other creative endeavors, the path to generating this energy is the same.

Many women go through life without paying much attention to the health of their reproductive system until they want to get pregnant. Hormonal birth control, oblivious to nature's rhythms, scrambles the messages from the artava mothership and cuts off awareness of natural cycles, which makes it easy to forget the moon flows and the natural shifts in energy that keep us balanced. The mind can become so busy that a period or ovulation comes and goes, and we hardly notice it. Preventing and supporting pregnancy can begin as a practice of self-awareness. With this knowledge, you are connecting to your creative potential, however you choose to express it.

## PREGNANCY PREVENTION AND YOUR FERTILITY BASELINE

Teaching young people how to avoid pregnancy without the use of chemicals is dear to my heart. I was uncomfortable with using hormonal birth control from day one and had to go outside what was offered by the mainstream to find more options myself. I learned how to track my cycle and got to know my cervical mucus. The sooner teens and young women learn to recognize rhythms and track their cycle, the more prepared they will be to manage fertility naturally when the time comes.

The hands-down best guide to natural birth control is *Taking Charge of Your Fertility* by Toni Weschler. This book was first published in 1995, and its updated editions are still a favorite for cycle tracking using cervical mucus and changes in body temperature. Once you discern your ovulation pattern and your window of fertility, you can choose to abstain or use birth control during this window. With a sound daily routine, you are more likely to have recognizable signs. Imbalances in the body that affect ovulation and menstruation can make fertility more difficult to track. I recommend devoting six months to observing ovulation and working with Weschler's book to get the whole picture of how the fertile stage of your body works. Once you have this knowledge, you are prepared to move toward, or away from, pregnancy. (Perimenopause bonus: when your ovulation cycles begin to change, this knowledge will again become very useful.)

## HORMONAL BIRTH CONTROL

I never *tell* a woman to get off hormonal birth control. However, if asked for Ayurveda's perspective on it, I do say that it masks our natural rhythms and clouds the vital signs of our cycles. That said, getting pregnant when one is not prepared (or wanting to) can be unhealthy in obvious as well as subtle ways. What I see, time and time again, is that women who have established an awareness of their natural rhythms end up feeling uncomfortable with using hormonal birth control. They want to transition away from it. It seems to be a form of intuition.

If you are transitioning from hormonal birth control, it could take six months to a year to begin to know when you are fertile using natural methods. When you are coming off hormones, ovulation may be irregular for several months. Add to that six months to get an accurate sense of when you ovulate. That makes nearly a year before you can count on a natural approach to fertility management. Timing is important in managing fertility: be sure you are ready to commit to other methods of birth control or to abstain from sex as you take on the project of learning your body's ovulation cycle, if you wish to avoid pregnancy.

In a culture that elevates solar energies, a lunar-like slowdown—listening to the body's messages and managing fertility without drugs—runs contrary to the go-go-go paradigm. One of the many issues with the prevalence of hormonal birth control as a therapeutic is that it invites women to mask signs of imbalance in the cycle by "correcting" it without addressing a root cause. Women can blaze ahead without resolving what is causing problems in the generative system. In the Ayurveda view, causative factors that are allowed to linger will become more problematic. Not taking hormones, and relying on a knowledge of your body's rhythms, has many other health benefits as well.

Given all this, if you need to use hormonal birth control to control painful symptoms or avoid pregnancy, think of it as a stopgap while you work at establishing the kind of balance that will heal your cycle or take time to become comfortable with natural birth control methods.

# FERTILITY MEDICINE (VAJIKARANA CHIKITSA)

Fertility is an expression of deep wellness. Sexual vigor is life vigor. Even if you do not want to become pregnant, this branch of medicine still supports vitality and builds ojas. *Vajikarana chikitsa* (aphrodisiac therapy) is one of the eight branches of Ayurveda and focuses on fertility, semen, and the enhancement of sexual vigor. "Aphrodisiac," which you may think of as a substance that enhances sexual desire, is not the definition of *vajikarana*. Having a healthy libido is a result of this kind of therapy, but vajikarana seeks to strengthen the entire body by strengthening the generative system and its tissues and functions. A healthy person trying to promote ojas, to feel full-power and deeply nourished, is a good candidate for this therapy.

Vajikarana is primarily nutritional therapy. Many sexual rejuvenators are also used for tissue rejuvenation. We know that shukra is sweet, unctuous, and cool, and foods and medicines that have these qualities—shatavari, milk, ghee, *amalaki*, and *rasala* (sweetened yogurt)—are used in this context. Deep nutrition doesn't take its seat in the body in a day or two, and you must work with this therapy consistently over time. You can find a table of aphrodisiac foods in appendix B.

## Top Herbs for Fertility

*Shatavari* translates literally to "woman who has one hundred husbands," so you can see what that is pointing at. See Sexy Cacao (page 249).

**Aloe**, or *kumari* (its Sanskrit name), means "like a virgin" as this plant is said to impart youthful health to the female system. See Aloe-Pom-Cran Tonic (page 254).

**Lotus** roots, seeds, leaves, and flowers are used as a tonic for the heart and reproductive system. See Lotus Root Curry (page 279).

*Amla* is the best rejuvenator for pitta-type women. See Chyawanprash Herbal Jam (page 256).

**Chasteberry** may support healthy ovulation, and it's an herb to try when ovulation is absent or irregular.

# Recipes for Fertility

In addition to the recipes already mentioned, these contain cooling and building qualities:

Date Shake (page 243)

Moon Milk (page 247)

Kate's Tahini Treat (page 309)

*Sheeta virya*, the cooling potency, is very important in aphrodisiac therapy, and most of the substances listed in the box are cooling. Hot and dry reproductive tissue is not ideal and can result from too much stress, depleted ojas, overexercising, alcohol and smoking, or an excessively hot and sour diet. People with more fire in their constitution will be more prone to heat. Heat will, over time, dry out tissues. It takes time, but it is inevitable. Slowing down for self-care is an important part of remedying this trifecta of heat, dryness, and depletion. Notice the mention of cool underground caves, bodies of water, and the refreshing scents of cooling flowers in the following passage on aphrodisiacs from the *Ashtanga Hrdayam*:

Big ponds with lotus flowers frequented by honey-intoxicated bees,
fragrances of jasmines and blue lotuses and underground rooms which are cold,
rivers with waves of foam, mountains with blue peaks, onset of dark clouds,
pleasant moonlit nights, pleasant wind with smell of the pond full of kumuda (water lily),
nights that are agreeable for sexual enjoyment.

—*ASHTANGA HRDAYAM,* UTTARASTHANA, 40, 42–45

# In the Bhav

Fertility energy certainly has a feeling: calm and cool, lunar. Cool colors like deep green, blue, purple, pale pink, white, and silver and gemstones like pearls and opal all create what I like to call "the bhav." *Bhavana* is a meditation technique where one visualizes oneself as the divine or a divine characteristic. The Sanskrit word *bhavana* means "calling into existence," which is exactly what preparing for pregnancy is. To get in the bhav with fertility, visualize shukra, the essence of nourishment that is called forth from the bones by sexual desire (review this on page 31). Wear white, silver, and pearls; bathe in the moonlight; and drink moon milk. Definitely stop and smell the roses.

## SHAKTI VERSUS STRESS

Stress is the enemy of ojas, so stress is the "anti-vajikarana." The irony of this is how women are surrounded by stress-inducing suggestions of things that can go wrong with fertility, and the Western medical approach of compartmentalizing and medicating does little to address a woman's health. The best practice for enhancing fertility is to build the strength of the tissues, yes—but also of the self.

Think about all the things you do to be healthy, all the positive affirmations you offer to the universe every time you sit down to a good meal or do your dinacharya routine. Take a life-affirming approach to enhancing fertility. Seek out others and listen to their conception stories. Access the network of humans who have walked this path before you; build faith and wisdom in a natural process. Build a relationship with nature and with the building blocks of matter. It is from this realm that new bodies take shape. Follow lunar rhythms and rest in a flow of energy that is bigger than you.

Rituals for connecting and digesting emotion are incredibly important if you are having trouble getting pregnant. Work with ritual and lunar rhythms in tandem with Western interventions, if you are using them.

## REFLECTIONS ON INFERTILITY

In cases of complications with getting pregnant, one can feel devastated and inadequate, in a yo-yo of hope and grief. This is a real and true aspect of achieving pregnancy for many women. Ayurveda's view on grief is that it needs time and space to be digested, like any stimulus or impulse. We tend to focus on "fixing" things like infertility, and while there are many targeted healing practices for *physical* infertility, grief and other emotions are likely to be a deep part of the process. I'll let the following Woman's Story do the talking about the importance of grieving as part of self-care.

## A Woman's Story: Grieving Infertility

Anna's is a story of grief, infertility, self-care, and miracles. She was my client for about a year and embraced her Ayurveda diet and lifestyle completely. What struck me about her is how she folded grieving into her self-care. You can find a link to Anna's full story, and a ceremony she created for grieving infertility, in appendix C.

After years of fertility charting and five failed IVF cycles, I was physically, emotionally, and spiritually exhausted. I had been diagnosed by a reproductive endocrinologist with poor egg quality, an amorphous diagnosis for which Western medicine does not have a solution (only to try a lot of eggs to see if you get lucky or to use another woman's eggs).

I began working with Kate on Ayurveda rejuvenation after my third IVF cycle. I was lacking in the grounding kapha necessary to nurture a pregnancy. To boot, the IVF cycles themselves greatly aggravated vata. My path to rebalance involved eating tons of ghee and being conscientious with dinacharya practices: abhyanga, twenty minutes of Nadi Shodana breathing with the warm oil on my skin, followed by gentle yoga, and keeping up my vata-pacifying diet. All this made me feel fantastic and more grounded. My fourth and fifth IVF cycles were better, but I didn't get pregnant. Along with the devastation, I felt deep relief knowing that I would never subject my body to a hormone-stimulating cycle again. I grieved profoundly.

Six months later—when we were exploring a prospective egg donor—I got pregnant. Along with the emotional clearing from openly grieving our losses, I credit the two years I'd put into physical and emotional rejuvenation with Ayurveda. I believe it created the foundation I needed to get pregnant. (And my second child was also a wonderful surprise!)

## MAKING SPACE FOR FERTILITY

Something I have noticed in my practice is the body's need to move more prana toward the activity of reproduction. As we have seen, survival wins over reproduction when there is a shortage of resources. I have seen women needing to carve out space for the activity of fertilization and gestation *before* the body will make the space to allow pregnancy. For example, a woman who manages a lot of people at work and "mothers" her team members may be creating a sensation in the system that there aren't enough resources for another being to mother.

Building up physical stores of strength in the tissues is one thing, but in a system on the edge of overload, mental factors may need to shift as well. Think of this as a redirection of prana. Life energy follows attention, and the energy and attention needed to grow a new life sometimes need to be present before the body feels safe to support a pregnancy. This doesn't mean the body is weak; it means it's smart. Some women are more sensitive to subtle energies than others (usually those with space, air, and fire elements in the constitution) and may find the mind plays a large role in fertility.

The recipes and practices for the new moon (page 92) usher energy down and in, slow the stimulation of the senses, and turn attention inward to supporting generative functions. Use any of these practices as a ritual to redirect prana from everything going on "out there" to paying attention to the "in here." Bodies love this! Redirecting prana inward allows its counterpart, full-power fertility on the full moon (or when you ovulate), to express more freely.

## BUILDING OPTIMAL OVA

Ayurveda places great importance on the quality of the ovum and sperm, as they are the primary fertility components and genetic substratum for the baby. Practices for building optimal eggs include all the basic routines from part two and the use of fertility-enhancing foods and herbs, as we've just discussed. Digestive care and balanced qualities in the diet ensure the nutritive factor, rasa dhatu, is smooth, cool, and unctuous and makes its way to artava dhatu. Focusing on general self-care before trying to get pregnant is ideal. Everything, including your pregnancy and postpartum period, will be smoother if you are optimally nourished.

A key point to note here is that fertility medicine is advised *before* trying to get pregnant for building optimal ova and sperm. Eggs take about three months to grow to the point of being fertile, and Ayurveda's way of optimizing a healthy ovum, when possible, is to do a preparatory cleanse, then rejuvenate for three months before conceiving.

# When Cleansing Qualities Are Needed

With all this talk of nourishing qualities to optimize fertility, in some cases, it is the opposite that is needed. When they have too many heavy, sticky qualities or ama in rasa dhatu, women may experience kapha imbalances such as water retention, cystic pimples, lethargy, and PCOS. Rather than introducing more nourishing qualities, they need to purify rasa dhatu with blood cleansers like turmeric, *musta*, red clover, tulsi, and burdock. See the recipe for Cleansing Herbal Infusion on (page 222), and find more about balancing rasa in chapter 3.

This rejuvenation using aphrodisiac substances for three months *before* conception is a traditional Ayurveda preparation for both partners. The couple is advised to abstain from sex during the three-month period. It takes this long for shukra to build from food and for the sperm and egg produced to reach maturity. The intention of the cleanse is to balance accumulated doshas, so they do not build into the fertility components, and to build a reserve of strength that is funneled into the reproductive tissues. Once you are pregnant, head over to chapter 14, and never undertake any cleanse when you are pregnant.

The traditional Ayurveda ideal is to attend a panchakarma for deep cleansing and rejuvenation (see the list of centers in appendix C). If you don't have the resources, and you are healthy but looking to optimize further, a preconception home cleanse is possible. Do what you can to be as balanced and strong as you are able and feel good about it.

# PRECONCEPTION CLEANSE

Plan to begin your cleanse between ovulation and menstruation, and clear your calendar, to the extent possible, for a period of five to seven days. While you may have obligations, such as childcare and work, seek any ways that you can make your days more spacious. Enlist the help of friends and family. This first phase of preparing to conceive gives the body the chance to process ama and pacify doshas by eating a simple diet. You will be surprised by how profound it feels to prepare for conception with intention.

Phase 1 should improve your appetite and metabolic fires, and when you enter phase 2, focus on eating rejuvenating foods and recipes from this book for a one- to three-month period. You may choose to continue to eat this way for longer, and remember the body takes three months to prepare a fertile egg. Taking ghee on an empty stomach improves digestion of this ojas builder, and over the course of the following weeks, you will continue to nourish the artava by taking ghee on an empty stomach daily. Emerge feeling strong and deeply nourished.

**Do this first:** If you have signs of ama (see chapter 7), follow the guidelines to get your digestion on track before moving into phase 1.

**Then:** Look over the Home Cleanse Program on page 84. Take note of the "Things to Consider" section. If you are underweight or recovering from injury, illness, or imbalance, cleansing may not be the best course, and you would do well to consult a practitioner instead about a personalized program.

Follow the gentle Home Cleanse program on page 84, adding in the following extras.

Phase 1 (five to seven days)
- Time this phase between ovulation and menstruation.
- Eat a diet of primarily New Moon Kichari (page 286). Choose from the menus in the program if you need more options.
- In the morning, after tongue scraping, take shatavari ghee* on an empty stomach. You may start with 1 teaspoon and increase to 1 tablespoon gradually when you feel it digests easily.
- Do not eat until you are hungry, at least one hour.
- If you are very sturdy, this phase may continue for seven days. If you have low body fat or are not so sturdy, keep it to five days or less.

**Phase 2 (one to three months)**

- Begin to work in other foods slowly, but continue with the ghee in the morning for up to three months.
- Use ghee, warm spiced milk, meat soup, eggs, and small legumes such as lentils and mung beans. Avoid all processed food, especially trans fats. Build the body with natural, whole foods.
- Enjoy a Date Shake (page 243) or Moon Milk (page 247) regularly.
- If you need cooling, have Aloe-Pom-Cran Tonic (page 254) daily.
- Ensure that your period is flowing well and regularly. You can promote this with practices from chapter 11.

*You may use shatavari ghee (see appendix C for suppliers, or find a recipe for making your own in *The Everyday Ayurveda Guide to Self-Care*) if you have a hot, light, or dry constitution. Shatavari contains phytoestrogens, and the safe bet is not to use it if you have a family history of breast cancer. Use plain ghee instead.

Fertility is an aspect of overall health. The ideal approach is to focus on your health first. Just take care of you. Later you will see how the qualities that support fertility are on the rise in your body and mind. The glorious thing is that the path to feeling deeply connected to your creative power, maintaining a firm and stable vessel to hold this potential, and the focus to harness it into manifestations of any kind are all results of living in nature's flow.

# 14

# Pregnancy
# and Childbirth

*A pregnant woman is to be treated as if one is walking with a pot of oil, without letting a drop to fall.*

—*CHARAKA SAMHITA,* SHARIRASTHANA 8:22

As the body, heart, and mind expand to create, nurture, and raise babies, how do we move through life like a pot of oil, smoothly and gently, so no drop will fall? What changes can we make to our foundational practices for digestion, good food, and healthy natural rhythms to support us through this time of life?

General daily practices lay the groundwork for womb and overall health throughout the massive physical demands of the grihastha period, including gestation, birthing, and the active householding that follows. This pitta time of life requires calming, grounding, and slow qualities, many of which can be provided by a nourishing diet and simple self-care. The irony of this time of life is that self-care can easily be eclipsed by caring for others. The most important lesson of grihastha is to learn to integrate self-care into the matrix of family life.

Ayurveda's guidelines for pregnancy begin even before conception, as we saw in our last chapter. Regimens for the pregnant woman seek to create ideal circumstances for healthy babies and mothers. The health of the baby is entirely dependent on the health of the mother, as the fetus is produced from the mother's rasa. Maintaining strong and healthy rasa dhatu during pregnancy, as we will see, is key to a healthy term, a healthy baby, and a sound recovery postpartum.

## THE PHYSICAL TRANSFORMATION OF PREGNANCY

During pregnancy, the mother's body is a waxing moon. The space of the womb and the circulating rasa, which brings nutrition to the fetus, then become the universe for this being. Together, food, agni, and kapha's building qualities transform nutrition into new tissue. According to Ayurveda, a fetus is built from rasa (the digested food of the mother), and everything we have

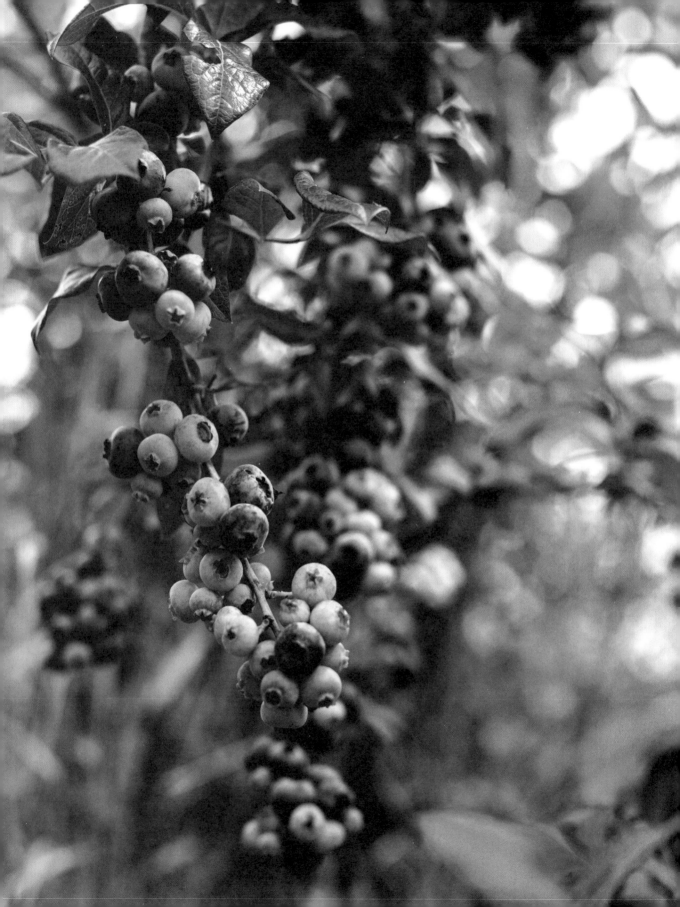

already learned about cultivating excellence of rasa dhatu contributes to ideal circumstances for nutrition of the mother and baby and the formation of breast milk.

Ayurveda texts provide clear dietary and lifestyle guidelines for pregnancy, as specific as month to month. The nine-month journey of a fetus—the development of soul, senses, and limbs—is carefully described by changes each month. Based on these developments, the monthly diet for a pregnancy is also carefully described. Central to the diet are milk, ghee, butter, honey, and rice. Preparations made of combinations of these staples are medicated with different herbs each month to support specific growth of the fetus.

While *garbini parichaya* (ideal protocols for the pregnancy) deserves its own detailed book, we will take a broad perspective on pregnancy, along with some basic diet and lifestyle factors to consider.

## GARBINI PARICHAYA

*Garbini* means a pregnant woman. Aspects of prenatal care in Ayurveda cover not only the physical dimensions, but also the psychological, spiritual, and social. Descriptions of embryology in the texts discuss the development of the soul, senses, and mind of the fetus, even before the components of the body. As food affects the physicality of the embryo, energy affects the subtle body. The energy you are surrounded by during pregnancy is as important as the food you eat. General principles of "wholesomeness," primarily a positive mental attitude of the mother, and a practice of prayer or gratitude practice, especially to the rising sun, provide healthy "food" for the senses and soul of the developing baby.

Other energetic practices include anointing the body with cooling scents, such as essential oils or pastes of lotus, sandalwood, rose, lavender, and jasmine, as well as moonbathing and wearing flowers (which could also mean keeping fresh flowers in the home if you are not keen to actually wear them).

## THE ROLE OF VATA IN PREGNANCY

The body's ability to "hold" a fetus for a full gestational term is an action of vata. While supporting fetal growth requires good food and the building nature of kapha, vata holds space for the baby and governs the timing of gestation and birth. The activity of birthing is the biggest movement apana vata makes in a lifetime, and birth can have lasting effects on the functions of apana: elimination, urination, menstruation, and circulation through the hips and legs. We will look more at that in the next chapter, but know that pregnancy is a time for balancing the qualities and strengthening the functions of vata for a smooth pregnancy, birth, and postpartum period.

Keep vata in balance by avoiding cold food and drinks, excessive travel and exercise, or too much stimulation of the senses. Oil massage is an important tool to keep vata in balance and is good to include in your pregnancy rituals. Take care to massage gently, as vigorous massage is not recommended when you are pregnant. Sit down to do your massage, and do not oil the bottoms of your feet for safety. Apply the oil to your body as described in the instructions on page 323, but do not rub or press hard. Simply apply the oil and let it rest on the skin for 10 to 20 minutes, then have a warm shower. The oil that you usually use on your skin should still be good unless you feel too hot, then use coconut oil or a pitta massage oil. Traditionally, a sesame oil base is favored, but again, this can be too warming for some during pregnancy. You may also add essential oils of the cooling fragrances mentioned earlier.

Regular oil massage during pregnancy reduces the likelihood of stretch marks and may improve sleep, digestion, and mood. Think of an oil massage as a calming, restorative treat. You may even treat yourself to Ayurveda bodywork on a weekly or monthly basis if it's available.

Do not do oil massage when you feel overheated or nauseous, have just eaten, or are having any complications with your pregnancy.

## WHAT TO EAT DURING PREGNANCY

I have noticed an interesting trend in my practice: when women find out they are pregnant, they want to know exactly what to eat and how to "do pregnancy right." Pregnant bodies are incredibly smart and have cravings for the right foods and activities at the right time. Tuning in to your body and giving it what sounds good at the moment is the first practice to adopt during pregnancy. The mind is likely to step in with a few words about this and that, but your pregnant body is on a mission: it will tell you what it needs. Take in the recommendations that follow, sit with your true cravings, and see if they align.

The general Ayurveda principle of not "snacking" may no longer apply when you are pregnant, as you may not feel well digesting big meals, or you may be unable to make it more than an hour or two without eating. This is normal, so do not worry about how often you are eating. The more frequent need for food is likely to continue as or if you breastfeed as well.

These guidelines describe the kinds of food that produces ideal rasa with enough juice for mother, baby, and breast:

- Palatable (this means appealing to you, which may change week to week)
- More liquid, like soups and stews
- Predominantly sweet in taste, like whole grains, fruits, and root vegetables
- Unctuous, containing natural oils
- Made with digestive spices

# A Woman's Story: Missed Miscarriage

Somewhere between 10 and 26 percent of pregnancies miscarry, according to the National Institutes of Health statistics, and the percentage in reality is likely higher.[8] As an Ayurveda practitioner, I may hear about women's miscarriages more often than friends and family. That they are statistically common makes miscarriages no less heartbreaking. It strikes me as a place in women's wisdom where, collectively, we could benefit from more stories, more sharing. My dear friend Stewart had a "missed" miscarriage last year, in which her baby's heartbeat stopped at ten weeks, and it was still fourteen days before her body released the fetus. This is her story.

I was not prepared for the grief that followed my missed miscarriage. I often felt like I was at the bottom of a hole and unreachable. I cried a lot, I felt the pain, I sank deep in it. My heart broke for everything I had imagined for that baby. My heart broke for the hopes, dreams, and excitement my family had. But in no way did I regret the celebration of this baby, the sharing of the news, the clothing I'd bought. It was all worth it, and I would do it again. Allowing myself the time and space to really be with the hard feelings helped immensely in the long run.

After a miscarriage, you suddenly find yourself in a body that had just been serving such a profound purpose, that changed and grew for pregnancy, and still shows those changes, but you are no longer pregnant. All were painful reminders of the purpose I'd just had but that is no longer. I found that trying to show love to my body gave me the most peace and healing. I arrived at a place where I could acknowledge that my body knew something wasn't right and did what it was supposed to do, even though it wasn't what I wanted. As I miscarried in my bathroom, I felt bound to all the women who had been in the same situation before me and to all the women who would go through it after me.

# Best Foods for Pregnancy

This group of building and cooling foods contains the best components for building rasa dhatu. They are primarily composed of water and earth elements, balanced with the sweet and slightly astringent dark fruits that support robust rakta dhatu. Preparations that are cool, liquid, milk-like, and unctuous have an affinity for rasa.

Some of these ingredients may not be available to you. Look in your area for foods with similar qualities. For example, jackfruit, which is abundant in India, is very similar to breadfruit and potato.

- Meat soup
- Mung beans (especially in a soup)
- Rice (especially red)
- Wheat (heirloom varieties)
- Butter
- Ghee
- Milk, if you digest it well

- Yogurt mixed with sugar and spices
- Honey
- Sugarcane
- Jackfruit
- Bananas
- Amla berries, gooseberries
- Black grapes, raisins, prunes

**A word about wheat:** Wheat is one of the most nutritious grains according to Ayurveda; it is a prime builder and is very important for vegetarians. Modern wheat, however, has been through a lot of processing, all the way down to the seeds and gluten, which has depleted its nutritional value and stymied the body's ability to digest it. Heirloom seeds, on the other hand, ground into flours or cracked as in bulgur wheat, are an excellent food and becoming easier to find in stores. Sourdough breads made with heirloom flours may be the best way to eat wheat, as the culturing predigests the wheat and makes it lighter. If you can find, or make, a bread like this, have it warm with ghee. It is an excellent rasa builder during pregnancy.

Milk, ghee, sweetened yogurt, and rice porridges cooked with milk are top among the recipes mentioned in classical texts. If you do not digest milk well, don't worry. You can use plant milks (homemade), and if you do not eat meat, you can make mung bean soups instead of meat soups and use ghee, yams, and other roots. Being completely plant-based during pregnancy may not be appropriate for some women, and it is good to remain open to cravings. Your body may be communicating a deficit or imbalance it needs addressed. Here I share a woman's story on this topic.

# Woman's Story:
# Vegetarian Diets and Pregnancy

A lot of women feel conflicted about eating meat. Being a vegetarian can be difficult for light body types and doesn't work for many women, regardless of constitution, when they start growing babies. I asked my colleague Adena Bright, a women's health Ayurveda specialist, to share her story of using animal foods in the diet.

I was vegetarian for two years before conceiving my first child. I wanted to be a "good" Ayurveda practitioner, and I wanted to have a "perfect" Ayurveda baby. Only a few weeks into this first pregnancy, I went out to dinner and surprised myself by ordering a burger—topped with blue cheese and bacon! I had craved meat since becoming pregnant, yet the mental battle with myself around regularly consuming animals continued throughout that pregnancy and into my first year postpartum.

Postpartum, I struggled with severe blood sugar challenges, energy, motivation, and mood. I had trouble sleeping, and I could not tolerate caffeine or alcohol at all—even a bit of dark chocolate or *kombucha*. My baby was strong, but my health was suffering. I wasn't the mother I wanted to be.

Animals of all sorts are listed as medicine in the classical texts of Ayurveda. "Meat soup" in particular is mentioned for healing vata imbalances. Meat is considered to be "guru" or heavy guna/quality. Guru guna builds the tissues. At what stage in a woman's life does she need more brmhana than in pregnancy and postpartum, when she is literally building a human, blood, bone, and brain?

Instead of leaning into more discipline, I learned to soften around dogma, honor personal truths, and see the reality of the situation. One of my deep inner knowings is the truth in blood for blood, dhatu for dhatu. I began eating meat soon after birthing my first child and continue to use animal foods now as a mother of two. In order to fulfill my dharma of motherhood, to give abundantly and hold space for others, I must be nourished on the deepest level possible. For me, sacred animal foods are now a vital part of my healing.

Find Adena's chicken soup recipe on page 276.

Spicy and overly sour foods are not recommended during pregnancy because increased hormone levels can cause high pitta, especially in the second trimester. As the baby grows and may constrict space for the stomach, hyperacidity is not uncommon, and sticking to soft, sweet foods keeps the acids calm. Gentle spices like cumin, cinnamon, cardamom, coriander, and fennel are excellent for improving digestion without increasing acidity. Too much meat, trans fats, old or stale food, and large beans that cause wind (such as kidney or fava) are not recommended. Any food that gives you gas is not a good idea, as space in your abdomen is already in use! Adding gas in the intestines will not feel nice.

In general, moving toward a diet of home-cooked soups, stews, and hot cereals, and incorporating ingredients from the earlier list will serve you and the baby well. It will also set you up to continue eating this way postpartum, when the building qualities of your rasa will go to breast milk and to healing and rebuilding your body during a demanding period. All the recipes in the Medicinal Foods section (chapter 23) are suitable for pregnancy. In addition, consider these:

> Creamy Coconut Breakfast Kichari (page 264)
>
> Chyawanprash Herbal Jam (page 256)
>
> Essential Mineral Vegetable Broth (page 272)
>
> Date Shake (page 243)
>
> Moon Milk (page 247)
>
> Rasala Medicinal Yogurt (page 311)
>
> Yogurt Rice with Pomegranate Seeds (page 265)
>
> Sesame Crunch Chutney (page 298)
>
> Black Sesame Balls (page 303)
>
> Pumpkin Seed Cilantro Pâté (page 293)

Most of the foods and practices discussed for fertility (see chapter 13) also support pregnancy, as they are ojas builders. Take care, however, when using medicinal amounts of any herb or spice when you are or might be pregnant. Culinary use is absolutely fine, but drinking spiced waters or herbal infusions with certain substances all day may not be safe during pregnancy. Raspberry Leaf and Nettle Brew (page 223) is a safe and nourishing infusion that can be used freely when you are trying to get pregnant or during term. Ayurveda's medicines and preparations specific to supporting pregnancy are many, and seeking out a professional to work with will help you build on the dietary recipes you find in this book.

Being the universe for a baby is a cosmic enterprise and an opportunity to attune to a sense of your body as a planet. If you began practicing Ayurveda before pregnancy, lucky you. If you are coming to it in pregnancy, know that the diet and lifestyle you begin now will support you well beyond this time of life, and the principles of rhythms and nutrition will bring you smoothly through birthing and postpartum, manifesting strength in all that comes next.

# 15

# Self-Care for the New Mother

I continue to be amazed by the way women's bodies mobilize to support pregnancy, birth, and lactation. The reserves of inner strength in these bodies is a wonder of nature and something to hold in deep trust. In Ayurveda, the forty-two-day window of time after a birth is sacred. Taking the opportunity to rebuild your body supports the future of *you* as well as your family. Hold the bright image of tejas as a guide—imagine that you are gently feeding this flame with your intentions; your oils; and your sweet, warming foods. The act of rejuvenation is as clear as it is profound. Women's bodies are built to sustain life, for self and others, and this magical time of self-care is a service to all those who are in your care.

## AYURVEDA'S PERSPECTIVE ON POSTPARTUM

Postpartum is a six- to eight-week period that begins after the birth of the baby. In Ayurveda, this is a time to calm the air and ether elements of vata. The new mother is said to be "afflicted by emptiness,"[9] which makes this a vulnerable time, and she requires special care to rejuvenate. While the traditional perspective on postpartum describes management of vata and rejuvenation through rest, kindness, nutrition, and oil massage, the mental and emotional factors of the postpartum time are not addressed much in the texts. They are clear that the family and partner of the woman must provide positivity and tenderness. Yet complete healing after pregnancy is very much an internal journey that requires a good amount of time, space, and digestion of emotion. All this while sleeping little! Being afflicted by emptiness can feel lonely, despondent, and exhausting. From Ayurveda's perspective, healing at this time is a filling of space, with heavy, warm, oily, stable qualities. The pillars of healing to provide these qualities are food, oil, herbs, and rest.

Ayurveda recommends a forty-two-day window of special care for the mother. Traditionally, this care was often administered by family—grandmothers, aunts, and mothers. It is still common for a mother to live with her daughter during this period, to make traditional recipes, give oil massages, and assist with her daughter's healing. While complete recovery from birthing takes one to two years (not just forty-two days!), an opportunity like this six-week window only comes once. This is the *most important time* to strengthen the body and to rejuvenate vata and agni. Proper postbirth care results in emerging stronger, while an improper regimen can cause weakness that lingers for years and likely leads to imbalances, usually of a vata nature.

I have been lucky enough to observe the benefits many women experience from an Ayurveda postpartum regimen. These days, Ayurveda-trained doulas, who can help by providing vata-pacifying meals and regular oil massages in your home, are becoming more available all the time. Look in your area for an "ayur-doula." The difference in this stage when supported by Ayurveda versus without Ayurveda is like night and day.

## REJUVENATING PRACTICES FOR POSTPARTUM

Vata is aggravated by the immense movement required during birthing, as well as the amount of space present in the body in a very short time. Postpartum oleation is the primary therapy to restore a healthy vata. This is achieved by carefully reintroducing foods for a strong digestive fire, working up to eating plenty of ghee and other fats, and doing oil massage daily during the postpartum period. It's important to note that while the Western clinical view of postpartum expects a woman to be fully recovered in six weeks, this is not realistic, and true rejuvenation takes months, possibly several years. This is normal.

### OIL MASSAGE

A vata-pacifying regimen is indicated after delivery (and during pregnancy, as we saw in the last chapter). Massage with sesame oil during this magical postpartum window will have lasting effects.

After an oil massage and a shower, you can wrap your abdomen in a cloth to calm the space element. The ancient practice of abdominal wrapping, or "belly binding," is like a hug for your abdomen and provides physical stability. Today, you can purchase belly bands, which you may find easier to use than a cotton cloth. If it causes you any pain, discontinue use; otherwise, wrap your belly for anywhere between two weeks and two months, but not when you are sleeping.

If you do not have access to the resources for this care, call on your community. Help them understand what kind of food you need to eat, and you may even find someone to do a massage or support you in finding time to do this yourself. To do your own massage, follow the instructions on page 323. A favorite herbal oil for postpartum is *ashwagandha bala* (suppliers are listed in appendix C). Don't give yourself a hard time if you don't have an oil massage every day during this forty-two-day period! Even a few times each week will have far-reaching benefits.

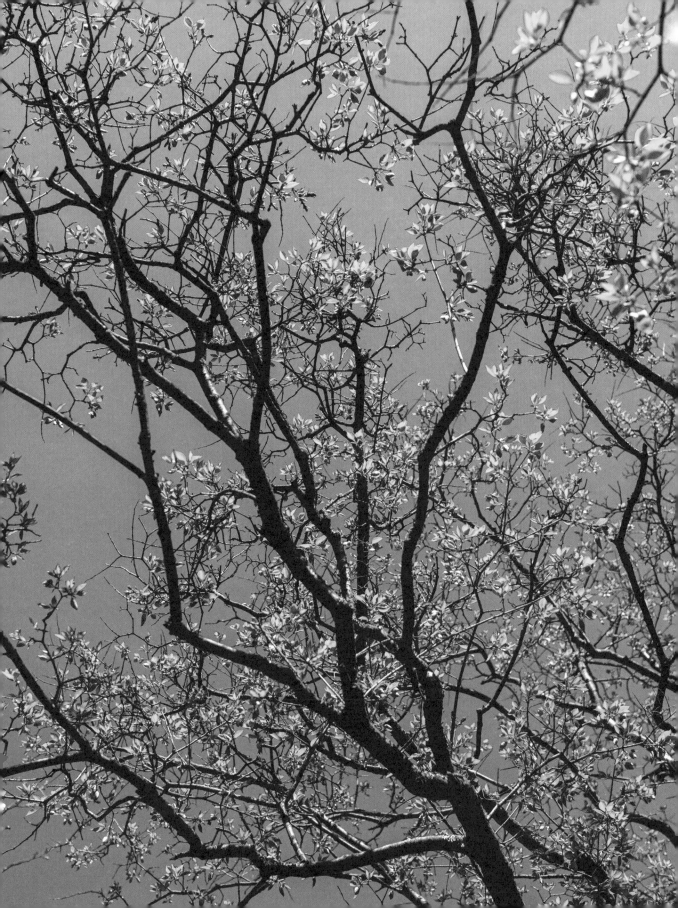

# A Woman's Story of Postpartum

Jessie is a client who has been working with Ayurveda for many years. After a premature delivery, her thoughtful postpartum plan had to shift suddenly. It was beautiful to observe her work through the loss of how it might have been, the difficulties in releasing years of measured daily routines, and embrace and benefit from the simple practices of food and oil. Here she shares a bit about her experience, and words of encouragement.

My baby came seven weeks early, so I wasn't able to prepare for this phase in the way that I wanted. Immediately, I experienced increased gas. I also experienced increased worry and anxiety (the postpartum hormones are real). The thing that helped me cope was to eat food. Any food. If you are feeding yourself, you are winning!

I was in and out of the hospital to visit my baby and carried a jar of coconut oil with me and would just stick my hands in it and oil when I could. It was easier to manage than sesame oil in the hospital. If you have time, oil the head and whole body to make both feel supergrounded. I was eventually able to see my massage therapist and get weekly abhyanga treatments. It feels so nice to be touched and cared for during this time.

Eventually I took chyavanprash daily. After four months postpartum, I still did these routines, and they made me feel grounded and like myself. If I could give one piece of advice, I would say: be as kind as humanly possible to yourself during this exceptionally vulnerable time. All thoughts are okay! Know they will pass, and if not, that's okay too. Know there is help out there, and dear momma, know you are not alone!

## POSTPARTUM DAILY ROUTINE

After childbirth, your time will not be your own, and daily routines will be set by the baby. However, continue to start your days with tongue scraping and sipping hot water or Essential Spiced Water (page 231). Maintaining this simple morning routine every day will have a grounding influence.

Sleeping more than a few hours at a time when breastfeeding a newborn is a gift. Try to sleep when the baby sleeps, and establish a schedule with your partner or a caregiver to allow you time to sleep when possible. It may be helpful to simply accept that you are tired during this time, and trust in the fact that women have survived and thrived through this stage of life for millennia.

Get a bit of sunlight every day, even just standing in the sun, and taking gentle walks when you are ready.

If you can't do oil massage, do Oiling the Ears and Feet instead (see page 65).

Stay warm. It's natural to feel cold when vata is aggravated. Sleep with a hot water bottle, wear cozy socks, and be sure to keep warm, even if your environment doesn't seem cold.

Take it one day at a time. It is easy to have big postpartum plans for your self-care and then feel exhausted and emotional. It's natural! Go slow, take space, and take your time in everything you do, when possible.

## POSTPARTUM NUTRITION

Agni will be irregular during the first month or so after birth. Rehabilitate your digestive fire by beginning postpartum with watery soups made of mung beans, mild spices, and a little ghee; Red Rice Kanji (page 271), or Warming Wheat Soup (page 268). Gradually increase the thickness of the soups over a few days to a week, beginning to add root vegetables as your appetite improves and you feel less gassy. Some amount of bloating and gas is unavoidable, especially in the first week or two. Notice if eating makes it worse, and do not increase the heavy nature of foods until the gas decreases a bit. Add cooked green vegetables later, as they contain a lot of air and ether elements. Milk and dairy (except ghee, which can come sooner in small amounts), then meat, are the last foods to add in. This process may take a few weeks; let your agni be your guide.

After this agni-boosting period, continue to eat soupy, warm foods with plenty of ghee, especially meat soup and kichari, and builders like Medjool dates and sesame tahini, as well as recipes from the second box on page 172. If you are setting up a meal train for your community to help provide you with fresh food, consider sharing these recipes. Try to eat 2 tablespoons or more of ghee daily, when your appetite allows (see the first box on page 172 for ideas).

Raw and high-fiber foods may increase wind at a time when winds need calming. Avoid large beans and salads, and make sure whole grains are cooked with plenty of water and tossed with ghee. Date shakes, warm spiced milk, white basmati rice, and kichari are smooth and nourishing go-tos that will likely appeal to you and not cause any imbalances. Overall, eating according to your appetite is best. Gravitate toward what you're craving. If you can, stock the pantry with the foods discussed here before your baby arrives. If you breastfeed and as you heal, your appetite will increase, and you will gradually feel more up to the task of digesting heavier dishes.

Drink Essential Spiced Water (page 231) to aid digestion, and favor fenugreek, turmeric, cumin, coriander, fennel, and ginger in your cooking.

# How to Get Your Ghee

Ghee is the cleanest burning fuel for the lamp of your luminosity and supports metabolic fires and inner strength. The flame of agni can literally be blown out for a short period, and it is important not to begin nutritional oil therapy until your appetite has returned. Once hunger resumes, ghee can be added by the tablespoon in porridge, in soups, in a date shake, in a cup of warm spiced milk, in sweets (see Almond Cardamom Diamonds, page 306), and slathered on warm sourdough bread, to name just a few. Have a goal to consume one 16-ounce jar of ghee each month for the first three months after delivery. Keeping three jars dedicated to this task alone will help you keep track and notice if you are falling behind.

If ghee feels too heavy to you, try making it from cultured butter, or purchase cultured ghee (see appendix C for a supplier).

# Recipes for Postpartum

These recipes include foods that are warm and smooth, but not too light, and contain healing therapeutic ingredients for postpartum. When in doubt, add a bit of cooked meat, sea vegetables, and mung beans to round out a meal. Remember to build up agni first with lighter foods, as described earlier.

Raspberry Leaf and Nettle Brew (page 223)

Warming Wheat Soup (page 268)

Essential Mineral Vegetable Broth (page 272)

Beets and Barley Stew (page 284)

Red Rice Kanji (page 271)

Umami Kichari (page 288)

Date Shake (page 243)

Creamy Coconut Breakfast Kichari (page 264)

Every Body Dal (page 280) with basmati rice

Yellow Dal Supreme (page 273) with basmati rice

Chicken Soup with Coriander and Lemon (page 276)

Rasala Medicinal Yogurt (page 311)

Almond Cardamom Diamonds (page 306)

# Herbs and Spices to Support Lactation

Incorporating the following herbs and spices into meals and herbal waters may support lactation. You will find a lot of these ingredients in our recipes. Consult a practitioner for more information about therapeutic use.

Ajwain, caraway, and celery seeds

Fenugreek

Nettle

Raspberry leaf

Urad dal

Vidari (wild yam)

## A FEW THOUGHTS ON POSTPARTUM CHALLENGES

It seems like there are a few sneaky, but fairly common, postpartum issues that women encounter, and many feel unprepared. First of all, we need to share more stories about hemorrhoids, postpartum indigestion, and other unglamorous changes. I continue to be surprised by the stories women tell about postpartum experiences when asked. "How did I not hear about this from you sooner?"

Although you may "bounce back" after the first birth, the recovery period is not always as smooth after the second. It's normal to have a more difficult postpartum time for subsequent births. I'd like to shine light on a few things I commonly see, so you can focus on healing rather than feeling confused or compelled to "just live with it." Awareness of potential challenges before your child is born can help you recognize signs and symptoms sooner if you feel you aren't getting back on track as quickly as you'd like. Healing the signs your body is giving you leads to healing on all levels, and living with pain and discomfort isn't always necessary. In general, if something—especially in the apana regions, like elimination—doesn't feel quite right after a birth, Ayurveda can help. This section is an overview, and this book provides some first-tier recommendations, but never hesitate to seek the perspective of a practitioner to get a more personalized plan.

## THE PELVIC FLOOR

The pressure of downward movement during birth is a huge event for vata, and even in the case of a cesarean delivery, it will still be disturbed. Like any physical trauma, both require a rehab period. This is a normal requirement for the body and does not indicate a weakness. Apana imbalance can affect the bladder, colon, uterus, pelvic floor, sacroiliac joints, and abdominal muscles. This can result in a weak bladder, hemorrhoids, uterine prolapse, increased gas, bloating, and constipation, among other symptoms.

Vata pacification, care of apana vayu through the recipes mentioned earlier, oil massage, and a breathing practice to redirect the flow—such as Nadi Shodhana or Sama Vritti Ujjayi in appendix A—are the first line of healing.

Two therapies that target apana regions and pacify vata with warm, moist qualities are Yoni Steaming and sitz baths. Yoni Steaming (page 318) can help in toning and strengthening the uterus and is useful in instances of prolapse, as well as in healing the generative organs. A Herbal Sitz Bath (page 316) is extremely soothing as well as healing for hemorrhoids, which can result from the pressure of birth and can come and go for some time. Hemorrhoids are exacerbated by constipation, so be sure to reduce refined foods and follow the postpartum dietary plan described earlier to get your colon back on the right track.

Targeted pelvic floor and core training strengthen the supportive role of abdominal muscles and the holding function of the bladder, and they make back injuries less likely later. Pilates and yoga can be good for this, but when an area that was strong is now weak, going back to the movement routines you did before birth can be tricky. So many times I have seen women ambitiously "get back to exercising" and suffer injuries, especially those resulting in sciatic and back pain. Working with an instructor in the beginning, or working with a program specifically for postpartum considerations, can ensure that you are doing movements correctly to target and strengthen your pelvic floor and abs. You will be so grateful for any effort given to rehabilitating your core.

Simple actions, such as contracting and engaging the pelvic floor muscles for a few seconds and working up to longer times, can begin as soon as one week after birth, but you must honestly assess your energy and rest for longer if needed. This kind of pelvic floor work is called Kegels, and it's a good idea to learn how to do it from an instructor.

Waiting too long (more than three months) to strengthen your pelvic floor makes recovery more challenging, and it will take longer to build your strength. If you've had a C-section or any complications with birth, consult your health care provider about the best timing for exercise of any kind. In the event you start working with your pelvic floor and experience back or pelvic pain, talk with a physical therapist or personal trainer.

## ASKING FOR HELP

When we say that it takes a village to raise a child, we're not just referring to the child: all parents need support as well. I want to emphasize how helpful it can be to have support, whether it's asking for food delivery or finding a pelvic floor specialist. I see a lot of women who pride themselves on being self-sufficient, which is an amazing accomplishment, but they get used to working too hard. Gestation and birth are the most demanding physical activities your body will undergo, and the path back to full strength can take a year or more. Plan for this and do not overextend yourself. Be patient in your recovery. Lining up help, and asking for it when you didn't expect to, are OK. Even if you do have what it takes to go it alone, save your reserves.

Open the lines of communication with women who have walked this path before you. Joining a prenatal class that continues to meet, in person or online, after you have delivered is a great way to find support and be with others in the same stage of life. Postpartum is an overwhelming time, and social interaction can too easily get put on a back burner. Being with other new parents having similar experiences can help you feel a part of a whole, supported by a life stream. Consider keeping in touch as part of your self-care routine.

Ask family and friends for their postpartum stories. And when your time comes, please share your birth and postpartum story, with details, as freely as you like. Your experience contributes to the weaving of women's wisdom.

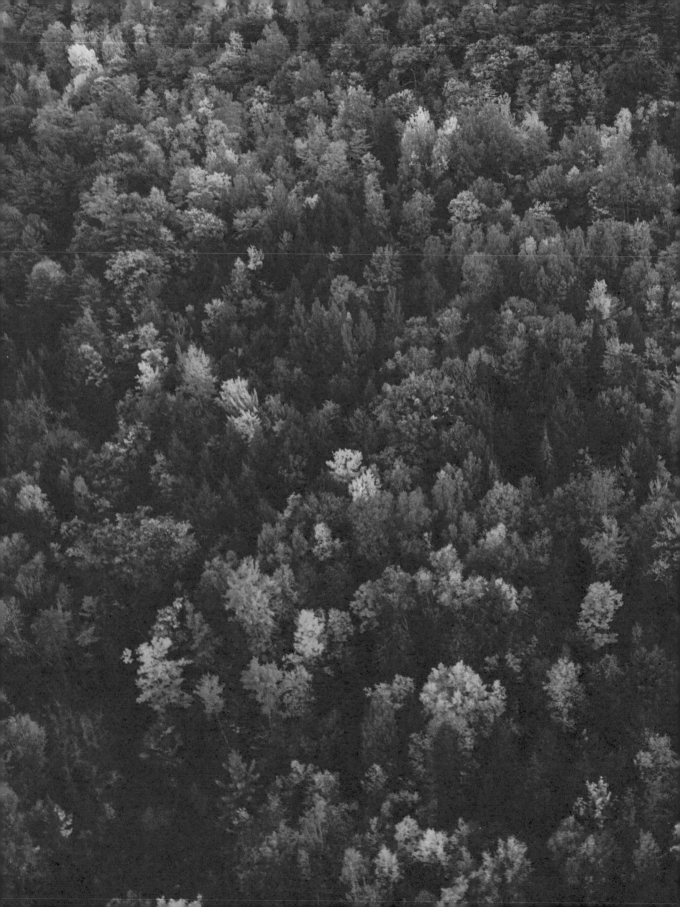

# 16

# Perimenopause

Ayurveda's spiritual and physical roots, specifically longevity medicine and vata pacification, are golden guides for transitioning to *rajonivrutti* (menopause), the cessation of menstruation. Modern medical research on menopause focuses on hormone replacement therapy (HRT) and began as recently as the late 1990s. The Western approach to this life stage (as with so many stages) has been to focus on "fixing" its symptoms with HRT. Research has shown that natural hormonal changes of menopause have been linked to disease processes, such as osteoporosis and cognitive decline. In this context, a woman's transition to menopause is often presented as scary, pathological, and needing to be managed with pharmaceuticals to avoid disease later.

But this transition is natural. The body is wired to direct resources away from maintaining fertility and gestation. Aside from puberty, menopause is the most dramatic reorganization of priorities and function the body will undergo. A woman shifts from the potential for creating new life to supporting life as it exists.

Perimenopause is a period of three to ten years when menstrual cycles become irregular as a woman approaches menopause. This is a time of restructuring in both body and mind, a time to start asking deep questions, such as what can each of us do to support and nourish younger generations while in our middle to later stages of life? As the body undergoes physiological changes, how do our desires and aims also shift? How are we called to serve the world in our later years—and how has this changed from when we were younger?

Through Ayurveda's model of life, we have a magnificent view of perimenopause and menopause: how to support smooth changes, maintain luminosity, and manage imbalances that may arise. Implementing lifestyle and diet changes *before* menopause provides the qualities needed for a smooth transition. If you are somewhere between the ages of thirty-five and fifty, it's prime time for fostering balanced habits.

The classical Ayurveda texts address vaginal and womb health, and menstruation in its healthy and imbalanced states. There is not much information about the period of life for women after menstruation, which is called *vridha* ("old age") and begins around age fifty. The texts offer information about managing early menopause, and they define menopause as a natural result of aging. Deep discussion in recorded texts stops after fertility, gestation, and postpartum. This is an unfortunate omission. These texts were codified in premodern times when mortality rates were higher, the need for procreation perhaps more pressing than it is now, and women's roles in the home and family primarily child-centered. In modern times, we are living longer and spending more years in the vata time of life. While there are certainly strong female figures in Vedic myth and living lineages of feminine power in India, from a *medicinal* standpoint, women's wisdom postperiods is hard to come by. We must share more experiences of living, and healing, as elder women.

## WHAT IS PERIMENOPAUSE?

Ayurveda describes perimenopause as a gradual decrease of brmhana qualities due to the aging process. As we move toward the vata stage of life, pitta and kapha reduce. Space and air elements slowly begin to predominate. With a reduction in building qualities in rasa, the body is no longer supportive of a monthly renewal of artava. This natural decrease begins around age thirty-five according to Western medicine and age thirty-two in the Ayurveda texts. Perimenopause is most likely to occur between the ages of forty-five and fifty, with many changes, like irregular periods and an increasing dry quality, being apparent from about thirty-five onward (but likely more noticeable closer to forty-five). While perimenopause may last anywhere from three to ten years, the average is four.

Imagine a gentle and gradual easing of ambition or intensity, with interests perhaps shifting from career, motherhood, or accomplishment to contemplation, relaxation, and satisfaction of heart's desires that haven't yet had their time in the limelight—the vanaprastha stage of life. In conjunction with physical therapies, welcoming these subtle shifts will help provide for a smooth transition, while stress can, as we saw in chapter 1, make for a rocky road. Applying Ayurveda's view of the elements can teach us to temper changes. Introducing rhythm, earth and water elements through medicinal foods and herbs, and other practices can alleviate hot flashes, sleep problems, a metabolic slump, or feeling anxious or depressed during perimenopause.

# Woman's Story:
## Walking the Path of Perimenopause

My colleague Erin has been studying Ayurveda as long as I have; she is observant and aware. As she has been noticing signs of perimenopause and deep shifts in her approach to life, I invited her to share her experiences.

At age forty-five, I have clearly passed the threshold into perimenopause. I am aware of subtle changes in my menstrual cycle—it's longer, drier, and unpredictable. Emotions seem to flame hotter these days, and there were months I thought I would need one set of bras for my normal breasts and a new set of bras for my new period breasts. Coexisting with physiological changes is deep faith and trust—in everything. Trust feels like life is happening *for* me, not *to* me. Faith feels like I can let go into trust.

When I feel out of balance, abhyanga and shatavari are going a long way these days. This time of perimenopause is not just marked by the physiological changes. The most interesting and meaningful aspect of this phase of life is the existential questions and conversations I am having with myself and my friends. We are no longer asking, "What do I want to do?" but asking instead "How do I want to live?" We are exploring in community how we define work, what we want to manifest, and what we are grateful for. We are defining this newfound wisdom.

I hope to be a person who helps the next generation through this initiation, normalizing and celebrating it all. I am so grateful to the wisdom of Ayurveda that walks with me through all the stages of my life.

## HOW TO SUPPORT HEALTHY TRANSITIONS

Imagine a seaside cottage weathering a winter. If the siding or the roof is drying out and losing *snigdha* (unctuousness), it is more likely to degrade and expose weak spots to the elements. The changes bodies undergo at perimenopause, though gradual, are like a home weathering a season of wind. Ayurveda teaches us how to shore up our roof and siding, and prepare for the storm. Before the season is upon us, preferably. Symptoms become more noticeable and hormone changes more drastic, the closer one gets to menopause. Some may not experience many symptoms at all. Those with more earth and water elements in the constitution may "weather the storm" better than those with lighter constitutions of space, air, and fire.

Women of pitta constitutions may notice more signs of fire such as hot flashes and irritability, whereas vata types may feel more unstable and dry, and may fluctuate between hot and cold. Kapha types may enjoy a steadier transition but see more weight gain or fatigue with metabolic changes.

To reduce the symptoms of perimenopause, consider practices that align you with lunar rhythms, as detailed in chapter 9. If you are experiencing irregularities in body heat, mood, menstrual cycle, or sleep, establishing a stable flow of energy over a monthly cycle yokes the irregularity to nature's flow. Bodies love this; they seek stability. With *irregularity* being the hallmark of perimenopause, simple and patient *routines* around sleep, meals, play, work, and rest are the medicine. A little routine goes a long way.

## MANAGING COMMON SYMPTOMS OF PERIMENOPAUSE

The decline in sex hormones is gradual in perimenopause, so noticing and addressing any of these signs sooner rather than later can make this stage easier and support a healthy menopause later. In addition, there are targeted ways of working with vaginal dryness, hot flashes, sleep, metabolism, and mental fluctuations that may show up during this transition.

### VAGINAL DRYNESS

As brmhana goes down, vata increases with its dry, mobile, rough qualities. Some women may not notice this change until menopause. Being furthest down the line of dhatu nourishment, artava may experience dryness first, showing up as vaginal dryness. You may also notice dry skin, dry stool, anxiety, or difficulty focusing.

To alleviate dryness, shatavari, an unctuous herb, is favored for targeting artava dhatu. Take 1/2 teaspoon daily with a little hot water or milk. You should notice a change within a month if it's the right therapy for you. Aloe, another option, is best for pitta types. Drink 1/2 cup Aloe-Pom-Cran Tonic (page 254) daily between meals.

Mitigating dryness anywhere in the body is helpful. Increase avocado, sesame seeds, ghee, and olive oil in your diet if you digest them well. Practice oil massage, head massage, or oiling of the ears and feet as soon as you notice a dry quality. To apply moisture directly to your vagina, try a nightly application of coconut oil around the opening and on the vulva.

## HOT FLASHES

Ayurveda describes hot flashes as heat from the busy years of heightened activity—both mental and physical—compounded by the heat of stress hormones, moving in errant ways due to aggravated vata and resulting in flashes of upward-moving heat. For some, reducing spicy foods and ferments and heating substances like red wine, especially at night, can curb this heat. Adding in breathwork, like Nadi Shodhana (page 321), and weekly oil massage (page 323) settles the vata that carries the heat up. Together, these two actions often reduce hot flashes. If not, you may need to call on herbal remedies with the help of a practitioner. Find a few beginning herbal remedies in the box.

## Recipes for Reducing Hot Flashes

Reducing pitta almost always has a mental component. Nervines, relaxants that support the nervous system, are especially useful for calming the mind. Combined with pitta-reducing cool and astringent qualities, certain nervine herbs such as brahmi, sage, and rose are ideal for reducing hot flashes.

Cool-the-Flash Tea and Spritz with Rose and Sage (page 226)

Golden Mind Milk (page 248)

**Note:** It's okay—and natural—to be hot and sweaty. Sweat is a passage for release, and a smart body may just be doing its job during a hot flash. If you experience intermittent hot flashes during perimenopause and they do not interfere with your daily life, you can manage the symptoms for comfort, but it is likely they are temporary. In the meantime, pack an extra shirt, avoid wearing synthetic fibers (which stink when they get sweaty), and keep a sense of humor about that pitta off-gassing.

## DIFFICULTY SLEEPING

Sleep problems (at any stage) can be caused by vata and/or pitta disruptions. During perimenopause, vata may be increased due to a general increase of space and air elements in the body. This may cause difficulty falling asleep, waking up intermittently, or waking in the early morning hours. Pitta can disrupt sleep by waking you up in the middle of the night, between midnight and 2 A.M., often accompanied by heat and sometimes itching sensations. To ease these symptoms, review the sleep routines in chapter 6, and never underestimate the power of an evening oil massage to help you sleep. Pitta-type sleep problems are often associated with food choices or metabolic changes, so the recommendations in the following section and the "Hot Flashes" section are helpful.

## MANAGING METABOLIC CHANGES

For those with high pitta or stress hormones, wining and dining may not have the same appeal when you can't sleep (or wake up sweating) after. During this time of change, substances that are exceedingly light and sharp—qualities of pitta dosha—may increase the discomfort of hot flashes, especially when consumed at night. During the pitta time of night, 10 P.M. to 2 A.M., the body removes wastes from the bloodstream and digestive tract, and these wastes include excess stress hormones. Having food in your stomach at this time will compromise this metabolic process. Putting additional hot substances into the bloodstream close to this time will also complicate things.

Consuming pitta-aggravating food and drink close to 10 P.M. isn't a great habit at any age, but you are likely to notice how your body tolerates it less and less in your forties and fifties. It is natural and results from changes in the brmhana/langhana balance.

Consuming alcohol is especially problematic in perimenopause. Its qualities are very lightening, and at a time when the body is going through an exponential increase in light qualities, it contributes to imbalance that can, over time, affect the organs.

Alcohol has a distinctive ability to penetrate the bloodstream quickly and is incredibly heating and sharp in its qualities (have a sip of spirits on an empty stomach to experience this). A small amount of alcohol consumed earlier in the day may be "burned off" by physical activity, so there is less for the agni to do overnight. Drinking at the end of the day will definitely affect sleep and digestion. The interaction of alcohol and stress hormones can't be ignored. Ironically, alcohol is often used for stress relief, when over time it blocks the liver's ability to remove stress hormones from the blood!

Old habits need to be replaced with new rituals for winding down and celebrating. An oil massage, a walk outside, a craft or creative hobby, and may I suggest a champagne flute of Pomegranate Lime Mocktail (page 255) at happy hour?

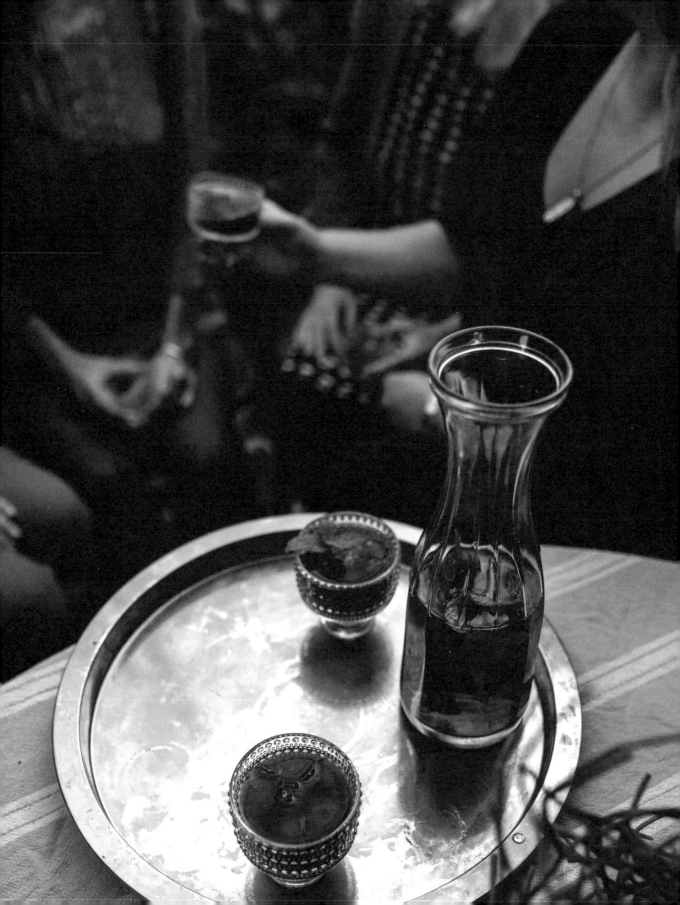

# The Role of Ojas in Perimenopause

The body's top factor for weathering changes is ojas. Ayurveda's ongoing prescription for preserving and building ojas is through optimizing digestion, getting enough rest, and avoiding overdoing it.

Ojas is also enhanced by subtle factors, such as sharing nourishing moments with nature and other beings and encouraging energy to circulate to the deep tissues. Everything we do to set ourselves up for smooth changes is about building inner strength and tissue integrity. For more on ojas, review chapter 3.

## THE MIND FACTOR

The enemy of ojas, our inner strength, is stress. Many women allow stress to eclipse self-care during the active stage of life. The effects of this compromise are not easily undone when one approaches the mid- to late forties. Perimenopause symptoms in mind and body will be most challenging when a woman has been under a lot of stress for a long time. The body in this case has learned to prioritize stress hormones, and as sex hormones naturally reduce in this stage of life, stress hormones do not have the same buffer of their cooler counterpart, estrogen. Grounding qualities in the physical body, which support the body-mind and ojas, wane as we age. Factors of stress, emotions, or activity levels that you maintained easily prior to perimenopause may begin to feel overwhelming. Your life's stress factors may be the same, but your nervous system's ability to manage them is changing.

This process may cause feelings of irritability, anxiety, sadness, and other mental fluctuations. According to Ayurveda, the mind, like rasa, permeates the entire body and colors our experience. The body's ability to cope with stress underlies many of the mental fluctuations women experience in perimenopause. At this point, we have the opportunity to see the interconnection between hormones, mind, rasa, and stress instead of compartmentalizing the mind. The great news is that you can see overall improvements in body and mind with general practices. For example, mental fluctuations may be soothed by an oil massage, which calms fluctuations in the nerves, or eating ghee, which also has an affinity for *majja dhatu* (the nerves).

The most important factor for coping with fluctuations in perimenopause, however, is to embrace doing less. Doing less reduces mental pressure, increases mental space, and opens the flow of the channel of the mind. Give yourself permission to ease up.

## IRREGULAR PERIODS

As hormones fluctuate, intervals between cycles can become longer or shorter in perimenopause. Periods can become inconsistent in the amount of blood: you may have spotting before or between periods, or experience heavy or longer-than-normal periods. The best medicine for irregularity is routine. If you are traveling a lot or finding yourself too busy to sit for a meal or do an oil massage and your periods are irregular, it is even more important to establish grounding routines. Consistent mealtimes, a consistent bedtime, or a new moon rest period will all provide stability for your body.

When daily routines do not remedy irregular cycles, working with herbs can help. Consult a practitioner who can suggest a mixture of herbs that will provide the qualities you need to return to balance. During perimenopause, some irregularity in the menstrual cycle is normal. If you consistently have spotting between periods, bleed for more than seven days, or experience a new onset of pelvic pain, see your health care provider.

## Spotlight on Chasteberry for a Smooth Perimenopause

Also known as vitex and native to India and China, chasteberry is a women's health panacea of sorts. This plant is used widely in teas, tablets, and tinctures for regulating women's hormones and shape-shifts to provide whatever action is needed. The plant seems to promote progesterone levels and ovulation and regulates irregular or absent periods. In tincture form, it is very strong and good for stubborn cases. Expect it to take as long as three months of consistent use to see changes.

A perspective check: Perimenopause is an opportunity to shift gradually into the vanaprastha stage of life. Allow ample space to accept, digest, and absorb changes that can affect your body and mind, as well as your sense of purpose. There's no need to crash headlong into battle with one of life's biggest rites of passage. Instead, take this time to fortify a strong vessel that can weather deep changes well.

# 17

# Menopause

The cause of menopause is aging. A body's release of fertility is not a disease, it is *parinama* (transformation). Menopause is the time when you get to collect the dividends on all your self-care investments from the previous decade. If you are reading this book before the age of transition to menopause, you can begin to look at the ways you can take some stress off your system, provide ideal nourishment, and optimize digestion. Lifestyle shifts take time and often require tectonic movements in how we "do" life and what motivates us. The more time you have to integrate Ayurveda into your lifestyle, the better set up you are for easy transitions.

Menopause is an opportunity to experience an embodiment quite different than in earlier stages of life. Due to hormonal changes, the elemental makeup of the body changes. With more of the clear, light qualities of air and space, we see a growing similarity between the qualities of the body and the qualities of cosmic space, providing an embodied substratum for spiritual evolution.

Menopause can be a time for gradually disengaging from worldly pursuits such as amassing wealth and accolades and managing the responsibilities of family, community, and professional life. As life expectancy grows, this stage can be quite long, even half of the total life span, so here we spend ample time on topics of life after fertility.

Your life may not always follow the flow described. Maybe menopause is not a time of renunciation. For example, I am often asked by grandmothers who are raising their grandchildren how to approach a slowdown and a release of responsibility when activity and responsibility are still a big part of their lives.

We can learn to differentiate between being called on in times of need by friends and family and seeking out new responsibility due to an attachment to busyness. In this time of life, health is about finding an appropriate balance of movement toward some amount of rest and away from so much activity. This is a natural law of aging. We live in a culture saturated with images of women in their seventies jogging. For some women, that may be a realistic goal. In the Vedic view of aging, where spiritual contemplation is the pinnacle, slowing the body and mind for health and balance is a fresh perspective (and one that will not be marketed to you!). For those who do not have the choice of slowing down, bolstering the system in other ways and being honest about what you can keep up with while creating healthy boundaries is the work of menopause.

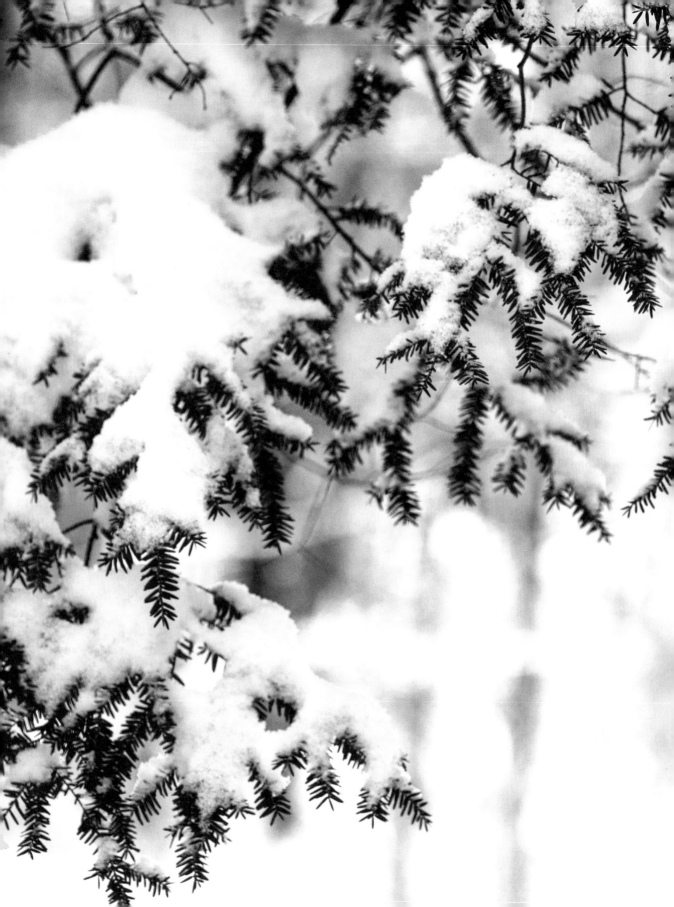

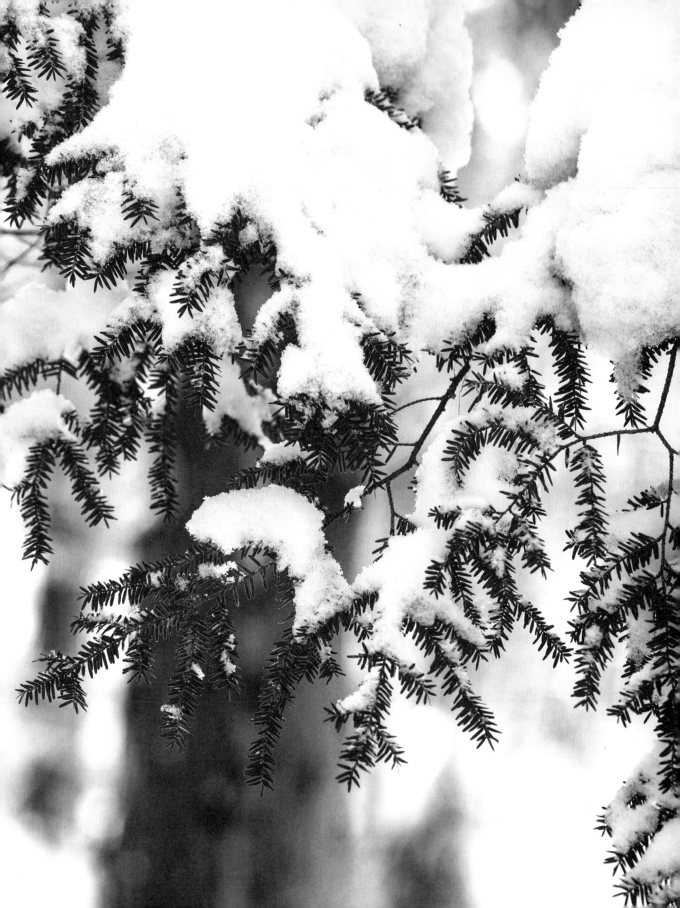

## WHAT HAPPENS DURING MENOPAUSE?

Menopause is defined as the time of life postmenstruation. When a person has not menstruated for one year, they are considered to be in menopause. Physiologically, estrogen drops at a faster rate than during perimenopause, and the ovaries will eventually cease to produce it, now that the body needn't maintain the potential to nourish another life. Some estrogen will then be produced in other tissues, namely adipose, and provide ample brmhana qualities when stress hormone levels are balanced.

Symptoms are most likely to appear in the first five years after your periods stop. This window is an important time to set up strong agni and ideal nourishment to protect your deep tissues, while working with stabilizing routines as the bedrock for dramatic change.

This vata time of life is characterized by increasing langhana qualities, such as rough and dry anywhere in the body (skin, hair, vagina, colon) and more space element in the mind, which may affect focus and memory. Many of the signs and symptoms of menopause, and how we address them, are the same as in perimenopause but less gradual, so please also reference the previous chapter for additional details. Always keep in mind that reducing stress hormones mitigates menopausal symptoms better than any other intervention.

Implementing lifestyle and diet changes *before* menopause will get the best results. If you are already in your late forties, know that common symptoms of menopause, such as sleep difficulties and hot flashes, respond best to therapeutics when you address them at the first signs. Take note if, for example, you wake up sweating in the night, possibly after eating a big dinner, or keep popping awake with anxiety at 4 A.M. Integrating small, beneficial changes in diet and lifestyle can smooth the transitions before early signs are affecting your day-to-day. Shifting to an earlier dinner or establishing a daily breathwork practice, for example, can improve digestion, detox, and sleep. When diet and lifestyle aren't managing your symptoms, herbal remedies can provide concentrated qualities needed for balance and nourish or clear the artava.

Some women—especially those with naturally resilient constitutions, balanced bodies, and/ or balanced stress levels—will not experience much discomfort at all in menopause. Integrating cyclic activity and rest, as described in our lunar rhythms in chapter 9, is one effective pathway to setting up and maintaining this kind of balance. Change aggravates vata, our light and airy companion. Couple that law of nature with menopause's natural reduction in moist, grounded qualities from sex hormones, and vata accumulation is doubled. As you will see, healthy menopause practices are vata-pacifying ones.

## MOON CYCLES FOR THOSE WHO NO LONGER MENSTRUATE

The question of following lunar rhythms in menopause is an interesting one. Women often ask me if their bodies still have a monthly cycle after menstrual bleeding and ovulation stop. The answer is, of course! The external and social energy of the waxing moon and the quieting, inward movement of the waning moon remain influences. With an increased affinity for the subtle during this stage of life, the influence of the moon may even feel stronger. This is a bonus of menopause.

## HOW TO SUPPORT HEALTHY MENOPAUSE

The body shows its intelligence when it shifts its resources away from fertility and childbearing. As the body shifts, the hormones are redirected into new expressions. With less estrogen on hand, maintaining bone health, supple skin, and regular moods may require some targeted self-care. Remember that the body can steal from the reserves of sex hormones to generate stress hormones, so any diet and self-care practices need to act in tandem with stress reduction.

### OIL MASSAGE

Oil opposes aging and promotes moisture via the largest organ in the body. Oil massage calms the winds of vata and lends plumpness to the skin, which directly supports rasa. Regular oil massage, at least weekly, mitigates the dry quality. And oil benefits more than just skin. The qualities of oil maintain the status quo in the tissues by holding things together, opposing breakdown, and softening tissue, which the aging process hardens. Favor warm, heavier oils in menopause—sesame is the favorite. Using an herbal "vata oil" integrates vata-pacifying herbs into your massage practice (find a recipe in appendix A and online suppliers in appendix C).

## MAINTAINING HEALTHY BODY WEIGHT

A healthy amount of body fat buffers the aggravation of vata caused by decreasing estrogen. Ayurveda describes "plumpness" as beauty and the fullness of rasa dhatu as the most desirable state at any age. Dry and light qualities entering the rasa contribute to the drying out of the body in general, including skin, vaginal tissues, and mucous membranes. Over time, deeper tissues like bones, marrow, and nerves will also dry out, leading to less mental resilience and conditions that can lead to osteoporosis. Being too thin at any stage of life will have this effect, but during the change to menopause, moisture is essential for protecting the body. The body produces estrogen and stores moisture in body fat. Heading into menopause with a healthy body fat buffer is ideal.

## SUGAR AND METABOLIC FIRES

On the other side of feeling happily plump is unhealthy weight gain, which can congest rasa and cause ama. For most women, the metabolism slows down at menopause. As earth and water elements decrease and air and space increase, the fire element can slow down or become erratic, affecting digestion and metabolism. As in all stages of life, eating sit-down meals and avoiding eating between meals is an excellent practice for keeping agni balanced.

One of the prime instigators of weight gain during menopause is the body's slow metabolizing of simple sugars. Even white rice can become sticky and heavy in the body at this stage of irregular agni. Before trying anything else for managing unhealthy weight gain, first reduce sugary foods, especially white sugars like candy and conventional pastries. Relying on "burning it off" with exercise is not the ideal approach, an important point for those who need to protect their joints.

I have noticed that the agni slowdown comes on strong as menopausal changes begin and may balance out in a year or two. There's no need to think, *I have to give up sweets for the rest of my life*. Rather, imagine this transition as a pocket of time where certain shifts will be most beneficial. Stabilizing the agni during change is supported by grounding routines like consistent mealtimes. You may find your agni fortifies itself. To encourage it, when having a treat, have some ginger tea alongside to boost the metabolic fires.

## BEST FOODS FOR MENOPAUSE

The best foods to eat during menopause are warmly spiced, oily, moist, dense, and mineral-rich. You will find many recipes in part four that use ingredients from the following list. While vata is on the rise, eating more cooked foods and less raw food is a good rule of thumb. Even cook your fruits! Employ digestive spices, to boost absorption, in your food and your water. Draw from recipes that rejuvenate and sustain you. Add another spoonful of ghee to your meal if you find you are often hungry before the next one. Try Sesame Crunch Chutney (page 298) in place of crunching on chips and crackers, which contribute to the dry quality.

- Seeds, such as pumpkin, flax, sesame, and hemp
- Sesame seeds, butter, and oil
- Whole grains and legumes

- Almonds (especially in homemade almond milk)
- Ghee, avocados, and olive oil
- Seaweed
- Bone broth (page 277) or Essential Mineral Vegetable Broth (page 272)
- Urad dal
- Cooked fruits
- Nourishing Herbal Infusion (page 218)
- Demulcents that bring moisture, such as licorice, slippery elm, marshmallow, flax, and chia
- Herbs such as ashwagandha, brahmi, shatavari, and vidari (wild yam)

## What Is Wild Yam?

Wild yam is a Western sister to Ayurveda's herb vidari; both are sweet, unctuous, a little heavy, and cool. This combination is, like the even juicier herb shatavari, similar in qualities to estrogen. Using wild yam or vidari during the menopause transition counters excess heat and supports shukra, artava, and longevity.

## MAINTAINING BONE HEALTH DURING MENOPAUSE

During this stage, bones need more earth and water elements to balance the porosity of the air element. Metabolizing good fats is paramount! Bones are essentially built of minerals, so mineral-dense foods become equally important. We know that rasa dhatu, the first tissue layer, carries the nutrition that will feed each successive tissue in turn. The deep tissues—bone, nerve, marrow, and generative—are the furthest from the moist, lubricative qualities of rasa and the first to show signs of excess dry, rough qualities. While it's easy to say, "Eat good fats and get your minerals," what about when they aren't reaching those deeper tissues?

Everything we learned in chapters 7 and 8 about digestion and metabolism remain potent ways to get nutrition to those bones. Favor high-quality cooking oils, especially ghee and sesame oil, and reduce sticky, hard-to-digest fats like cheese, ice cream, and fried foods. As a targeted therapy for bone health in menopause, let's look at some medicinal foods and how to use them.

## MEDICATED GHEES

Bone is the only deep tissue that is composed of earth and air. Bones, despite their structural function, are actually a seat of vata. They are naturally porous and hollow, yet filled with marrow, a cool, unctuous liquid that supports them. When Ayurveda addresses the bone tissue itself, minerals and medicated ghees are the way to go.

Ghee is the best fatty substance to deliver medicines to the deep tissues due to its penetrating quality. For bone health, ghee is medicated with bitter herbs, as they have an affinity for the light aspect of bones and are anti-inflammatory, which may slow down the degenerative process. One classic formula of bitter ghee is *brahmi ghrita*, which can be ordered from one of the suppliers in appendix C. You can find a recipe to make your own brahmi ghee in *The Everyday Ayurveda Guide to Self-Care*.

You can imagine that bitter ghee may not taste great on toast. There are several options for using this herbal ghee that not only increase palatability but optimize absorption as well. The practice of using herbal ghee can be done daily for those who digest it well, continuing for a few months in the cold, dry time of year, or more often for those who experience dryness. More is not better, however! For doses larger than 1 tablespoon, consult a practitioner for proper guidelines.

Take brahmi ghee first thing in the morning on an empty stomach. You can mix this with a bit of hot water and take between 1 teaspoon and 1 tablespoon, depending on the strength of your digestion. Wait until you are hungry and the ghee has passed through your stomach to eat anything else for optimal absorption. Sip hot water during this time. If you are burping up the ghee when you have a sip of water, try a smaller amount until your stomach begins to process it easily, then increase slowly to reach at least 1 teaspoon. Be sure to wait to eat until you can sip water without a ghee burp. It may take a few weeks, but your agni will get the hang of it.

If you do not digest fats well, consider doing a Home Cleanse Program (page 84) before beginning an herbal ghee protocol. This process optimizes absorption.

If taking it straight is not palatable, use the Longevity Bone Tonic recipe on page 253, preferably two hours or more after dinner. This technique can be used in the morning as well, on an empty stomach if that digests better.


## BONE BROTH

The most direct way to support any tissue, blood, fat, or bone is to seek out similar qualities in food form. This makes bone broth the closest in qualities to bone and the best way to nourish them, especially for those with weak digestion. Bone broth can make a big difference in how you feel through the first years of menopause.

Bone broth naturally contains collagen, a building block of bone tissue. From the Ayurveda perspective, it is simply bone-for-bone. Vegetarian sources of bone builders, such as ghee and sesame seeds, require a strong agni to digest. In cases where one is still encouraging strong digestion, or for those with digestive health concerns of any kind, bone broth mainlines nourishment, and its oily quality actually heals digestive linings. (Vegetarians can drink my Essential Mineral Vegetable Broth recipe on page 272.)

Ayurveda tells us that animal products are the most beneficial when they are local and fresh. Procuring bones from your own cooking with local, grass-fed meats or from a local butcher and simmering bone broth yourself is the best way. You can find a recipe for this on page 277. Avoid buying packaged or powdered forms of bone broth and collagen.

## DEMULCENTS

Substances that are slimy have a unique ability to protect and heal tissues from dry, rough qualities. During menopause, when these qualities can come on fast, using demulcents is very balancing. Here are some ways to work them into your diet.

- Add ground flaxseeds to cereals.
- Soak 2 tablespoons of chia seeds in 10 ounces of natural fruit or vegetable juice for one hour, then drink through a straw.
- Make chia pudding by soaking 2 tablespoons of chia seeds in 1 cup of plant milk overnight; add sweetener and spices for a treat.
- Drink teas or herbal infusions that contain licorice, marshmallow, and slippery elm daily.
- Drink aloe juice.
- Add kombu to your legumes.

## Demulcent Recipes

You won't *know* there are slimy foods in these dishes, but they will serve you well!

Raspberry-Ginger Secret Smoothie (page 260)

Strawberry Rose Smash (page 259)

Homemade Flax Milk (page 242)

Spicy Black Gram Soup (page 281)

Aloe-Pom-Cran Tonic (page 254)

Warm Arame and Kale Salad (page 292)

## SPIRITUALITY AND MENOPAUSE

Today, many of the women I see in the menopause stage of life are seekers. Maybe we are magnets for each other, or it's a cultural shift. It is as though a veil is lifted, and an innate desire for spirituality bubbles up when responsibility to family, work, and community subsides. In mainstream culture, spiritual seekers don't receive a lot of positive reinforcement. It seems we've been taught to feel concerned with being relevant and self-sufficient as we age, as opposed to the Vedic model, which empowers connection to the spirit. Both of these are important, but I see a blossoming spirituality in menopausal women. To the part of you that wants to explore, to study the nature of self and cosmos, to *expand*, I say congratulations! This is a natural phenomenon.

Space is expansive, and it increases in our physiology in the vata time of life (and in home life if you are an empty-nester). It's natural to gravitate toward spaciousness and expansiveness during menopause. The grounded nature of the body itself is changing, the direction of energy is moving up, the stars are aligned for accessing higher states of consciousness. How do we celebrate this? Many of us are missing the cultural structure for celebrating these deeper states. Modern culture promotes secular values.

From the view of the ancients, every body contains an experiential pathway toward spirituality: the breath. If you are in a later stage of life and find you are seeking but not sure what or where, breathwork may yoke you to a sense of that which you seek. Spending time with prana by attuning to your breath awakens the subtle aspects of your body. Give breath practice a season, and it will bear fruit. Nadi Shodhana (page 321) is an ideal practice for moving energy.

As space and air elements increase in the body, you may encounter something that feels like anxiety, changes in the content or pace of your mind, mood swings, even headaches. A daily practice of Nadi Shodhana, even for a few minutes, can centralize the energy.

# A Woman's Story:
# Menopause Notes from an OB-GYN

Elizabeth is a full-time gynecologist of thirty years. I'm pleased to include her professional observations as well as her own story of walking the path in vanaprastha.

> I am sixty-four years old. I discovered Ayurveda around the time of menopause, and to be honest, I initially thought of it as a way to remain the nubile maiden. The messages we receive as women, from very early in our lives, are often messages of valuing an ideal *out there* that someone else defines rather than an ideal *inside* defined by self and universe. By a Western medical provider, menopause is often treated as a time when women become irrelevant and treatments offered are to keep this transition from being difficult for those around us. Often, these treatments come with many side effects and are temporary fixes.
>
> My goal now is not to be more or less of anything, but only to be. My goal is not to live forever, looking like I am thirty. My goal is to embrace the transitions of life in a way that allows me to age and die well, while being a part of this world. In this vanaprastha time of life, I am still professionally productive, working forty-plus hours a week, but my focus now is sharing the wisdom I have learned over these decades. I spend more time on spiritual pursuits and the study of Ayurveda. This is part of my process of letting go, getting ready to move on. In my personal life I feel both a pulling in and an expansion of who I am.

Menopause is not an imbalance; it is an opportunity. There is nothing more natural than this change in your body, and with that, the changes that may come in how you relate to life, in what you want out of it, and where you are going next. The shift from fertility to cosmic connectivity is magical and full of grace. When we shift our gaze to aging well and maintaining vigor, may it be with an aim toward self-evolution.

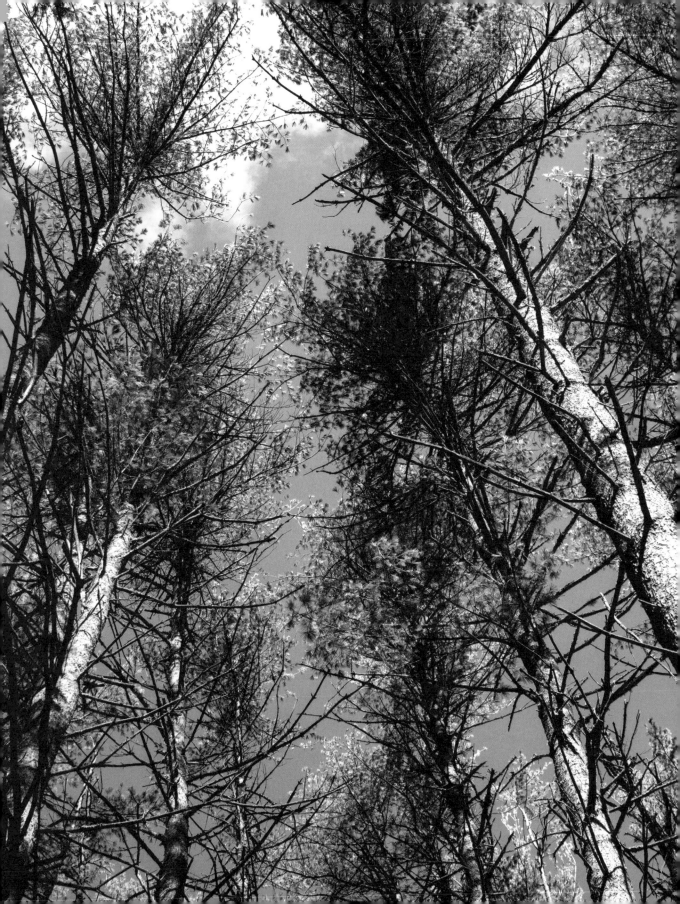

# 18

# Longevity and Healthy Aging

In my early thirties I spent a few weeks vacationing at a country inn that, to my surprise, was booked up by elderly guests. I sat at group dinner tables with couples in their seventies and eighties and listened to their stories. What struck me more than their stories, however, was how they interacted with life. In general, I noticed that everyone was easygoing. They weren't sweating the small stuff, as though they had seen so much in life, it would take a lot to rock the boat. At the time, I was stressed out. Being around these folks was a balm for my anxiety. I was spending so much time worrying about things that hadn't happened yet, while these people had seen it all, been through it, and were still chugging along and enjoying the simple things.

In my late forties, I now know I can practice being present for the now, while doing self-care to preserve the longevity of this body. I pace myself, then go full-steam ahead at intervals. There is a way to hold the present moment within the big-picture context that enriches the present. Ayurveda is a longevity science, after all, and I might as well walk the talk.

In Vedic philosophy, the longer one lives in good health, the more time one has for spiritual evolution. The kind of self-purification that leads to evolution is considered most appropriate in the later stages of life, when it is assumed there are fewer daily responsibilities. Ayurveda offers the viewpoint of turning our attention and energy to contemplation and self-purification in our old age.

Old age is the time of life when we do our most important work. This view is antithetical to the cultural messaging that we become useless and irrelevant once our "productivity" decreases. Leaving the planet and its peoples better than we found them, making sukha (good space), is the mission of old age, as described by the ancients. (Heading into retirement to squander the resources of future generations is not the goal.) As responsibilities to parents, children, and career make way for simpler days, mentorship and volunteer work are a meaningful way to share a lifetime's wisdom and skills.

After age fifty, Ayurveda considers the mind to be more important to our health than ever. We carry with us the conditioning of all we have learned in a half-century. Purification of the mind, whether through practicing rejuvenating mental attitudes, breathwork, meditation, or prayer, becomes the most important aspect of the sannyasa stage of life, roughly seventy-five until death.

While it seems that true health results more from a sound vantage point and purpose than anything else, physical concerns as the body degenerates are very real. Concerns around aging generally include osteoporosis, maintaining joint and connective tissue mobility, libido, and mental acuity. For disease manifestations in later stages of life, such as high blood pressure, diabetes, and the like, Ayurveda can help, but it's best to work with a practitioner on an individualized plan. Physically, Ayurveda recommends a path of rejuvenation through juiciness born of fire, earth, and water elements. While all the rhythmic factors in this book, practiced over a lifetime, support healthy aging, let's discuss particular practices, foods, and herbs for targeted support.

## LONGEVITY THERAPIES FROM AYURVEDA

*Rasayana* is the eighth branch of Ayurveda medicine. It can be translated as "path of juiciness" or "anti-aging." Aging is inevitable, and there is truly no anti-aging. We can, however, counteract the ailments associated with aging, and longevity is indeed a science of aging well. In general, rasayana bolsters the health of the body, and vajikarana (the science of strengthening generative tissues) is a subset of rasayana. Rasayana therapies can be dietary, medicinal, or behavioral. Substances that rejuvenate provide building blocks for ojas and excellence of all the dhatus. Strong tissues are more resistant to disease and aging. In modern terms, rasayana therapies are considered immunity boosters, and most have antioxidant properties.

If aging is an oxidation process, a slow degeneration, then rasayana is generative, directly opposing dry, light, rough, mobile qualities. It fills and bolsters the bones, nerves, marrow, and nervous system, keeping the sense organs and mind keen, and rendering the body resistant to fractures and pathogens. This is done through herbs, foods, and lifestyle.

Beware the tendency to add things all the time, like food and herbs, when sometimes—especially these days—healing needs *space*, and rejuvenation and satisfaction often result from doing less, thinking less, and talking less.

# REJUVENATING FOODS AND HERBS

*Dravya rasayana* are rejuvenatives in the form of food and medicine. Opposing the effects of aging through heavy, moist substances is not a definite physiological "cure" but a delay. Rasayana puts time on our side. There are scores of medicinal formulas, many named after their primary herb, such as triphala rasayana or ashwagandha rasayana. Certain foods are also mentioned as rejuvenators, and these can be included in the diet regularly for those who digest them well. The following lists are not exhaustive but give examples of the rejuvenative foods and herbs we use in this book.

I think of rasayana as deep nourishment. To me, it is administering loving care to the deep tissues, and this takes many forms in different circumstances. Even rest is a rasayana, and being in the bhav, visualizing that which you wish to create, can make almost anything take on rasayana qualities. Reflecting on feeling deeply satisfied and getting to know this feeling is a part of rasayana medicine.

## Rasayana Foods

| | | |
|---|---|---|
| Almonds | Dates | Pistachios |
| Aloe | Ghee | Rice |
| Amla | Less refined sugars | Turmeric |
| Bananas | Licorice | Walnuts |
| Coconut | Milk | |

Chyawanprash Herbal Jam (page 256), made of amalaki, honey, sugar, ghee, and spices, is the most widely used formula. Many of the rasayana follow this type of preparation for an herbal jam and use ghee, sugar, and spice. The amount of rasayana is generally between 1 teaspoon and 1 tablespoon daily, licked off a spoon, and can be used continually in old age.

The foods listed here can seem confusing, as milk and sugar are often named among inflammatory foods that create problems in the body. Keep in mind that Ayurveda texts were conceived in times where malnourishment was common, as opposed to the present when many health problems arise due to overnourishment. Even at a healthy body weight, we have to consider the purity of our foods, especially dairy. In undernourished bodies, cow's milk will be the best source of rejuvenation, but almond and coconut milks have similar (if lesser) qualities and can be used for rasayana purposes. For any substance, you can find something similar, local, and best suited to your personal constitution.

Remember the essential balance of langhana and brmhana. Rasayana, if it tips the scales too far into building without a proper balance of cleansing qualities, may cause problems instead of heal them. Certain substances may be rasayana for you and not for your neighbor. For example, aloe is especially good for rejuvenating pitta, because it is cool and slows inflammatory processes. Haritaki is especially rejuvenating for vata because it acts on the large intestine and keeps the bowels moving. Tulsi is good for kapha because it works on the lungs and circulatory system and can fend off illnesses like bronchitis and the common cold.

Rasayana can also be integrated into the diet with milk-based tonics (see chapter 23). Sweet and creamy foods can be your medicine! Medicinal hot cacao is a great example of crafting an appealing formula that actually satisfies the system and is made of real cacao, almond milk, a little maple syrup, and ashwagandha (see Sexy Cacao, page 249). A shift from eating refined sweets to taking a spoonful of chyawanprash daily for your "sweet tooth" makes the sweet taste medicine instead of poison.

Using rasayana foods and formulas after a period of eating light foods, as described in chapter 8, will prepare the agni and ensure you get the most out of these supportive foods. When agni is strong, these foods are best digested in the form of liquids and jams, prepared with digestive spices. Examples include Golden Mind Milk (page 248), Longevity Bone Tonic (page 253), Date Shake (page 243), and Chyawanprash Herbal Jam (page 256).

## LIBIDO AND LONGEVITY

In terms of feeling sexy, which is a concern I hear from women of all ages, look to the aphrodisiac medicines that were discussed in chapter 13. In general, when looking to strengthen sexual function, fulfillment, desire, *and* fertility, the medicine is the same no matter the age or stage of life.

In addition, I find that following lunar rhythms helps women attune to times in a cycle when it may be more natural to feel sexy, or not, due to the direction of energy moving out versus in. It is normal to have ebbs and flows in sexual desire and normal to feel sexier on a full moon, when soma is high. Being ceremonious about calling this energy in when the moon is round by moonbathing or making Moon Milk (page 247) will funnel your prana to your libido. (Draw on the full moon practices from chapter 9 for inspiration.) Directing life energy toward any expression, whether libido, agni, or mental acuity, requires attention and cultivation.

# A Woman's Story: Jann

Jann is an elder Ayurveda student who has continued to inspire me with the honesty and humor of her journey. She is energetic and introspective, and I want to be like her when I grow up.

I was seventy-one years old at the time of writing about my postmenopause, and I hope it brings glimpses of what may occur as well as resonate with those who have been through all the stages. I am grateful Kate chose to bring these too often taboo topics into a book.

[As I transitioned through menopause,] slowly little ups and downs occurred. My hair started drying out and then later went from straight to curly! My neck was a turkey neck. A few times I would feel a flaming hot sensation from head to toe and the sweat poured out of me. I actually liked those hot flashes; they were a quick tingle, and I felt a surge of feel-good down-yonder sensations.

My gynecologist tried to persuade me to do hormone replacement treatment (HRT) and I vehemently disagreed. This was a rite of passage for me, and I was going to embrace it with love and grace. Then, the periods stopped. After a year or so of dry kinky curls, my hair came back to fine and soft. My dry neck softened. My libido surged and I purchased a sexy thong for nighttime wear. It will get discarded in the heat of passion.

Now the good and not-as-good news. Vaginal dryness came—although a number of years later. My skin is starting to dry again, but I am working on that with an Ayurvedic lifestyle. Well, it will greatly improve once I stop drinking the pinot grigio. This may be too much information, but surprisingly, something is still working, and I can have spontaneous, how-did-that-happen orgasms. That's good news for you younger ones. The other good news is that I have mellowed even more in many ways—anxiety-provoking stuff has eased as I let go.

—EXCERPT FROM JANICE DOLK'S "MY STORY OF A JOURNEY FROM MENARCHE TO POST-MENOPAUSAL,"[10] ORIGINALLY PUBLISHED ON *ELEPHANT JOURNAL*

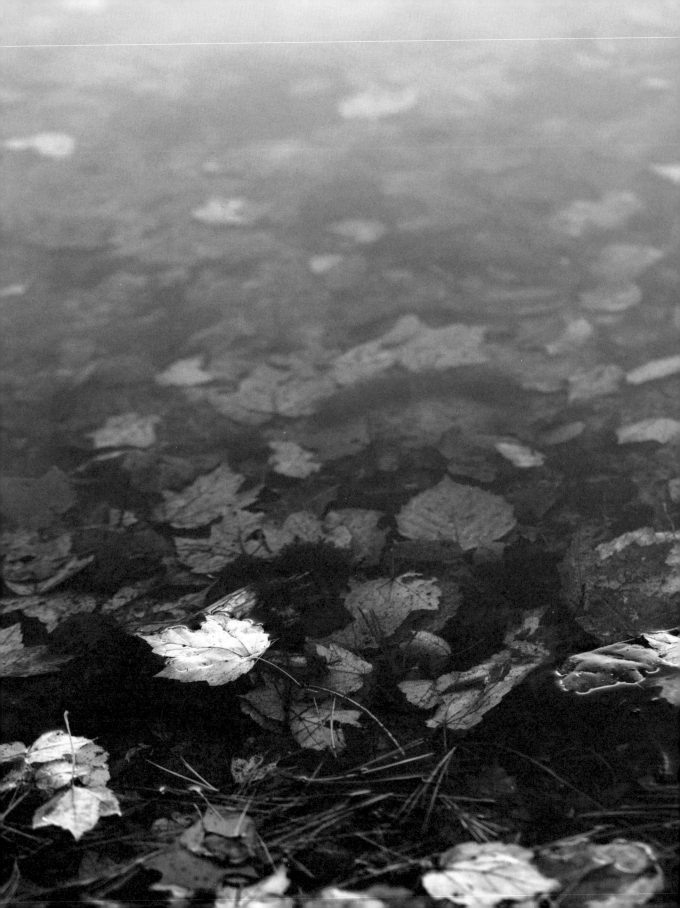

## CIRCULATION AND EXERCISE

In the vata time of life, enhancing free-moving prana is important. The constricting, hard qualities of vata can cause blockages in the flow and hardening of tissues. Allowing any area to be cut off from the flow consistently makes that area vulnerable. Moderate, weight-bearing exercise just to the point of sweating, five days a week or more, is good to keep up. Breathwork moves prana and softens hardness perhaps better than any other therapy, and learning how to breathe freely while moving (and anytime) will carry you well through old age. In cases of injury affecting your exercise routine, breathwork circulates, and even if you are laid up, you can still practice. Sama Vritti Ujjayi (page 322) is a good place to start establishing a rhythmic and conscious breath.

Consider a daily routine that includes 20 minutes of something brisk, 20 minutes of weight-bearing with breath, and 20 minutes of breathwork in whichever order you prefer. Be open to the day and its ways as you tailor your movement routines. If you feel lethargic, do the brisk part first. If you feel anxious, do the breathwork first. When you don't have an hour, prioritize based on the qualities you are feeling that day. Physical therapies for softening hardness and constriction also include oil massage followed by steam, whether it's a steam room, moist sauna, or hot shower or bath; drinking warm water; and eating warm foods. If you aren't able to do movement, these therapies will keep circulation strong.

## REJUVENATING MENTAL ATTITUDES

Rasayana is not just food. The limb of rejuvenation therapy called *achara rasayana* (rejuvenating attitudes) is a particularly potent longevity technique. The mind is a force to be reckoned with at any age, but one has likely built skills of self-influence over time. If not, it's never too late to start. All the choices we make, the body's response to stressors, and how we approach our current stage of life and unavoidable death, are influenced by mental attitudes.

The attitudes to strive for are as follows:

- Truthfulness
- Anger management
- Moderation of sense pleasures (alcohol and sex are especially mentioned in the texts)
- Nonviolence in thought and action
- Avoidance of excessive worry
- Indulgence in creative activities
- Pleasant speech
- Spiritual practice
- Good bodily hygiene
- Stable thoughts and straightforward actions
- Charity
- Self-study

While it's easy to become set in your ways, mental plasticity supports juicy, soft qualities in the body and brain. Changing your mind softens the hard quality that comes with age, and a bright outlook and influence on others enhances life. Seeking to rejuvenate the mental attitude tempers the effects of aging. In truth, we should all strive for these behaviors at any age. Whether you aim for self-evolution or another set of values, the point is to stay on a path of thoughtfulness. A youthful mind and attitude comprise an anti-aging technology that improves with age.

As we age, we are likely to move less and rest more. While the physical demands of the body lessen, including rejuvenating behaviors in our days is a clear path to juiciness. The juice, in this case, is a growing spirituality.

A knowledge of the effects of time on human bodies remains at the heart of Ayurveda's longevity wisdom. As we weather changes throughout the seasons of life, each stage and its changes are an opportunity for surrender, release, and renewal. As we wax and wane through each day, month, season, and stage of life, an arc of life emerges. Illuminating the life stages on the cosmic road map of Ayurveda provides the "you are here" approach to the present moment. Aging is always happening, and longevity practice isn't just for old age.

As we accept natural change and learn to recognize signs of imbalance, we are free to move through our days and seasons empowered with the wisdom and tools to be proactive, to build, to cleanse, and to heal. The Ayurveda path leads us with the integration of self, environment, and quality.

Substances from nature are the substratum for qualities, and next up we step into the Ayurveda kitchen to work with healing preparations and bring intentions for good health into our food.

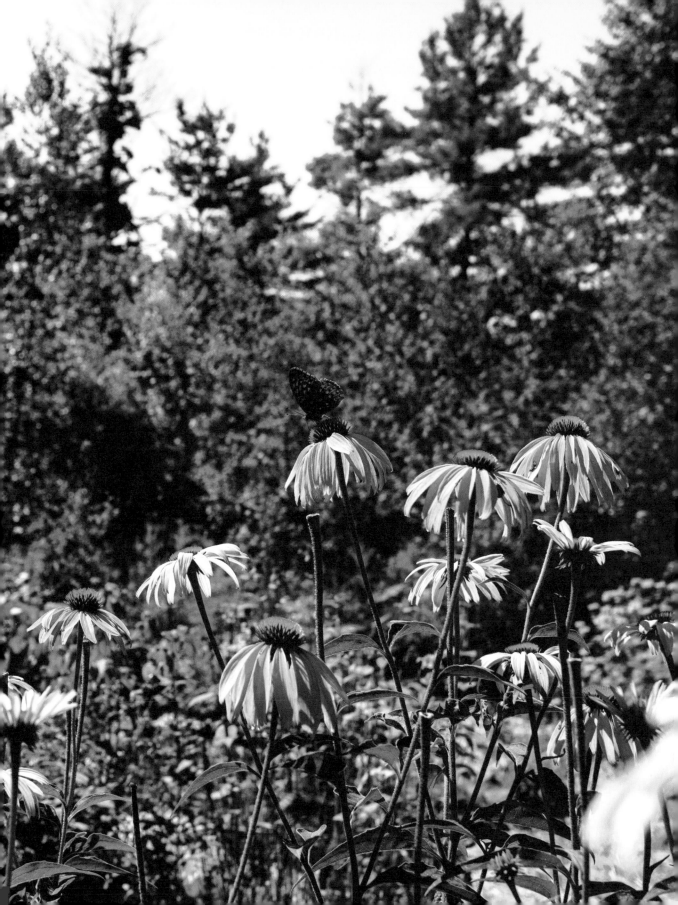

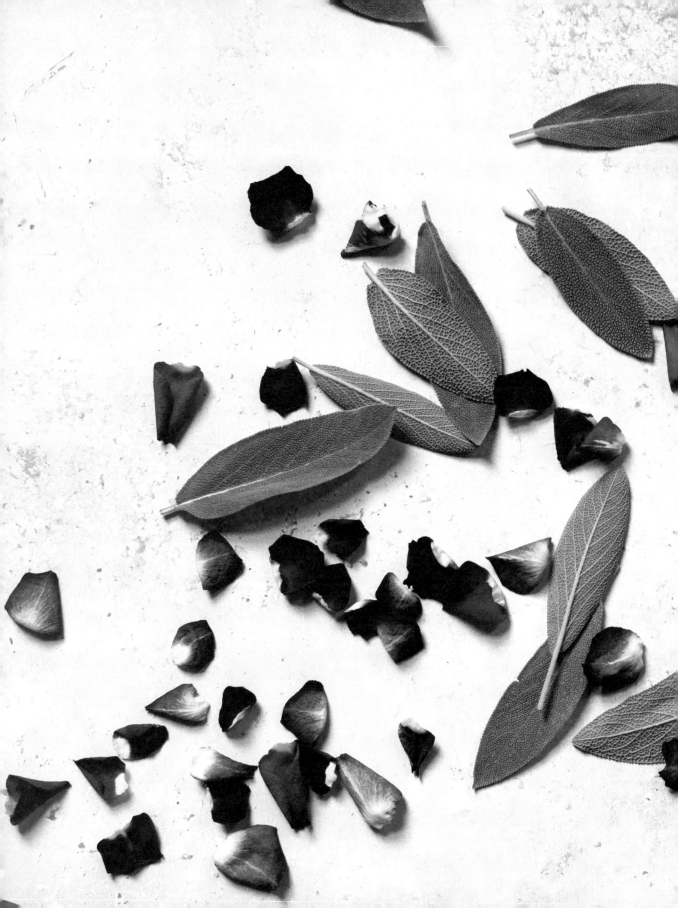

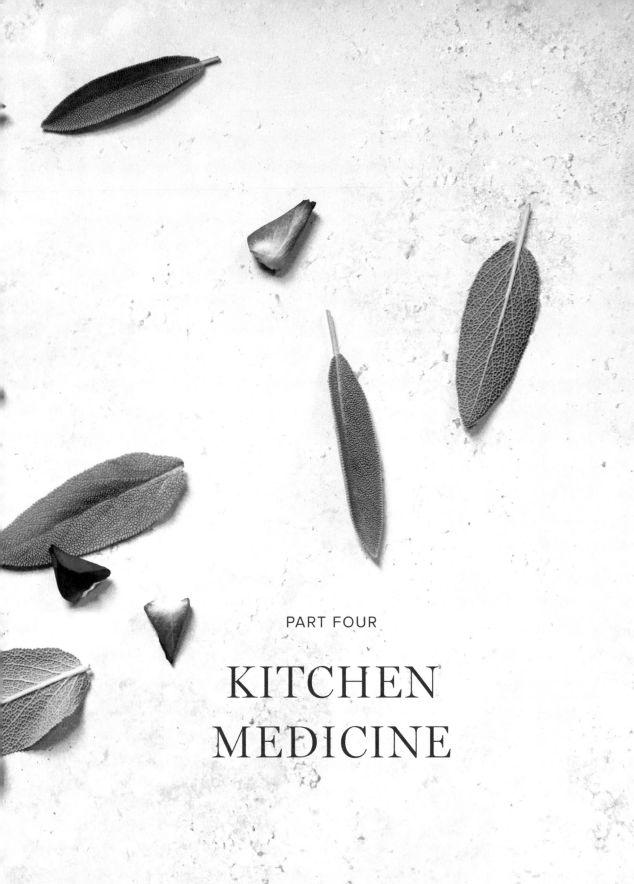

PART FOUR

# KITCHEN MEDICINE

Ayurveda is clear: get to know your food and herb allies. In this section, we discuss the in-depth therapeutic actions of herbs and spices and how to apply them in recipes. In Ayurveda's cooking, herbs and spices have concentrated qualities and actions that improve digestion and metabolism and target tissues and systems. In our case, we focus on the generative system.

Recipes are divided into several categories:

**Herbal infusions** are an easy, drinkable way to work with the healing power of herbs to both cleanse and nourish.

**Digestives** are often light and sharp to improve digestion and circulation.

**Tonics** are building in nature and target deep tissues.

**Medicinal meals** are dishes for daily fare—breakfasts, lunches, and dinners—rounded out by superfood condiments and a few treats.

I don't organize recipes by condition, such as "recipes for perimenopause," because most recipes serve many purposes. For example, a food that strengthens the generative system is composed of the cool, building qualities of earth and water elements. It is unctuous, oily, and stabilizing. Digestive spices are partnered with the builders to improve metabolism. This same preparation enhances fertility and libido, nourishes a pregnant or postpartum woman, counteracts aging, and pacifies vata. The primary overlapping principle in women's health in all stages of life is excellence of ahara rasa (see page 28). You will find this is true for all of these recipes.

Let's set up an Ayurveda kitchen to inspire and nourish you and those you care for. You will cultivate excellent rasa and all the life-giving attributes this brings to women and their communities.

# 19

# Therapeutic Spices and Herbs

Knowing how to use spices and herbs therapeutically gives you the power to cool blood, clear stagnation, enhance sexy juices, boost immunity, and build robust menstrual blood. Central to the science of Ayurveda is an understanding of the properties and effects, both beneficial and harmful, of what substances we take in. Herbs and spices have a higher potency than food and are effective healers. Ultimately, any substance is the result of its elemental constitution. The elements lend their qualities to the substance, and when that food, spice, or herb is digested, those elements affect the body. Something with a lot of air in it, like popcorn, will increase air element and decrease earth.

A substance's effects vary by circumstance and season. For example, a spicy pickle may fire up the appetite when it is slow but cause heavy, hot periods if taken in excess during the menstrual cycle.

The classical text *Charaka Samhita* describes a substance as a piece of cloth and the qualities and actions of that substance as the threads woven together to make the cloth. For example, rose—a mainstay of women's health—is sweet, cool, subtle, and slightly bitter. All of these qualities balance pitta, and rose gravitates toward rakta dhatu, a tissue dominated by pitta. A pitta pacifier in rakta dhatu curbs hot flashes, heavy bleeding, skin rashes, and headaches during the pitta time of the cycle. To target heavy periods, we may blend rose with other astringent and rakta-loving plants, such as in Hibiscus Rose Cordial (page 312).

## RASA: TASTE

Each of the six tastes is the result of a combination of two elements and the resulting qualities. What the taste buds perceive is the elemental constitution of the substance. A food or herb can contain more than one primary taste. Each of the tastes has certain actions on the body. Something astringent is dry and will reduce moisture in the body. Something salty is heating and will increase warmth in the body.

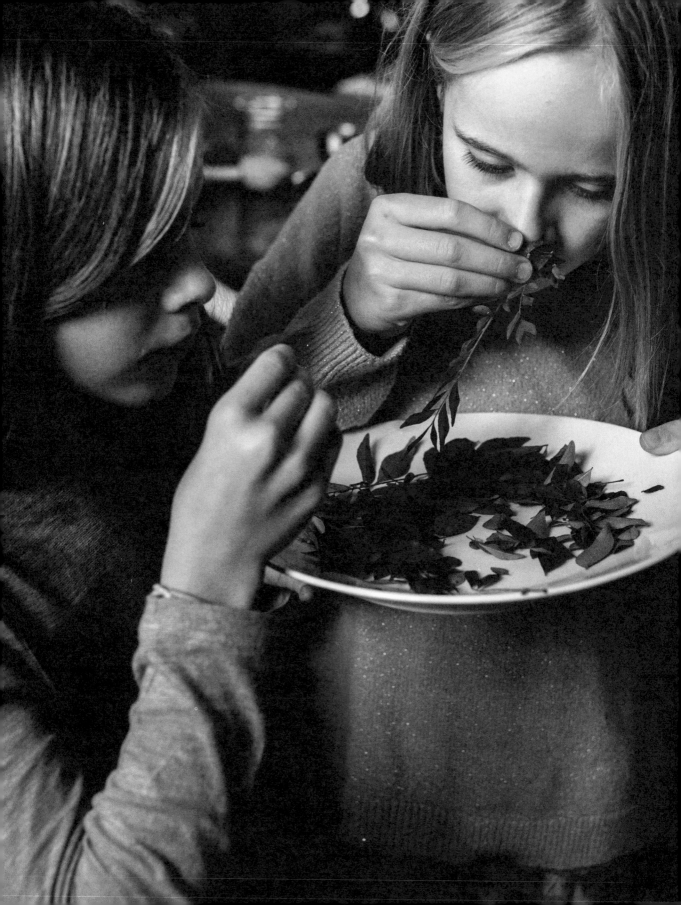

## Building/Nourishing Tastes

**Sweet (*madhura*):** Earth and water. Heavy, oily, sticky, and cool substances, such as bananas, milk, almonds, meat, and rice. Sweet taste builds tissues—especially rasa dhatu, shukra, and ojas—and nourishes bones, skin, hair, and generative tissues. In excess, it can clog channels and aggravate PCOS. Balances vata and pitta; aggravates kapha.

**Sour (*amla*):** Earth and fire. Heating, heavy, and moist substances, such as sour cream, yogurt, stinky cheese, citrus fruits, fermentations, and vinegar. Sour taste increases agni, warming, cleansing, and energizing the body's tissues and senses due to its light quality. In excess, the heat and moisture of sour can cause heavy periods, acne, irritation, and swelling. Balances vata; aggravates pitta and kapha.

**Salty (*lavana*):** Fire and water. Hot, heavy, and sharp substances, such as sea salt, rock salt, and seaweed. Salty taste holds moisture in the body, improves digestive activity, and lubricates and clears obstructions of the channels. In excess, salty taste can cause swelling and heavy periods and diminish shukra. Balances vata; aggravates pitta and kapha.

## Reducing/Cleansing Tastes

**Pungent (*katu*):** Fire and air. Dry, light, and hot substances, such as black and hot peppers, ginger, garlic, mustard, and onion. Pungent taste removes mucus and dries fat; it also dilates the channels of the body and gets blood moving, as in castor oil packs. In excess, the heat and sharpness of pungency can irritate mucous linings and contribute to heavy periods, while the dryness and lightness can deplete the rasa dhatu and overheat rakta. Balances kapha and vata; aggravates pitta.

**Bitter (*tikta*):** Ether and air. Dry, cool, light substances, such as coffee, dark leafy greens like kale and collards, matcha, fenugreek seed, and turmeric. Bitter taste is cold, reduces fat, cleans the blood of toxins, improves digestion, and reduces moisture. In excess, it can dry the body, make you feel cold, deplete the body, amplify aging, and contribute to vata-type period imbalances. Balances kapha and pitta; aggravates vata.

**Astringent (*kashaya*):** Air and earth. Dry substances with a diuretic action, such as cranberries, hibiscus, pomegranate, vegetable skins, tea, and honey. Astringency is cold and dry, tones tissues, cleans rakta, decreases sweating associated with hot flashes, and curbs heavy periods. In excess, astringency contributes to dryness and painful periods. Balances kapha and pitta; aggravates vata.

In normal healthy states, the elements in the body will stay balanced by enjoying mostly sweet taste with the other five tastes in smaller amounts. The doshas will be balanced. Using culinary herbs and spices regularly is the simplest way to establish this equilibrium.

When imbalances are present, calling on the therapeutics of either nourishing or reducing tastes can bring back an essential balance, as in promoting sweet, sour, and salty foods for a vata imbalance. Once the proper qualities are coming in through the diet, the stronger actions of herbs and medicinal spices may be used judiciously to further correct imbalances as needed.

## FOODS PRIZED FOR WOMEN'S HEALTH

The following groups of foods support women's health in different ways. All should be easily digestible and include some sweet taste so as not to aggravate vata, the instigator in many artava problems. Some foods have an affinity for the generative tissues or a particular ability to build the blood.

- Foods that are both unctuous and cool, such as milk, for shukra
- Foods that cleanse the blood (bitter and astringent, with an affinity for rasa/rakta dhatus), such as beets, prunes, and pomegranates
- Foods that nourish without clogging the channels, such as whole grains and mung beans
- Foods that are high in minerals and are blood- and bone-building, such as sea vegetables and urad dal
- Foods that are unctuous, building, *and* mineral-rich, such as dates and sesame

Favored Ingredients

| | | |
|---|---|---|
| Beets | Lotus root | Red rice |
| Cherries | Meat soup and bone broth | Seaweed |
| Dates | Mung beans | Sesame seeds |
| Eggplant | Natural cow milk* | Sweet potatoes and yams |
| Figs | Nuts, especially almonds | Urad dal |
| Flaxseeds | Oats | |
| Grapes and raisins | Pomegranates | |
| Heirloom wheat and varietals | Prunes and plums | |

You will find more information on these foods and how to use them throughout the recipes. *Goats drink less water and eat more bitter and astringent plants than cows do, therefore its qualities are lighter. For this reason, it is a little less building but is a good second to cow's milk for those who digest it better.

## Spotlight on Sea Vegetables

Women need minerals for building and nourishing blood and bones. Sea vegetables have higher concentrations of trace minerals than most other foods. For those who don't include red meats in their diet, sea veggies are a must. Sea vegetables are salty in taste, slimy, and jivana (enlivening). Jivana is a function of a robust rakta dhatu, which provides energy and a zest for life.

This powerhouse food source enters rasa easily, directly builds red blood, and has minerals such as iron and B vitamins, calcium and potassium, and iodine, which is essential to metabolic function. In the menstruating years, sea vegetables provide much-needed building blocks for replenishing the blood and keeping energy levels up.

Our recipes include nori, dulse, arame, sea moss, and kelp. Different types have different concentrations of minerals, and a wonderful way to get in a variety is my Triple Mineral Gomasio (page 299). See also Warm Arame and Kale Salad (page 292) and Raspberry-Ginger Secret Smoothie (page 260; now you know the secret!).

Working with food as medicine is exciting and empowering. Remember to sit down and slow down when you eat. Do your best not to eat and drink while moving, as this aggravates vata and inhibits digestion. Prepare and enjoy food with love and gratitude. Healing is loving-kindness. Aim to be in relationship with the substances that provide for you.

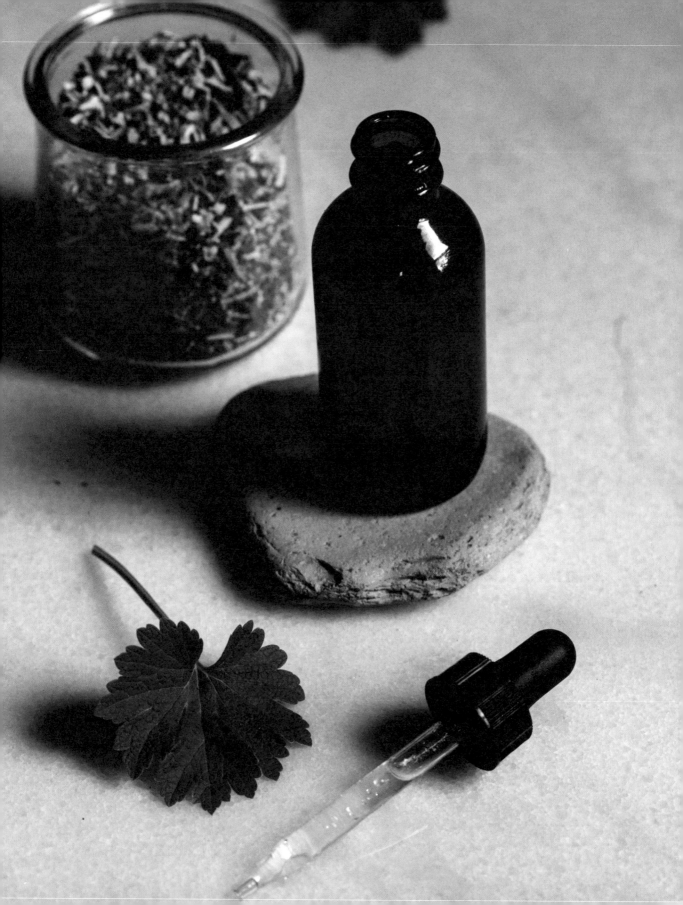

# 20

# Herbal Infusions

Nourishing herbal infusions are stronger than tea and can be drunk warm or cool. In the pharmacopeia of women's herbalism traditions, infusions are the simplest way to get the power of herbs into your life. Herbalists worldwide have extracted the qualities of plants with hot water for millennia. Liquid preparations are an effective way to provide hydration and nourishment that requires much less from the agni. When you're feeling stressed, hot, or lethargic, there is an herbal infusion for you.

Many different parts of the plant are used in herbal preparations: leaves, flowers, stems, seeds, and roots (sometimes called the rhizomes)—and in some cases, all of them. For example, with marshmallow, only the root is used. With lotus, the flowers, seeds, leaves, and roots are used. Raspberry leaves as well as the fruit may be used. Recipes will always indicate what part of the plant to use. Herbs may be harvested and used fresh, dried and ground, or dried and cut, depending on the season and what is available where you live.

Preparing herbal infusions is a rewarding self-care technique that heals and hydrates. In general, to get medicinal potency, try to drink 1 quart daily. If your agni runs colder, warm it up and keep it in a thermos. If you are in a hot climate, you may enjoy infusions cool (not iced!).

When initially working with most herbal medicines, try a very small amount to rule out any allergies. Then give it at least a month of consistent use before expecting changes.

To make an herbal infusion, you will need the following:

Two 32-oz (1-qt) mason jars, preferably with wide mouths

A tea strainer or cheesecloth

Herbs, fresh or dried (In general, you will use twice as much fresh as dried.)

The following three recipes are formulated to be tasty and effective. As you get to know the tastes of the herbs, or as your herb garden expands, you will begin to use herbs intuitively.

# Nourishing Herbal Infusion

## (BEST FOR VATA)

**MAKES 1 QUART**

This overnight infusion contains nourishing and hydrating plants. The demulcent quality of marshmallow and slippery elm protect the membranes of the gut and support healthy elimination. Oat straw is a famous rejuvenator and nourisher that also has nervine actions that support feeling calm and resilient. Nettles supply minerals and a purifying punch to balance this building formula.

> ½ cup fresh oat straw/milky oats (¼ cup dried)
> ½ cup fresh nettle leaves (¼ cup dried)
> 1 tbsp dried marshmallow root or slippery elm

Combine the herbs in a 1-qt mason jar and cover with almost boiling water. Cover and allow to steep overnight (8 to 12 hours).

In the morning, use a metal sieve to strain the infusion into another glass jar. Drink at room temperature, or warm gently to drink as a tea.

Sip the quart over the course of the day (always within 24 hours), and make a new batch in the evening for the following day.

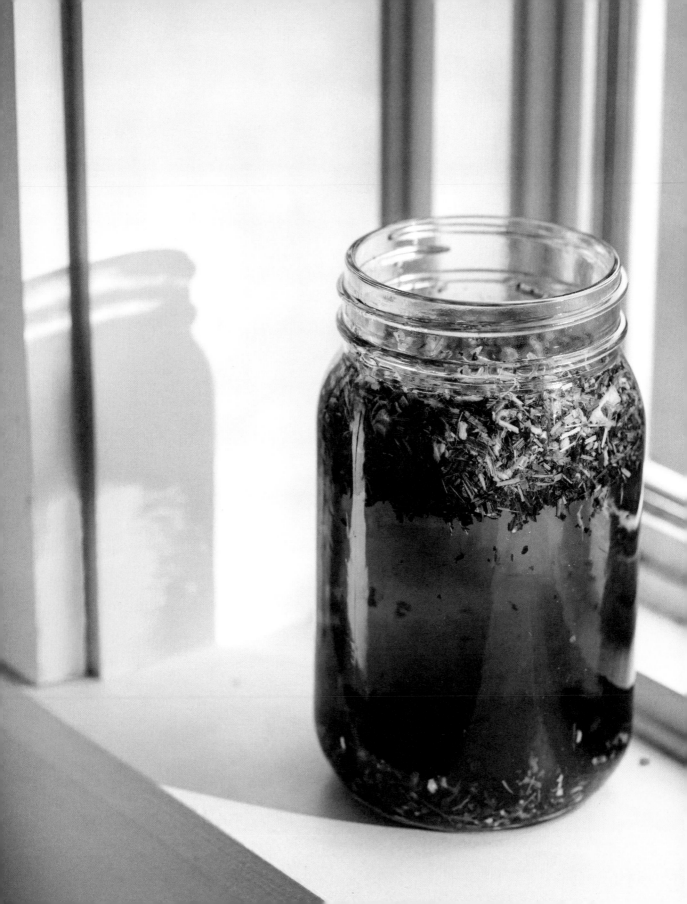

# Cooling Herbal Infusion

(BEST FOR PITTA)

**MAKES 1 QUART**

Rose is a famous pitta balancer that reduces heat and calms the mind and nerves with its soft and sweet taste. Both raspberry leaf and red clover purify the blood, remove toxins, and support healthy reproductive tissues. Together this trio is cooling, nourishing, and cleansing, and it targets the rakta dhatu and generative system.

> **2 tbsp fresh rose petals (1 tbsp dried)**
> **½ cup fresh red raspberry leaves (¼ cup dried)**
> **½ cup fresh red clover blossoms (¼ cup dried)**

Combine the herbs in a 1-qt mason jar and cover with almost boiling water. Cover and allow to steep overnight (8 to 12 hours).

In the morning, use a metal sieve to strain the infusion into another glass jar. Drink at room temperature, or warm gently to drink as a tea.

Sip the quart over the course of the day (always within 24 hours), and make a new batch in the evening for the following day.

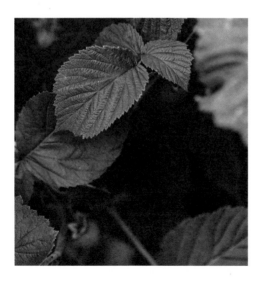

# Refreshing Phanta Infusion

## (BEST FOR PITTA)

**MAKES 1 QUART**

*Phanta* is an infusion made using cool water. This method is used for formulas intended to reduce heat or to infuse delicate plants that lose their properties in hot water. Chamomile, peppermint, and hibiscus hold up well in a cool infusion. All three are cooling: chamomile brings a softness to the mind, hibiscus cools the blood, and peppermint harmonizes acid and bloating. Hibiscus also supports healthy hair and skin by optimizing rasa and rakta dhatus. I love to drink bright red hibiscus infusions in summer; their astringency is especially refreshing in humidity.

> ¼ cup fresh chamomile flowers (2 tbsp dried)
> ¼ cup fresh peppermint (2 tbsp dried)
> ¼ cup fresh hibiscus flowers (2 tbsp dried)

Combine the herbs in a 1-qt mason jar and cover with room temperature water. Cover and allow to steep overnight (8 to 12 hours).

In the morning, use a metal sieve to strain the infusion into another glass jar. Drink at room temperature.

Sip the quart over the course of the day (always within 24 hours), and make a new batch in the evening for the following day.

# Cleansing Herbal Infusion

(BEST FOR KAPHA)

**MAKES 1 QUART**

This astringent formula is tonifying for conditions of excess moisture, as well as deeply purifying. Burdock and tulsi motivate the circulation and remove stagnation, while raspberry leaf and nettles lend a balance of cleansing and rejuvenating qualities. Each of these herbs also has a sweet taste—so pleasant to drink!

> 2 heaping tbsp fresh sliced burdock root (1 heaping tbsp dried)
>
> ¼ cup fresh red raspberry leaves (2 tbsp dried)
>
> ¼ cup fresh nettle leaves (2 tbsp dried)
>
> ¼ cup fresh tulsi leaves (2 tbsp dried)

Combine the herbs in a 1-qt mason jar and cover with almost boiling water. Cover and allow to steep overnight (8 to 12 hours).

In the morning, use a metal sieve to strain the infusion into another glass jar. Drink at room temperature, or warm gently to drink as a tea.

Sip the quart over the course of the day (always within 24 hours), and make a new batch in the evening for the following day.

# Raspberry Leaf and Nettle Brew

**MAKES 1 QUART**

Red raspberry strengthens and tones the uterus; it has been used for centuries to prepare women for childbirth and to rebuild the uterus postpartum. Nettle provides much-needed minerals, and oat straw bolsters the deep tissues and nervous system. Bring a few jars of this infusion—or sachets of the blended herbs for enjoying later—to your postpartum friend.

**2 tbsp dried nettle leaves**

**2 tbsp dried red raspberry leaves**

**2 tbsp dried oat straw**

Combine the herbs in a 1-qt mason jar and cover with almost boiling water. Cover and allow to steep overnight (8 to 12 hours).

In the morning, use a metal sieve to strain the infusion into another glass jar. Drink at room temperature, or warm gently to drink as a tea.

Sip the quart over the course of the day (always within 24 hours), and make a new batch in the evening for the following day.

## How Long Should I Use Herbs?

Nourishing herbal infusions are like food and can be enjoyed regularly, but stronger herbal medicines, like tinctures or powders, tend to be intense and targeted. Ayurveda's recommendation on using herbal medicines is generally three to four months. If it is the right medicine for the condition, you should see an improvement by this time.

# Triphala Tea

**MAKES 1 CUP**

*Triphala* is a mixture of three dried and roasted Indian fruits. This compound tones each of the digestive organs: the stomach, small intestine, and large intestine. Triphala's benefits cast a wide net: it optimizes the digestion, assimilation, and absorption of nutrients. This optimized nutrition then creates optimized body tissues. Triphala also ensures that waste moves out of the colon. Drink this tea 2 to 3 hours after dinner or before bed.

>  1 cup hot water
>  ½ tsp triphala powder

Place the triphala in the bottom of a mug. Pour the water over the powder; cover and steep for 10 minutes.

Strain the infusion, or simply leave the sediment at the bottom as you drink

## How to Use Triphala

For general health maintenance, taking ¼ to ½ teaspoon of triphala powder nightly is a reliable serving size. If your stool gets loose, switch to amalaki powder (see appendix B). If your stool is hard or not passing, increase to as much as 1 teaspoon of triphala. As with any herb, if your triphala is old, it won't work as well and you will need to use more. I have noticed a difference with using different brands of triphala, so be open to changes in your recipe.

Triphala may taste unpleasant in the beginning. The taste that is lacking in your diet will stand out—bitter, sour, sweet, and so on. As your body finds balance, triphala begins to taste milder. Your taste buds will tell you how it's working!

While triphala is relatively mild, if you have any doubt about taking herbs that may have a laxative effect, be sure to consult with your health professional, and do not use if you are pregnant.

# Double-Duty Sage and Salt Deodorant Spritz

**MAKES 4 OZ**

Aromatherapy engages the senses and can calm, cool, or invigorate. This armpit spritz couples clary sage with pink salt, which can neutralize the bacteria that cause stinky pits. Keep it on hand and ditch your store-bought deodorant.

Clary sage is an aromatic, sweeter variety of sage, an astringent and purifying herb. It can regulate menstruation and has an affinity for the lower abdomen. You can use other oils such as lavender or rose, but avoid sharp oils like eucalyptus or citrus, which may burn your skin.

> **3 oz distilled water**
>
> **2 tsp pink salt**
>
> **1 oz witch hazel**
>
> **10 drops clary sage essential oil**
>
> **4-oz amber trigger-style spray bottle**

Heat the distilled water in a small saucepan, and dissolve the salt in the hot water. Transfer the salt water to a glass measuring cup with a spout and let it cool completely.

Add the essential oil and witch hazel to the water and stir well. Pour it carefully into the spray bottle (the trigger style does not clog from the oils) and shake well.

Shake before each use, and rinse the nozzle with hot water if it clogs.

# Cool-the-Flash Tea and Spritz
# with Rose and Sage

**MAKES 1 QUART**

I asked Brighid Doherty, founder of Solidago School of Herbalism, if she had a most-recommended recipe for hot flashes. This was it! This infusion is composed of dried rose petals and sage leaves. Rose petals are energetically cooling and nourishing to women's reproductive and nervous systems. They taste floral and divine. Sage leaves are cooling and drying. Sage is an astringent herb that is known to dry body secretions from sweat to breast milk, making it ideal for counteracting hot flashes and high pitta.

This tisane can be enjoyed in the evening before bed to cool night sweats or sipped throughout the day from a water bottle to help cool hot flashes. It's most potent when made fresh daily, but it will keep in the refrigerator for up to five days.

To make a cooling face or body spritz, soak a washcloth with the tisane and rub it over the body, especially during night sweats, hot flashes, or reddening of the skin. Fill a spray bottle with the tisane and mist it on the face for cooling on the go.

> **2 tbsp dried rose petals**
> **2 tbsp dried sage leaves**
> **1 qt boiling water**

Place the herbs in a 1-qt mason jar or 4-cup teapot. Fill the jar or teapot with boiling water, and steep for 20 minutes.

Use a wire mesh tea strainer to strain the tisane into another jar. Enjoy it hot by the mugful or iced by the glassful, or carry it with you in a thermos—either hot or iced, depending on your preference—throughout the day.

Store in the refrigerator for up to five days in a mason jar with a tight lid.

---

Working therapeutically with herbs for women's health is surprisingly effective. I have witnessed herbal therapies heal all manner of imbalances—and been healed myself.

Many people have affinities with certain plants. Once you discover the ones that work for you, the relationship between self and plant only grows stronger. Keep in mind that herbs are precious resources, and use them judiciously. Do not overbuy and waste them or let them languish. Start small, buy half a pound at most, and establish a consistent herbal practice before procuring more.

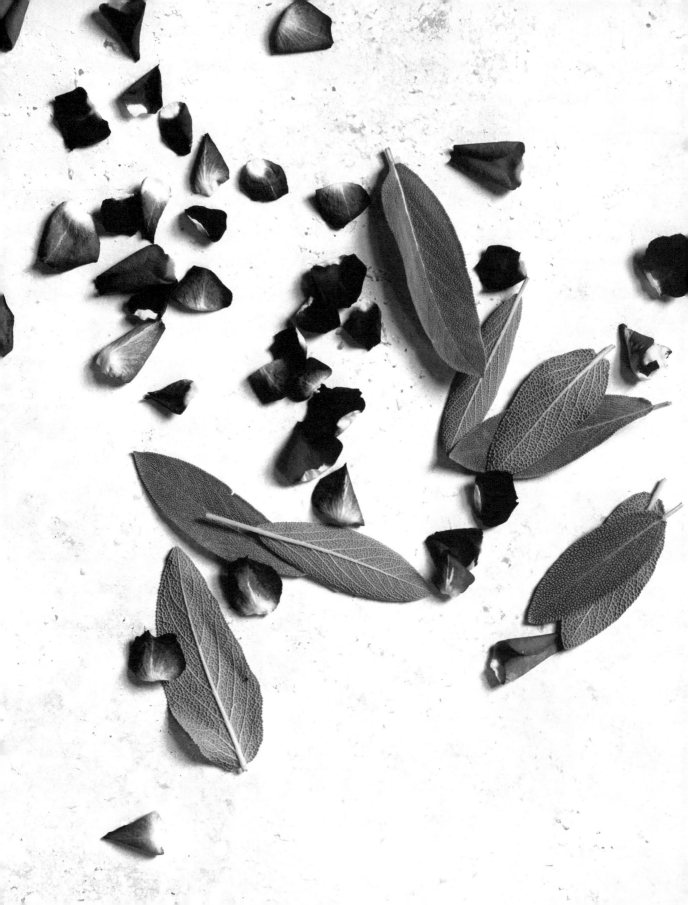

# 21

# Digestives and Culinary Spices

In Ayurveda, spices are most often used for improving the digestive fire and the absorption and assimilation of nutrition and medicine. Spices can improve the quality of ahara rasa, the nutrient precursor created from food, and the ability to digest ama. Some spices, such as rosemary and turmeric, also have effects on the blood and can purify rasa and rakta dhatus, reduce inflammation, and improve circulation. Spices are included in herbal medicines to improve the digestion of the medicine and its assimilation into the tissues.

Spices are often the seeds of plants (such as coriander, the seed of the cilantro plant). Each seed contains the potential energy to grow a plant and has more intensely concentrated qualities than food substances. Sometimes spices are roots, such as ginger; bark, such as cinnamon; or leaves, such as thyme and oregano.

These powerhouses are essential medicines when you suffer from acidity, gas and bloating, lack of appetite, malnutrition, or indigestion after eating. They can be incorporated into your cooking or the water you drink, or they can be ground finely and taken with a little hot water before or after meals. Working with spices makes a world of difference for me. I am so grateful for how they have healed and strengthened me over time.

While you will find spices incorporated into tonics, meals, and medicines, spiced waters and spice mixes for cooking are the easiest and best options. Just as with the herbal infusions from chapter 20, I offer recipes to get you started. Once you are in the flow with flavors and medicinal actions, you may invent your own.

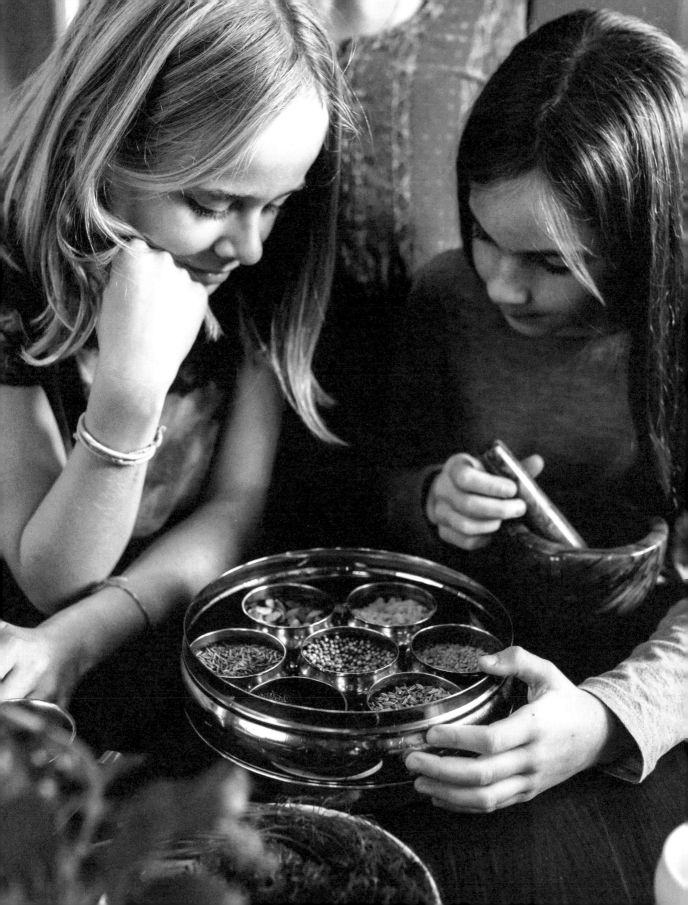

# Basic Cooked Water

**MAKES 1½–2 QUARTS**

Water is heavy and cool, and when there is ama or weak agni, water can actually be hard to digest. At these times, it feels as though water just sits in the gut. Adding agni to the water by cooking it lightens the heaviness, warms it, and renders it easier to digest. Cooked water is the first line of defense when ama forms in the stomach.

When you have that heavy feeling in your gut or mind, make a batch every day and drink only cooked water throughout the day until you feel better. Drink it at a temperature that is conducive to your environment. It can be taken hot in wintertime and room temperature in summer.

**2 qt water**

In a large saucepan, bring the water to a boil. Boil, uncovered, for at least 5 to 10 minutes. If you're experiencing water retention, excess mucus, or weak digestive fire, boil it for 15 to 20 minutes.

Drink warm or at room temperature.

# Essential Spiced Water

The panacea of spices is CCF: cumin, coriander, and fennel. Together they make a combination that is healing for all body types and each stage of digestion in the stomach, small intestine, and colon. It's a go-to when your gut feels off but you're not sure what's going on. With consistent use of a few cups daily, this mixture purifies rasa and rakta dhatu, which can improve digestion and the skin.

**1 qt water**
**½ tsp cumin seeds**
**1 tsp coriander seeds**
**1 tsp fennel seeds**

In a medium saucepan, bring the water to a boil. Add the seeds to the water and boil for 10 to 15 minutes.

Cool, then use a tea strainer to strain the water into a mason jar. You can drink it hot or room temperature. Make only what you need for one day, and avoid storing and drinking leftover cooked water.

# Ajwain Water

Ajwain (also known as bishop's weed or carom seed) has a pungent, lively flavor similar to that of caraway. This herbal water, also known as *oma* water, is slightly heating and has an affinity for the lower abdomen. It has a carminative effect and is often used for abdominal pain related to digestion, menstrual cramps, or PMS, and it is especially recommended postpartum to support agni. Regular consumption of ajwain water may boost the metabolism for those who need to improve the assimilation of nutrients or lose weight.

**1 tbsp ajwain seeds**
**1 qt water**

In a frying pan over medium heat, dry roast the seeds until you can smell them.

In a medium saucepan, bring the water to a boil. Add the seeds, cover, and simmer for about 10 minutes.

Allow the mixture to cool a bit, then use a tea strainer to strain the water into a mason jar. Drink it hot or warm, as needed. Make only what you need for one day, and avoid storing and drinking leftover cooked water.

# Cooling Coriander Water

**MAKES 1 QUART**

Helpful for reducing hot flashes, cleansing the blood, and supporting the liver, coriander water optimizes the quality of ahara rasa. It is tasty, versatile, and healing. This one is good for all body types and all seasons, and it improves digestion as well as blood quality.

**1 tbsp coriander seeds**
**1 qt water**

In a frying pan over medium heat, dry roast the seeds until you can smell them. Remove from the heat and crack the seeds with a mortar and pestle.

In a medium saucepan, bring the water to a boil. Add the seeds, cover, and simmer for about 10 minutes.

Allow the mixture to cool a bit, then use a tea strainer to strain it into a mason jar. Drink a cup hot or at room temperature throughout the day for hot flashes. Make only what you need for one day, and avoid storing and drinking leftover cooked water.

# Soothing Rose Sweet Tea

**MAKES 2 CUPS**

These sweet and warming spices are the most sattvic, which means calming for the mind. You'll find belly comfort and grounding calm in this tea, with the heat of ginger to stoke agni and the power of cinnamon to curb sweet cravings. Add the soft aromatics of rose, and this is a hug in a cup.

> **16 oz water**
> **1 tsp grated gingerroot**
> **½ tsp ground cinnamon**
> **½ tsp dried rose petals or buds**
> **Pinch of ground cardamom**

In a medium saucepan, bring the water to a boil. Add the rest of the ingredients, cover, and simmer for about 10 minutes.

Allow the tea to cool a bit, then use a tea strainer to strain it into a glass jar. Sip it hot, and add a bit of sweetener if desired.

# Cooling Fennel Soft Drink

**MAKES 1 QT**

In the Ayurveda tradition, a "soft drink" is a refreshing summer beverage made with spices, flowers, fruits, and sugar. Pitta dosha is hot and sharp, so it is balanced by cool and soft things. This fennel soft drink can be enjoyed to soften a sharp mood and is useful for those who experience hot flashes or premenstrual or natal heat. It's refreshing and balancing, and much better for you than what you might be used to calling a soft drink.

> **6 cups water**
> **2 tbsp fennel seeds**
> **2 tbsp coriander seeds**
> **¼ tsp ground cardamom, or 4 pods, cracked**
> **2 tbsp raisins**

In a medium saucepan, bring the water to a boil over high heat. Add the spices and dried fruit, and reduce to low heat. Cover with the lid ajar and simmer for 30 minutes. Four cups of liquid should remain.

Use a metal strainer to strain the mixture into a glass jar or pitcher, and cool to room temperature. Make only what you need for one day, and avoid storing and drinking leftovers.

# Sweet Rose Masala

**MAKES ¼ CUP**

Inspired by Persian cooking, this spice mix has the cool and calming sweetness of rose. Ayurveda texts recommend using flowers for flavor, aroma, and beauty. The nectar and aroma of flowers, a plant's reproductive component, increase shukra through the bhav of both flavor and smell. Use this mix to bring the blessings of roses to warm milk, baking, and even boiled water as a postdigestive tea.

2 tbsp ground cinnamon

1 tbsp coriander seeds

½ tsp ground cardamom

½ tsp ground turmeric

1 tsp dried rose petals

Pinch of ground cloves, or 1 whole clove (if grinding fresh)

Pinch of ground nutmeg

Combine the ingredients in a mortar and pestle, dedicated coffee grinder, or electric spice grinder and grind until uniform.

Store in a glass jar with an airtight lid. The masala will stay fresh for up to six months, but it will be more aromatic if you make it monthly.

## Make Your Own Masala: Working Therapeutically with Spices

In appendix B, you will find three tables that list spices according to their digestive actions. Consult these charts and try finding combinations that appeal to you. You are more likely to use spices consistently if you like their taste! Keep a balance of the six tastes in your mix by using the Essential Spice Mix as your base and adding one or more targeted spices from the tables.

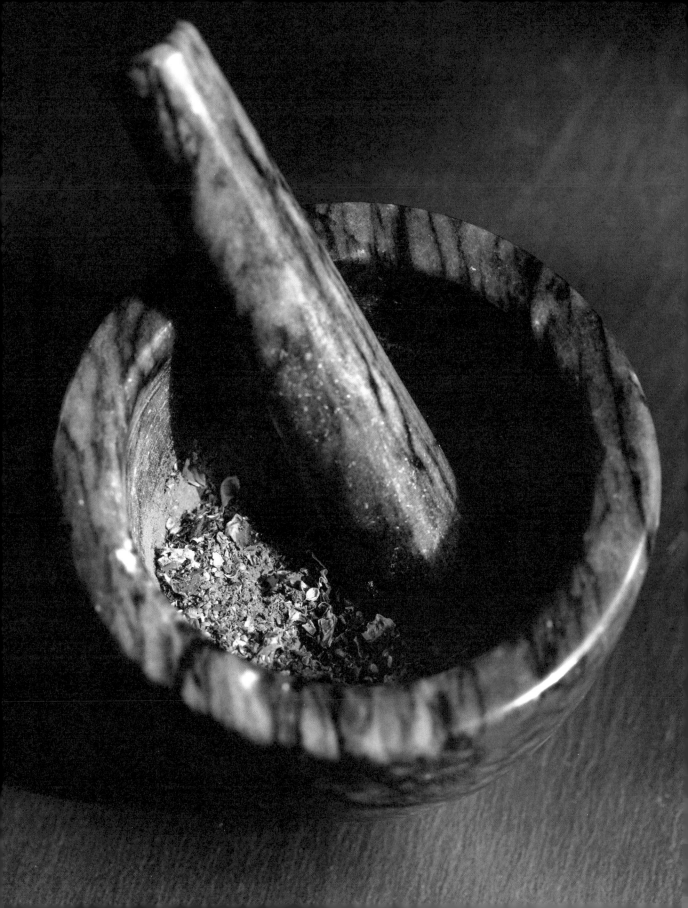

# Essential Spice Mix

**MAKES ¼ CUP**

Cumin, coriander, fennel, and turmeric comprise a common combination in Ayurveda cooking. Each of the spices has a targeted action to improve digestion, absorption, and assimilation. In addition to its use in savory dishes, this mix can also be added to boiling water as a tea to be sipped throughout the day for detoxification and digestion and to promote clear skin. Use this mixture as a balancing base, and then add from the chart of therapeutic spices (see appendix B) to personalize it.

> **1 tbsp coriander seeds**
> **1 tbsp cumin seeds**
> **2 tsp fennel seeds**
> **1 tbsp ground turmeric**

In a heavy-bottomed pan over medium-low heat, dry roast the coriander, cumin, and fennel seeds for a few minutes until you can smell them. Transfer from the pan to a wide bowl and cool completely.

Grind the whole roasted seeds in a spice grinder, or by hand with a mortar and pestle, to a uniform consistency. Transfer to a bowl and stir in the turmeric powder.

Store in a small glass jar with an airtight lid for up to six months.

# 22

# Women's Health Tonics

A tonic is a medicinal substance taken to increase vigor and well-being. Rejuvenatives stave off deficiencies and promote shukra by strengthening the generative system. Specific combinations are revered for their abilities to slow the aging process and/or improve sleep, brain power, or fertility. Foods that promote health can also be tonics, but I have described drinks and shake recipes here and placed meals in chapter 23. Use Women's Health Tonics to provide healing qualities in the morning or evening, as a light meal or to tide you over between meals. In general, these tonics work best when they aren't mixed with other food.

Many tonics in Ayurveda's medicine are milk-based, as milk has similar qualities to rasa and thereby targets rasa. Cow's milk is ideal for keeping the bones, nerves, and reproductive organs juicy. Almond and coconut milks are also rasayana. These nourishing tonics for the deep tissues are sometimes taken in the evening, close to bedtime, as it is during the quiet hours of sleep that the body can use energy to nourish such tissues. I often recommend these recipes for a light dinner if you get home too late to eat a meal, provided you enjoyed a good breakfast and lunch that day. A rejuvenation tonic is a great way to replace what your body has lost, give comfort and deep nourishment, and promote sound sleep.

For women's health, rakta dhatu (red blood) is also an important factor in health. A tonic for rakta may be aloe-based, as aloe is a rejuvenator for the female generative system. Dark fruits like raisins and pomegranates, as well as bitters that purify rakta, are balancing tonics when rakta is overheated, sticky, or oily.

# Basic Almond Milk

**MAKES 1 QUART**

Cool, sweet, and easy to digest, homemade almond milk is a go-to that is good for all doshas. Most store-bought almond milks contain very few actual almonds. This recipe is a base for many of the tonic recipes that follow.

> ⅔ cup raw almonds
> 4 cups water, plus more for soaking

Cover the almonds with cool water and soak for 6+ hours (overnight works, but no longer). If you oversoak the nuts, your milk will go bad faster.
Drain and rinse.

Add ½ cup of the water to the nuts and blend to a paste using a hand blender or carafe blender. Add the rest of the water and blend on high for 1 minute.

Strain through a fine sieve or cheesecloth. Reserve the pulp for baking and to thicken cereals and soups.

Store in a glass jar in the refrigerator. Milk will keep for up to five days.

# Basic Coconut Milk

**MAKES 1 QUART**

Milk made from coconut meat has a cooling nature. It is a lot more affordable than homemade almond milk. It is rich and delicious but can contribute to overnourished rasa, because it is both cool and oily.

> **4 cups water**
>
> **1 cup unsweetened shredded coconut,**
>    **fresh if you can get it, or dried if you can't**

Boil 1 cup of the water, then soak the coconut in the hot water for 5 minutes. I do this right in the blender carafe.

Blend on high to make a paste, then add the remaining three cups of water (room temperature) and blend on high for 1 minute.

Strain the milk through a fine sieve or cheesecloth. Reserve the pulp for baking and to thicken cereals and soups.

Store in a glass jar in the refrigerator. Milk will keep for up to 5 days.

**Note:** My favorite plant milk recipe is almond-coconut milk. Use $\frac{1}{2}$ cup unsweetened shredded coconut and $\frac{1}{3}$ cup raw almonds, soaked, to 4 cups water. Follow the recipe above, grinding the almonds and coconut together to make a paste.

# Homemade Flax Milk

**MAKES 1 QUART**

Flax milk has a wonderful café au lait color and a nutty taste. Flax is a demulcent, which balances the dry quality and improves elimination. It is said to be good for detoxifying the skin, and regular use will improve the complexion's luster. Made into milk, flax is especially nourishing for rasa.

It's better to start with whole flaxseeds, because like most seeds, they begin to lose their nutritional potency once they've been ground and packaged. Flax oil, like all seed and nut oils, has a low heat tolerance, so do not heat this milk to a boil or it will lose its efficacy.

**4 ½ cups water**
**½ cup flaxseeds**
**Pinch of salt**
**2 Medjool dates, pits removed and coarsely chopped (optional)**

Put the water in a blender. Add the flaxseeds, salt, and dates.

Blend on low speed to combine, then increase to high speed for about 1 minute. (If you're using a high-speed blender, 30 seconds on medium-high will do it. Do not blend on high as you may heat the flax.) Let the solution rest for 2 minutes, allowing the flax to absorb some of the water.

Blend again for 1 minute (30 seconds in a high-speed blender). Let rest for 5 minutes.

Blend again for 30 seconds (15 seconds in a high-speed blender).

Strain the milk using a nut milk bag. You can also use a strainer lined with cheesecloth. Gather the cheesecloth around the solids and squeeze as you would a nut milk bag to extract the milk. You can add the solids to yogurt or breakfast cereal.

Store in a glass jar in the refrigerator. Milk will keep for up to four days.

# Date Shake

This is a classic nourisher for women. Dates and shatavari are both aphrodisiacs, and they target artava when taken with milk and ghee. This is a fantastic treat for enhancing fertility and supporting both pregnancy and the postpartum phase. A warm Date Shake is also comforting and soothing in times of stress or at the end of a busy day.

**1 cup organic cow's milk or almond milk**

**1 tsp ghee**

**½ tsp Sweet Rose Masala (page 236) or ground cinnamon**

**½ tsp shatavari powder**

**2 Medjool dates**

Place the milk, ghee, spice mix, and shatavari powder in a small saucepan; warm over medium-low heat.

Pit the dates and chop into quarters. Place them in a blender, then add the warm spiced milk. Blend until absolutely smooth.

Serve immediately.

# Best Medicinal PSL (Pumpkin Spice Latte)

What a way to get your flaxseeds! All winter squashes promote strength, and pumpkin also provides a rich array of minerals. Ashwagandha warms and grounds the body and provides a buffer against stress. This cozy cup will satisfy a latte craving and give you the support you need for an active day.

> 1 cup Homemade Flax Milk (page 242)
>
> ¼ tsp pumpkin pie spice, or ¼ tsp each ground ginger and cinnamon
>
> ¼–½ tsp ashwagandha powder
>
> ¼ cup pumpkin puree
>
> 1 tsp maple syrup or honey (optional)

In a small saucepan, warm the milk over medium-low heat. (You do not want to overheat it.) Add the rest of the ingredients, and combine with a balloon whisk over the heat.

Scoop a bit out with a spoon and test for warmth. Remove the PSL from the heat before it boils.

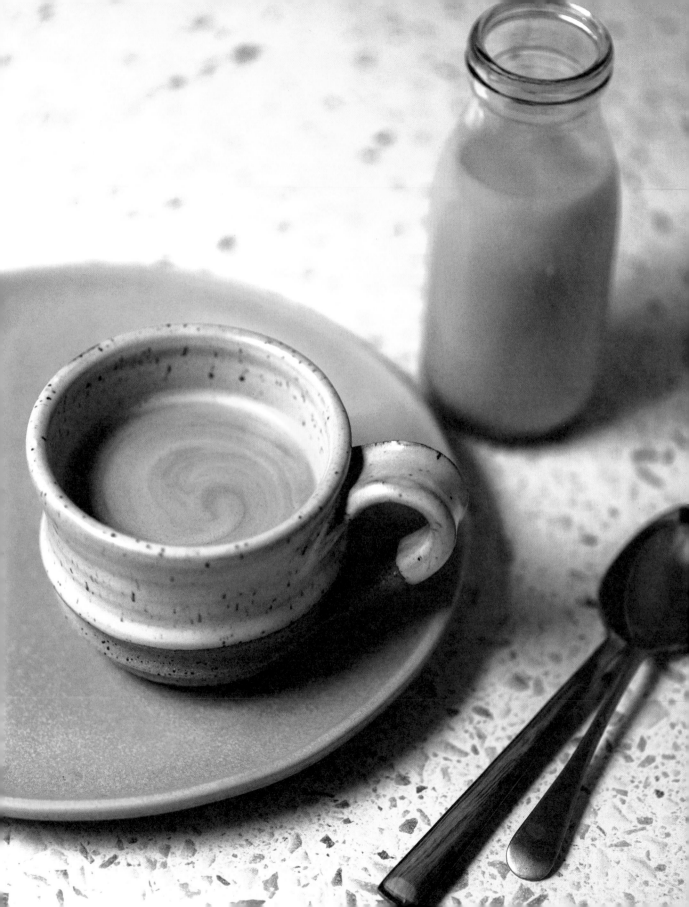

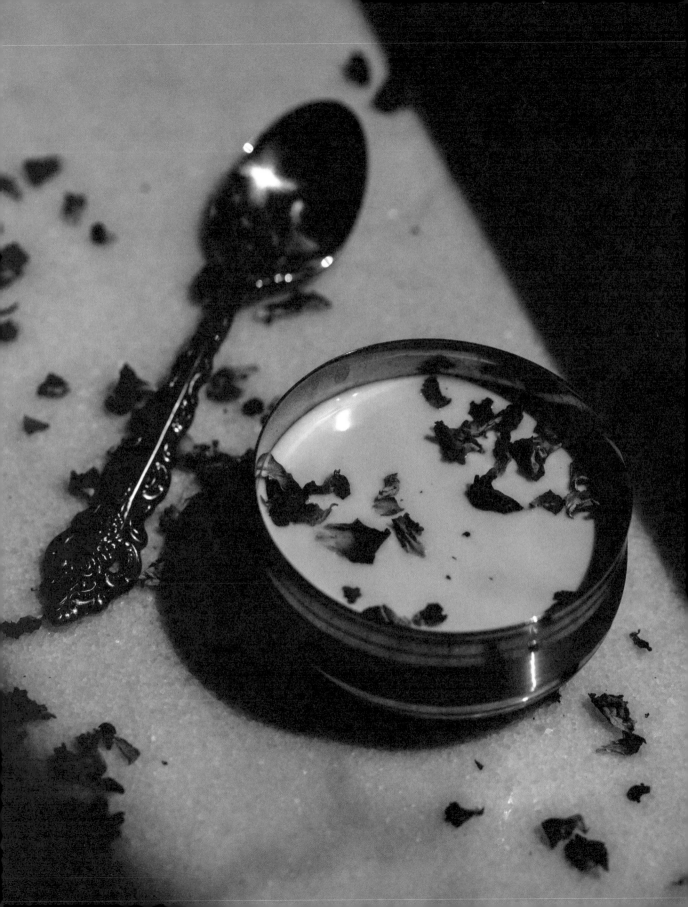

# Moon Milk

Imbuing milk with the energy of moonlight makes a targeted tonic for reducing excess heat and supporting reproductive tissue. Silver's luminescence aligns with the moon, and using a silver vessel, if you can, provides added shakti. Natural, organic cow's milk is the favored option if you have access to a trusted dairy. If this is not available, use Basic Almond Milk (page 240) or Basic Coconut Milk (page 241).

> 4 oz natural cow's milk or homemade plant milk
>
> Pinch of ground cardamom
>
> 3–5 dried rose petals

Pour the milk into a silver vessel, if you have one. (If you don't have something made of silver, use clear glass.) Stir in the cardamom, and crush a few dried rose petals into the milk.

Place the vessel in direct moonlight for a few hours (or even an hour—longer is better, but do your best). You should be able to see the moon's reflection on the surface of the milk.

This can be taken at night if the moon rises early enough. Or wait until morning and gently warm the mixture, but do not expose it to the sun.

Slowly drink the Moon Milk while sitting down and doing nothing else. Visualize the tonic entering your generative tissues.

# Golden Mind Milk

Brahmi is known for its ability to improve mental clarity, but this recipe's benefits go far beyond acuity. Ashwagandha supports the body's ability to adapt to stress, and combined with the nervine actions of brahmi and rose, this tonic strengthens both body and mind in the face of physical stress that results from work deadlines or travel. Mix in some turmeric and digestive spices to drive the herbal actions into the deep tissues.

½ tsp ashwagandha powder
½ tsp ground turmeric
¼ tsp Sweet Rose Masala (page 236)
⅛ tsp brahmi powder
½ tsp coconut or cane sugar
Dash of black pepper
10 oz milk of your choice

In a small saucepan over medium heat, warm the ingredients to steaming. Whisk to a uniform consistency with a balloon whisk or milk frother wand.

Drink immediately.

**Make Your Own Golden Milk Mix:** If you intend to make this tonic regularly, you can make a month's supply and use 1 heaping tsp per 10-oz serving.

Combine ½ cup ashwagandha powder, ¼ cup ground turmeric, 2 tbsp Sweet Rose Masala, 2 tbsp brahmi powder; ¼ cup coconut or cane sugar, and 1 tsp black pepper. Store in an airtight glass jar in a cool, dry place.

# Sexy Cacao

**SERVES 2**

The mineral content in cacao is why women crave chocolate before their monthly bleeding. Cacao is a blood builder. This recipe is heavy on the cacao to give you your fix. It is made medicinal by the addition of the unctuous, artava-building shatavari ("woman who has a thousand husbands"). Most plants that are used for women's health also have an affinity for the generative system, as does shatavari, whose cooling, sweet, and unctuous qualities are similar to those of estrogen. The aroma of crushed rose petals will put you over the moon with your first sip.

> **2 cups milk of your choice (almond, coconut, cow's)**
> **¼ cup cacao powder**
> **1 tsp shatavari powder**
> **1 tbsp sweetener (maple syrup, coconut sugar, raw cane sugar)**
> **1 tsp ground ginger**
> **A few dried rose petals**

Warm the milk in a saucepan over medium heat.

Add all the other ingredients except the rose petals. Whisk briskly until the mixture begins to steam.

Remove from the heat and pour into cups. For an extra gorgeous finish, whiz with a milk frother wand for a cappuccino-like foam.

Crush the rose petals in your fingers and sprinkle over the foam to garnish.

## Chocolate Cravings

If you get a strong chocolate craving every month, it means you are in need of minerals. See Spotlight on Sea Vegetables (page 215) to remedy this.

# Moringa Green Drink Three Ways

*Moringa* is a very special plant that is deeply purifying and has an affinity for rakta dhatu, removing excess heat and moisture. Its uniqueness lies in its ability to offer nourishment or purification, adapting to what the body needs. Have a taste and see—you'll notice a sweetness. Reach for moringa if you feel clogged, tired, or puffy.

Like matcha, moringa will separate from liquid, so whisk vigorously to make a smoother final drink.

## Nourishing Moringa for Vata                                       SERVES 1

½ tsp moringa
½ tsp maple syrup
1 cup almond milk, warmed

Whisk the maple syrup, moringa, and half of the almond milk in a 2-cup measuring cup. Use a fork if a whisk is too large for your cup.

Add the rest of the almond milk and whisk again.

## A Cooler Moringa Brew for Pitta                                   SERVES 1

½ tsp moringa
½ cup aloe juice
½ cup water

Whisk the moringa into the aloe juice in a 2-cup measuring cup. Use a fork if a whisk is too large. Add the water and whisk to combine.

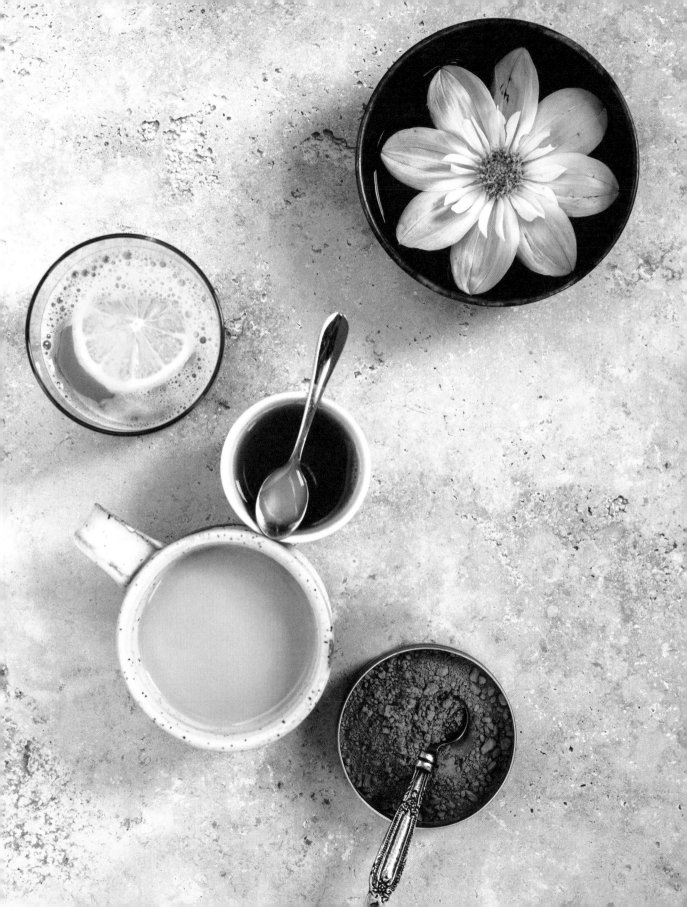

## Deep-Clean Moringa for Kapha

SERVES 1

**1 tsp honey**
**1 cup water**
**½ tsp moringa**
**1 tsp lemon juice**

Dissolve the honey in some of the water by whisking vigorously with a fork.

Add the moringa and whisk again, then add the remaining water and lemon juice and whisk for the last time.

## Clean Green Powders

I spent years pretending to enjoy the taste of "green powders" made of wheatgrass and spirulina in complicated smoothies, but now if I need the bonus from a bitter green like moringa, I prefer to keep it simple. It feels better in the gut, and I feel more connected to the medicinal plant without dousing it in bananas and almond butter. I just have it by itself between meals, kind of like a snack, or in the morning after exercise.

# Longevity Bone Tonic

Brahmi in milk is a classic formulation for enhancing both brain and bone. If you are having trouble taking brahmi ghee by itself, try this simple tonic as a palatable way of using this medicine. It is best taken in the evening, at least two hours after dinner, to allow the deep nourishment to work its way in while you rest, or on an empty stomach in the morning. The bitterness of brahmi may make this a stand-in for coffee!

**½ cup milk of your choice**
**¼ tsp brahmi powder**
**¼ tsp ground ginger**
**pinch of ground cardamom**

In a small saucepan over medium heat, warm the ingredients to steaming. Whisk to a uniform consistency with a whisk or a milk frother wand.

Drink immediately.

## The Amazing Brahmi

Brahmi is a light, sharp, and bitter herb that has an affinity for the brain and nervous system when used in a fat carrier such as milk or ghee. It calms, cools, and rejuvenates on subtle levels, while improving acuity and memory.

# Aloe-Pom-Cran Tonic

**MAKES 20 OZ**

This astringent mixture of cooling aloe and purifying pomegranate and cranberry has an affinity for the generative system and bladder. Daily use is helpful for reducing heat, cooling the menstrual cycle, and discouraging yeast and urinary infections.

> 1 cup pure pomegranate juice
> ½ cup pure cranberry juice
> ½ cup aloe juice
> ½ cup water

Mix all ingredients together in a mason jar.

Drink at room temperature, taking 4 oz after a meal one to three times a day. In hot weather, you can also enjoy a cool cup anytime. Store in a glass jar in the refrigerator for up to five days.

# Pomegranate Lime Mocktail

**SERVES 1**

Here is one of my favorite and prettiest mocktails, which can be enjoyed in a fancy way at any time of day. The deep color of pomegranate is also very satisfying for red wine lovers who are trying to replace the alcohol.

Pomegranate is a special pitta balancer, due to its sweet and astringent qualities, and it both purifies and nourishes the red blood.

**½ lime**
**¼ cup pure pomegranate juice**
**1 cup still or sparkling water**
**Handful of fresh mint leaves (optional, to make it a mojito)**

Slice the lime half into thin rounds. Put the slices in a glass, and muddle the lime gently with a long-handled spoon. If using mint, muddle the mint leaves at this step.

Pour the juice and water over the lime slices and stir gently.

For special occasions, pour the mixture over two ice cubes in a cocktail glass or serve with sparkling water in a champagne flute.

**Note:** It is best not to drink sparkling water along with a meal, as the bubbles will disturb good digestion. Consider it a happy hour treat before dinner. Or enjoy it when you toast a special occasion!

# Chyawanprash Herbal Jam

**MAKES 16 OZ**

This recipe is labor-intensive, but with this effort, you undertake true medicine making. Chyawanparash (pronounced "CHA-wan-praash") is a famous immune-boosting jam that combines *amla* berries with synergistic ingredients to boost digestion and absorption of the vitamin-rich berries. Herbal jams are taken daily by the spoonful. This medicine is strengthening to all ages and good for all body types, especially in winter.

The list of benefits and uses for chyawanprash is long. Benefits mentioned in the texts include sharpness of mind and senses, sexual vigor, and general longevity. This formula is also said to promote growth in children. I was first introduced to it in India, where it often appears on family breakfast tables and is used by all ages like a multivitamin. It is the most famous among the rasayana formulas for healthy aging.

> 3 cups fresh amla berries*
>
> 8 cardamom pods
>
> 1 tbsp whole peppercorns
>
> One 1-inch cinnamon stick, or ½ tsp ground cinnamon
>
> 2 tbsp fennel seeds
>
> 5 strands saffron
>
> 6 tbsp ghee
>
> 1 cup evaporated cane juice
>
> 1 cup local raw honey

Rinse the berries well. Steam them in a pressure cooker for 10 minutes or on the stovetop until soft, about 30 minutes.

Grind the spices together in a spice grinder.

Remove the berries from the water, setting aside a few tablespoons of the water. Allow the berries to cool, then remove the pits.

Puree the berries in a blender until smooth, adding a tablespoon or two of the steaming water if necessary.

In a large saucepan, warm the ghee over medium heat.

Add the puree to the ghee and cook for 10 minutes, stirring occasionally.

Add the sugar and honey; stir until thick and sticky.

Add the spices, and stir over the heat for 5 more minutes.

Allow the jam to cool completely, and store in a sterile glass jar. It will keep on the shelf for at least one month.

Take about 1 tablespoon daily in the cold season. Always use a clean spoon when dipping in.

\* **Tip:** If you don't live in a place where amla berries are grown fresh, you can order them online or purchase them frozen, if that's what is available. Do not use dried fruits or amla powder.

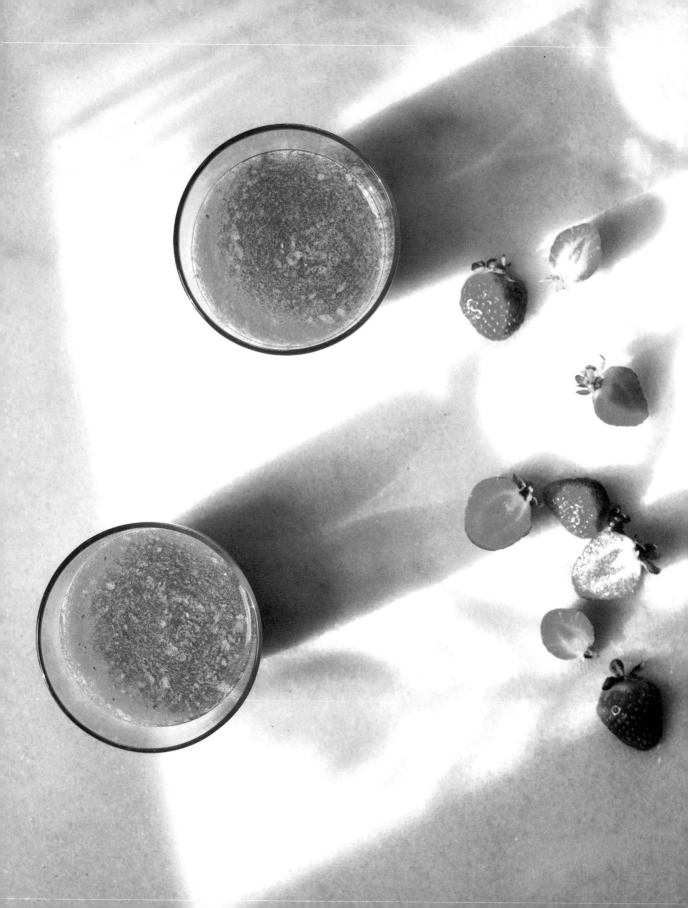

# Strawberry Rose Smash

**SERVES 1**

Who doesn't like a pink drink? Starting out the day with something bright, sour, and sweet provides a balance of building and purifying. This is a light and simple way to enjoy seasonal berries—you can use raspberries here if you prefer. This is a great way to incorporate chia seeds, a demulcent that moisturizes the digestive tract and supports elimination. This smash is best consumed in the morning before other foods.

> **1 tbsp chia seeds**
> **1½ cups water**
> **½ cup chopped strawberries**
> **1 tbsp Hibiscus Rose Cordial (page 312)**

Soak the chia seeds in ½ cup of the water for 5 minutes. Stir well.

Place all of the ingredients in a blender and blend on high until smooth.

Serve in a tall glass.

# Raspberry-Ginger Secret Smoothie

**SERVES 2**

What's the secret, you ask? Seaweed. Sounds crazy, I know. But sea moss (or Irish moss), a seaweed native to Ireland, contains 92 out of 102 trace minerals. It has the highest iodine content of any substance, which is essential to your thyroid and makes sea moss especially supportive to metabolic changes during menopause. This sea veggie is a demulcent, which lubricates and protects mucous membranes. Chocolate and raspberries provide the flavor.

Note that the sea moss must be prepared the night before for this recipe. Sea moss gel lasts up to one week in the refrigerator.

> 2 tbsp dried sea moss
>
> 2 tbsp water, plus more for soaking moss
>
> ¼ avocado
>
> 1½ cups raspberries
>
> 1 tbsp flaxseeds
>
> 2 tbsp cacao powder
>
> ½ tsp ground ginger
>
> 1½–2 cups almond milk
>
> 2–3 deglet noor or Medjool dates, pits removed and chopped into quarters

Place the sea moss in enough water to cover and leave to soak overnight.

Next morning, drain the sea moss and rinse well. Combine the sea moss and 2 tablespoons water in a blender and blend to make a gel.

Add the remaining ingredients and blend until smooth.

Pour into two glasses, and garnish with a few raspberries.

You can make this thicker with an extra tablespoon of sea moss and eat it like a pudding, or add more milk to make it a smoothie. Frozen raspberries will make a smoother final product.

# Raisin Mantha

**MAKES 1 QT**

Black raisins are "best among fruits" in Ayurveda. The dried black grape is sweet, cooling, and a little unctuous. *Mantha* means "mashed," and a mantha can be made with a combination of raisins, dates, and figs. Raisin mantha is an excellent medicine for reducing pitta in rakta dhatu and for nourishing rasa. This raisin mantha also promotes shukra. With its slight laxative effect, this drink alleviates bloating and constipation. Raisin water was a recommendation from my first Ayurveda doctor to give me energy and focus without taxing my digestion. Raisin mantha, strained, is useful for fasting and cleansing, as it keeps your energy up without challenging agni.

If you live in a country where prunes (dried plums) are available, these fruits have qualities and actions more similar to *draksha* than do "table grapes."

> ¼ cup black raisins or chopped prunes
>
> 1 qt water

Soak the dried fruit in the water for 1 to 3 hours. (I do this right in the blender.)

Blend well at high speed to puree.

Pour through a strainer into a glass jar. Discard the solids.

Drink between meals. This will keep in the refrigerator for up to three days.

**Note:** You can skip the straining step if you don't mind the raisin pieces.

# 23
# Medicinal Meals and Condiments

Any meal becomes medicinal when you tune in to the qualities of your food to foster balance. Your rasa, the liquid part of blood that circulates and nourishes your body, is responsible for your strength, satisfaction, and enthusiasm. Rasa directly builds all other tissues in the body; supports immunity; and makes babies, menstrual blood, and breast milk. Women need robust rasa. Since rasa is a direct result of well-digested food, the capacity of your meals to nourish, purify, and satisfy are intimately linked to your health and happiness. (For more on rasa, review chapter 3.)

The foods showcased in these recipes target the female generative system and boost the blood. Some meals nourish, and some cleanse. The introductions tell you how each recipe works, but feel free to make and eat something simply because it sounds delicious. Bodies are smart and will gravitate toward what they need. These meals are balanced in the six tastes, digestible, and pretty quick to make. The best homemade meal is the one you make without feeling stressed.

The chapter starts with lighter, breakfast-style dishes, but you can eat them at any time of day they appeal to you. Many of these light dishes are also indicated for cleansing and postpartum recovery. The recipes then move into main dishes: soups, curries, and kicharis of all kinds that you can rely on to support you in any stage of life. Finally, the end of the chapter presents super-food condiments, which are an ideal way to round out your meals with color, flavor, and qualities.

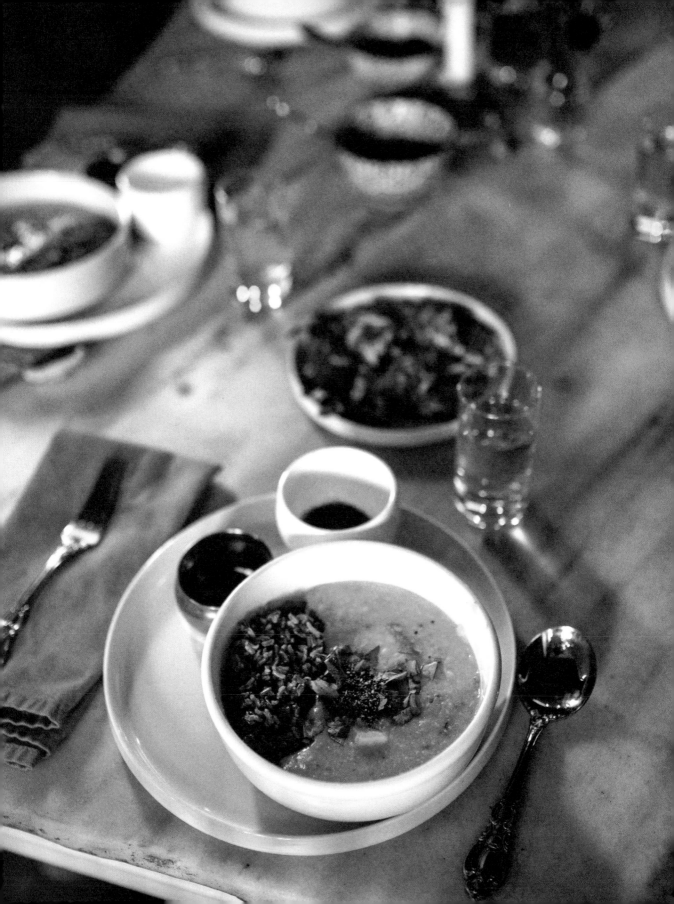

# Creamy Coconut Breakfast Kichari

**SERVES 2**

When you have a hankering for a sweet and creamy, wrapped-in-a-blanket kind of experience, here it is. This meal-worthy porridge is made with our big-time builder, urad dal. High mineral content from sugarcane and urad dal make this a filling and satisfying breakfast, and it can also be enjoyed in a warm ramekin as a dessert.

This recipe is a spin on a traditional preparation recommended in pregnancy and to support shukra, called *payasa vajikarana*. Payasa is a porridge-type sweet made of rice cooked with milk and sugar that has many variations.

> ½ cup urad dal
>
> ¼ cup basmati rice
>
> 2 cups water
>
> ½ tsp salt
>
> 2 tsp Sweet Rose Masala (page 236) or ground cinnamon
>
> ½ tsp ground ginger
>
> ¼ cup coconut sugar or evaporated cane juice
>
> 1 cup coconut milk

Soak the dal and rice in the saucepan in fresh, cool water for a few minutes, then rinse the dal and rice in a mesh sieve until water runs clear.

Place the water, rice, dal, salt, and spices in a medium saucepan over high heat. Bring to a boil. Reduce the heat and simmer, covered, for 30 minutes.

Remove from the heat and mash the mixture with a potato masher.

Stir in the sugar, then the coconut milk. Add another ½ cup of hot water if the mixture is too thick.

Serve warm in a soup bowl or a large mug.

# Yogurt Rice with Pomegranate Seeds

**SERVES 2 AS A MEAL OR 4 AS A SIDE**

Curd rice, or rice mixed with yogurt, is a South Indian staple. It is served at room temperature and feels refreshing at the end of a meal, in lieu of dessert, as a light breakfast, or at any time of day. This comes together quickly and is so light and satisfying that I often go for it as a meal in hot weather. You can go easy on the spices and try this as a quick meal for kids.

> **2 cups cooked basmati rice, cooled to room temperature**
>
> **2 cups fresh whole-fat yogurt**
>
> **2 tbsp finely chopped cilantro leaves**
>
> **2 tsp minced fresh ginger**
>
> **1 tsp salt**
>
> **2 tbsp pomegranate seeds, for garnish**
>
> **FOR THE TEMPERING**
>
> **2 tbsp sesame oil or ghee**
>
> **1 tsp urad dal**
>
> **1 tsp mustard seeds**
>
> **6 curry leaves, finely chopped**
>
> **¼ tsp hing powder**

In a large mixing bowl, mash the cooked rice with a fork or potato masher until the grains are partially broken up.

Add the yogurt and mix until uniform and smooth.

Stir in the cilantro, ginger, and salt.

*(continued)*

## MAKE THE TEMPERING

In a small frying pan, warm the oil over medium heat.

Add the urad dal and fry until they splutter.

Add the mustard seeds, curry leaves, and hing powder. Fry, stirring gently, until the curry leaves just begin to crisp.

Remove from the heat. Add the tempering to the rice immediately and stir to combine.

Serve garnished with fresh cilantro and a sprinkle of pomegranate seeds.

**Note:** Yogurt increases moisture in the body when eaten at night and is not recommended as dinner fare. Due to its sour taste, it is heating and aggravates pitta when eaten regularly. The fresher the yogurt is (more sweet and less sour), the less heating it is.

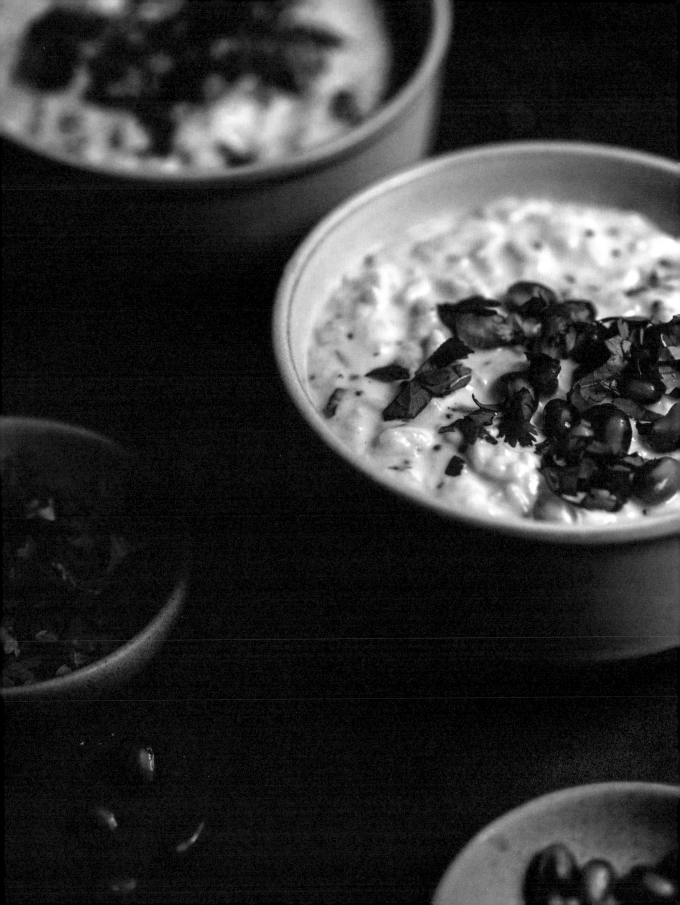

# Warming Wheat Soup

This drinkable soup, called *raab*, is a sort of cream of wheat. Primarily sweet in taste, with pungent digestive spices, this recipe brings hydration and nourishment and improves the digestive fire and immune system. This recipe is traditionally used to nourish the body and improve weak digestive fire, such as when you are sick or in early postpartum. Raab can also support lactation. This cuppa will likely appeal when more complicated things do not, and it is quick to make.

- 1½ tbsp whole-wheat, millet, or buckwheat flour
- 1 tsp ghee
- 1¼ cups water
- 2 tsp maple syrup, coconut sugar, or evaporated cane juice
- ⅛ tsp ajwain seeds
- ⅛ tsp ground ginger

In a deep frying pan over medium heat, sauté the flour in the ghee until it browns, about 1 to 2 minutes.

Add the rest of the ingredients and cook for 3 minutes, stirring constantly with a whisk.

Drink immediately. (The flour will begin to clump, or sink, if it sits.)

# Spiced Barley Soup

**SERVES 4**

Barley is a dry but hearty grain with an affinity for the uterus and bladder. Barley reduces excess moisture in the body and cleanses the bladder and uterus. A thin cereal made of barley and long pepper is a traditional formula for the first postpartum days. This soup is also good for clearing congestion and reducing fever.

> 10 cups water
>
> 1 cup barley, soaked overnight and strained
>
> 1 tsp salt
>
> 1 tsp ground cumin
>
> 1 tsp ground turmeric
>
> 1 tsp ground ginger
>
> ½ tsp ground black pepper or long pepper (*pippali*)

Combine all ingredients in a large pot and cover partially. Bring to a boil over medium heat, then turn down to simmer for 1 hour or until the grains break up and the soup appears creamy.

Stir well before ladling into soup bowls.

Serve warm as a light meal, or drink it throughout the day to hydrate and nourish when fasting. Add more hot water if necessary when reheating.

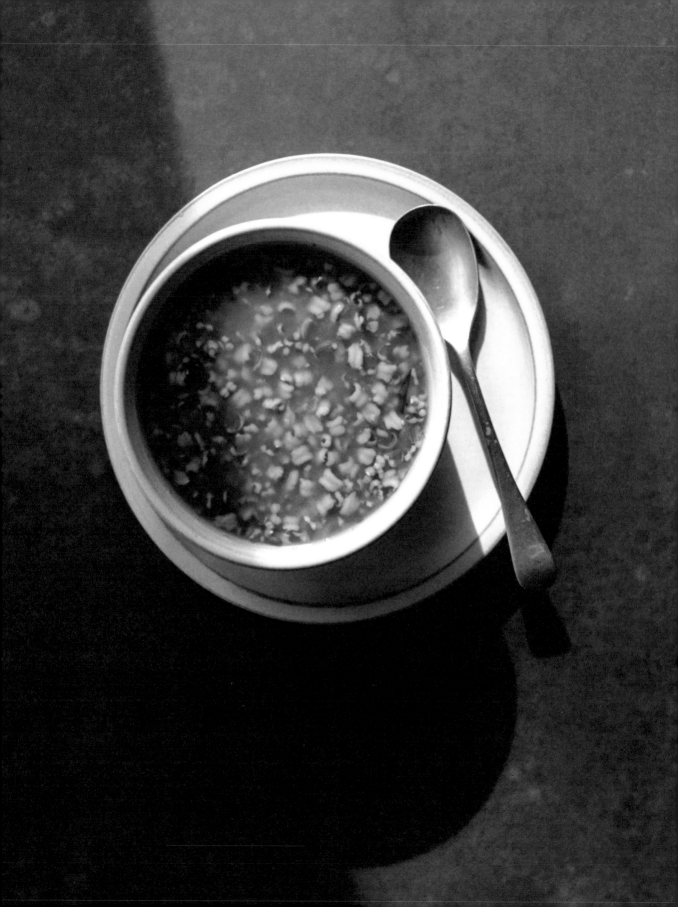

# Red Rice Kanji

**SERVES 2–4**

*Kanji* is a medicinal porridge used to rehabilitate the appetite after cleansing or illness, or when agni is low. Traditionally, it is made with highly nutritious red rice, considered the most nutritious among rice varieties. If you can't find red rice, brown rice will do. This is a great meal on heavy days of your period when you don't have much appetite or any time your digestive fire feels down. You can even fast on kanji for a half-day, full day or until the fire returns.

- ½ cup red rice
- One 2-inch strip of kombu
- 4 cups water
- ½ tsp ground ginger
- ½ tsp ground cinnamon
- ½ tsp salt

Rinse the rice well. Cover the rice and kombu with 1 cup of the water to soak.

Bring the rest of the water to a boil in a large saucepan over high heat.

Add the rice, seaweed, soaking water, and spices to the boiling water. Reduce the heat, cover, and simmer for an hour.

Remove from the heat and stir well.

Ladle the liquid into a bowl or mug, adding in some of the grains of rice. Add coconut milk if desired.

**Pressure/slow cooker variation:** Pressure cook the kanji for 15 minutes, then allow the pressure to release naturally (at least 10 minutes).

# Essential Mineral Vegetable Broth

**MAKES 3½ CUPS**

This broth recipe is incredibly nutritious and easy to digest. Its uses for women's health are many, due to its ability to provide excellent rasa dhatu. Vegetable broth can be enjoyed as a beverage with a meal, between meals, or while fasting, and it is used as a base for soups and in cooking grains and beans to add flavor and nutrition. Try keeping a bag of vegetable scraps (like kale stems and sweet potato skins) in the freezer so you can simmer them with herbs and sea vegetables to make your own vegetable broth. You can start from scratch, but I love being able to use scraps for this.

> 5 cups roughly chopped vegetables (carrots, potatoes, leeks, kale, parsnips,
>   fennel, washed organic vegetable skins, winter squash rinds)
> ½ cup burdock root pieces, chopped into thin slices
> 2 tbsp ghee
> Handful of fresh herbs (thyme, oregano, parsley, cilantro, etc.), stems included
> 1 bay leaf
> 1 bunch scallions or garlic scapes, sliced
> One 6-inch strip of kombu
> ⅓ cup dried dulse or wakame, cut into small pieces
> ½ tsp salt
> Pinch of ground black pepper
> 7 cups water

In a large, heavy-bottomed pot over medium heat, cook the vegetables and burdock root in the ghee for 10 minutes, stirring occasionally, until they begin to soften. Add the rest of the ingredients and bring to a boil. Reduce the heat to low, cover partially, and simmer 1½ to 2 hours.

Remove from the heat and strain through a metal mesh sieve into a glass bowl or other heatproof container, pressing on the vegetables with the back of a spoon to extract as much flavor as possible.

Allow the broth to cool completely, then transfer to glass storage jars. Keep in the fridge for up to one week, or freeze and use within one month.

# Yellow Dal Supreme

**SERVES 4–6**

This is my favorite summer soup! The astringency of summer squash tones down excess water element. This recipe is thinner and lighter, but you can cut the water down to 4 cups for a thicker soup if your appetite is hearty. If you're on your period or have variable agni, go lighter. This mung bean soup is meant to help your body get rid of ama (unwanted toxins) while nourishing your tissues and keeping up your strength.

1 cup yellow split mung beans

One 1-inch strip of kombu

5 cups water

1 tsp ground turmeric

1 tsp ground coriander

1 tsp Essential Spice Mix (page 238)

½ tsp salt

2 small or 1 big yellow summer squash

FOR THE TEMPERING

2 tsp coconut oil

1 tsp cumin or ajwain seeds

1 tsp mustard seeds

Big handful of curry leaves

Juice of ½ lime or lemon

2 tbsp chopped cilantro

Rinse the split mung beans under cold water until the water runs clear. Soak the beans and kombu in 4 cups of the water in a large saucepan overnight, or for at least a few hours.

Bring the soaked beans and kombu to a boil in the saucepan over medium heat. Add the spices and salt to the pot.

Chop the squash into half-moons (you should have about 2 cups) and add to the pot.

When the mixture comes to a boil, reduce the heat to low, and simmer for 30 minutes with the cover slightly ajar. If you want a thin soup, add the remaining cup of water after about 20 minutes and re-cover. No need to stir.

Heat the coconut oil in a pan over medium heat. Add the cumin, mustard seeds, and curry leaves, and sauté until you can smell them, just 2 or 3 minutes.

Add this to the dal and simmer uncovered for the last 5 minutes.

Remove from the heat and add the lime juice.

Serve with a topping of fresh cilantro, Mixed Greens Chutney (page 297), or a side of grain or cooked veggies.

## Speaking of the Supreme

Rinsing beans and grains well will remove most of the residual impurities left after harvesting, but some will remain. In Hindu legend, a poison, *hala hala*, was created when demons and devas churned the ocean to obtain the nectar of immortality (*amrita*). Early in the process of cooking grains, a foam gathers on top of the boiling water. Skimming off some of the foam from the sides of the pot is a good practice. I like to think of my food as amrita while I purify my dal, skimming the hala hala with a large spoon.

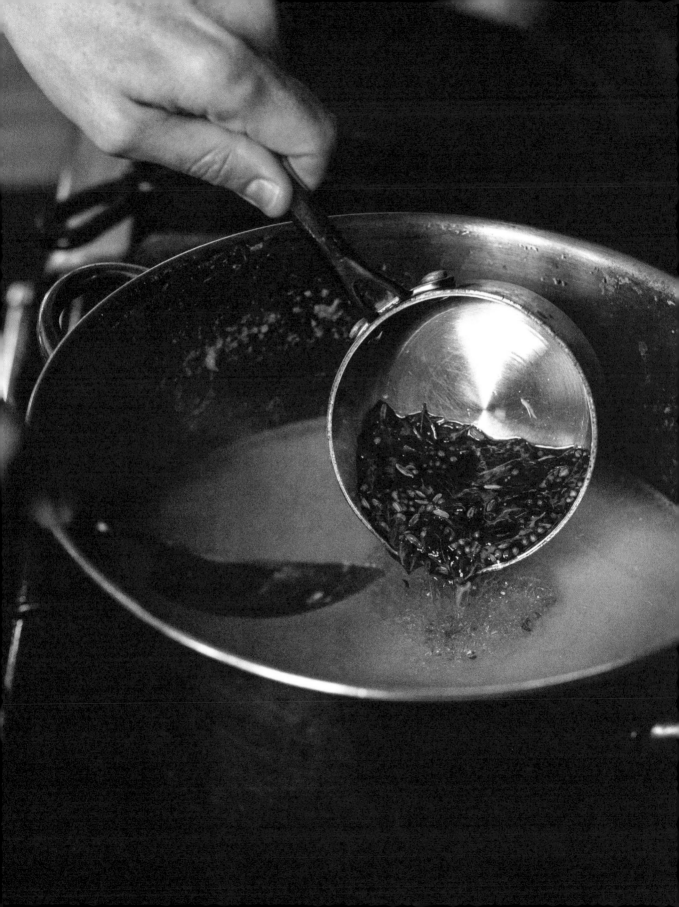

# Chicken Soup with Coriander and Lemon

This recipe was contributed by my friend Adena, an Ayurveda practitioner who specializes in women's health. In her story on page 165, she speaks to the sometimes controversial choice between vegetarian and nonvegetarian foods during pregnancy and postpartum. I chose to include a meat soup recipe because Ayurveda texts share many details about the medicinal uses of meat. Flesh is earth element and the most direct building food available. Meat is a reliable choice for remedying vata imbalance and to stave it off when the body needs the grounding of earth element, such as during pregnancy, breastfeeding, and menopause.

In Ayurveda, the dense quality of meat is always diluted in a soup. The larger and slower an animal is, the heavier the meat, and the more grounding and slowing it will be in your body. For example, chicken is light compared to red meats.

Further, the qualities of domesticated animal meat are considered heavier than those of animals raised in the wild. Domesticated animals tend to be less active, and their meat increases kapha more than that of wild game. If you feel strong eating vegetarian foods, there is no obligation to introduce animal substances. Keep up with your sea vegetables, and if the demands of childbearing or aging (or life!) begin to cause imbalances, consider that meat soup is a traditional medicine.

| | |
|---|---|
| 1 tbsp coconut oil | 4 cups chicken broth (recipe below) |
| ½ red onion, thinly sliced | Juice of 1 lemon |
| 1 tbsp chopped fresh gingerroot | ½ tsp salt |
| ½ tsp ground coriander | 2 tbsp kelp powder |
| 1 tsp curry powder | ⅓ cup roughly chopped cilantro |
| 1 bunch of broccolini, cut into 1-inch pieces | 2 cups cooked and diced or shredded chicken (roast chicken recipe below) |
| ½ cup grated carrot | ⅓ cup coconut milk |

Melt the coconut oil in a large, heavy-bottomed pot over medium heat.

Add the sliced onion and ginger, and sauté until the onion softens.

Add the coriander and curry powder; stir. Add the chopped broccolini and the carrot; stir to coat the vegetables with oil.

Add the chicken broth, lemon juice, salt, and kelp powder; bring everything to a simmer uncovered for 5 minutes.

Add the cilantro, chopped chicken, and coconut milk and heat through for a maximum of another 5 minutes.

Remove from the heat and taste for salt. Serve by itself or over a cooked grain.

## To Roast a Chicken

**Juice of 1 lemon**

**2 tbsp ghee, melted**

**Salt (¾ tsp per pound of chicken)**

**1 tbsp dried thyme**

**One 4- to 5-lb chicken**

One 4- to 5-lb chickenHeat the oven to 400°F.

Combine the lemon juice, ghee, salt, and thyme in a small bowl; whisk to combine.

Wash the chicken, pat dry, and remove the giblets from the cavity. Tie the legs with a piece of twine or use a small pan to keep them together.

Place the chicken in an ovenproof dish.

Rub the lemon mixture over the chicken, and drizzle any remaining mixture over the chicken to use the entire bowl. You may choose to put half of the lemon rind inside the chicken.

Place the chicken, breast side up, in a roasting pan. Bake for about 90 minutes, uncovered. Test for doneness by piercing between the drumstick and thigh, and make sure the juice runs clear, not pink.

Remove from the oven, cover with foil, and let rest for at least 20 minutes.

## To Make Simple Chicken Bone Broth            MAKES ABOUT 2 QUARTS

Remove the skin and meat from the chicken carcass.

Reserve 2 cups of the meat for the preceding soup recipe, and save the rest for another use.

Place all the chicken bones in a large stockpot and cover with 12 cups of water. Simmer covered on low for 10 to 12 hours, or pressure cook for 3 hours.

Remove the bones and discard. Use a fine mesh sieve to strain the broth into a large mason jar for the fridge or freezer.

Use within one week, or freeze and use within one month.

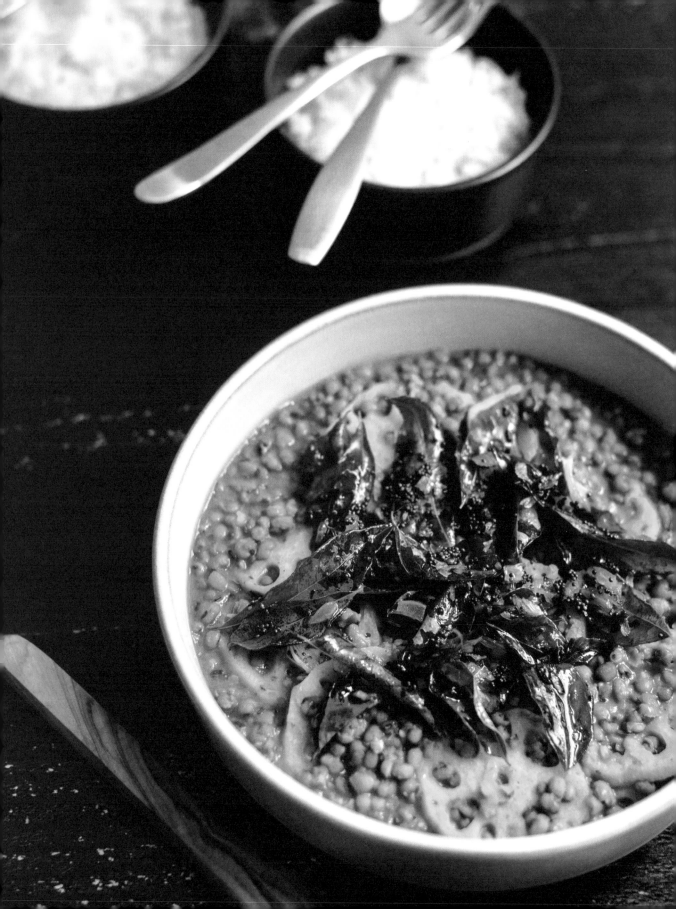

# Lotus Root Curry

Lotus root is cooling, sweet, and astringent. Lotus is a symbolic flower prevalent in images of Lakshmi, the goddess of abundance. The flowers rise up from swamps like phoenixes and are symbols of renewal. Lotus is favored for women's health, not only for its associations with the goddess, but especially as a pitta reducer and purifier of rakta dhatu.

In addition to healing conditions of heat in the bladder and blood, lotus root calms agitation of the mind. All parts of the lotus plant are used medicinally, but the root is delicious, like water chestnut, and enjoyed in cultures throughout Asia. Due to its astringency, the lotus root is a bit dry, so prepare this recipe like stew, with extra water or broth.

| | |
|---|---|
| 2 cups lotus root | 1 tbsp Essential Spice Mix (page 238) |
| ½ cup green mung beans, soaked overnight | 1 tbsp ghee or sesame oil |
| | ¼ cup chopped onion (optional) |
| 2 ½ cups water (or more to taste) | 1 tsp mustard seeds |
| ½ tsp ground turmeric | Small handful of curry leaves (optional) |
| ⅛ tsp hing powder | 1 tsp salt |

Wash the lotus root and mung beans. Chop the lotus root into ½-inch chunks.

In a medium saucepan, bring the water, mung beans, and lotus root to a boil over high heat. Add the turmeric, hing powder, and spice mix.

Cover and reduce the heat; simmer for 45 minutes. Check at about 30 minutes, and add more hot water if needed.

In a large frying pan, warm the ghee over medium heat.

Add the onion, if using, and sauté until soft. Add the mustard seeds and curry leaves (if using), and sauté until they splutter.

Add the salt and seasoned oil to the cooked mung and lotus root mixture; stir to combine over low heat.

Simmer covered until the curry thickens, or add more hot water if it is too thick.

Serve thicker, as a vegetable side, or stew-like over rice.

**Note:** You may have access to fresh lotus root, or you can find this frozen and already sliced.

# Every Body Dal

SERVES 4

I recommend this as your new go-to fast meal. Small beans like lentils are tridoshic and easy for most people to digest, whereas large beans can cause wind, which we should avoid during menstruation and postpartum. This dal cooks fast and is very versatile because you can add all kinds of different spices and vegetables. Dal builds and detoxes; in Ayurveda, it is a perfect food. In cool weather, I add cubed winter squash at the start of cooking. In summer, I add chopped zucchini for the last 10 minutes. And I always add kale!

**4 cups water**

**1 cup red lentils**

**1 tbsp (or more) Essential Spice Mix (page 238)**

**1 cup chopped kale or other vegetables of your choice**

**1 tbsp ghee or coconut oil**

**Chopped cilantro to garnish**

Bring the water to a boil in a soup pot over high heat.

Add the lentils and spice mix, and return to a boil. Reduce the heat and simmer for about 20 minutes.

Add the kale, and more hot water if needed; simmer for 10 minutes more.

Remove from the heat, stir in the oil, and sprinkle with cilantro. Serve with grain, bread, dosa, or a vegetable side.

## Time-Saving Tips

Red lentils are a fast-cooking legume. They don't need to be soaked beforehand, but if you do, the dal will be creamy in less than 30 minutes. This recipe is so quick and easy you can make it fresh each time and avoid eating leftovers

# Spicy Black Gram Soup

**SERVES 4**

The black gram legume becomes cream colored when skinned and split; then it is called urad dal. Along with a high mineral and protein content, urad has a slippery quality that gives it a laxative action. Ayurveda texts describe this legume as strength-promoting, especially for muscle tissue (making it a good choice for vegetarians), and it increases shukra and breast milk.

This decadent recipe is ideal for vata types who experience constipation in cold, dry weather because the soup will warm and moisten. This style of dal is more commonly found in northern India, where the weather can be colder and drier. It may remind you of *dal makhani* from Indian restaurant menus. Urad is heavy and slower to digest, which is why I paired it with lighter mung dal.

½ cup split urad dal

½ cup split mung dal

4 cups water

½ tsp ground turmeric

1 tbsp Essential Spice Mix (page 238)

2 tbsp ghee

1 cup tomato puree or tomato sauce

1 tsp garam masala

¼ tsp hing powder

1 tbsp fenugreek leaves (optional)

1 tsp salt

4 tbsp heavy cream or coconut cream (optional)

Rinse both types of beans well and soak together overnight.

In a large saucepan, bring the 4 cups of water, beans, turmeric, and spice mix to a boil over high heat.

Reduce the heat and simmer covered for 45 minutes. Use a hand blender to blend the dal partially in the pot, leaving it chunky but creamy.

In a medium frying pan, warm the ghee over medium heat.

*(continued)*

Add the tomato, garam masala, and hing. If using fenugreek, crush the leaves into the mixture with your hands. Sauté for 5 minutes.

Add the tomato mixture to the dal. Add a little hot water if the soup is too thick. Simmer covered over medium heat for 10 minutes.

Remove from the heat, and add salt to taste.

Pour the soup into wide bowls and swirl 1 tablespoon of the cream, if using, over each bowl before serving.

Serve with a cooked vegetable and a grain.

**Pressure/slow cooker variation:** Pressure cook the beans, turmeric, and spice mix for 10 minutes, then allow the pressure to release naturally. You don't need to soak the beans first if you're using pressure. You can use the slow cooker on sauté to continue with the recipe after you cook the dal. This is a great option if you are using the whole bean.

**Dosha note:** Due to the spices, tomato, and the heating nature of urad, this soup can aggravate pitta. The heavy, moist qualities can aggravate kapha, so kapha people are better off with other legumes, such as chickpeas and, of course, mung beans.

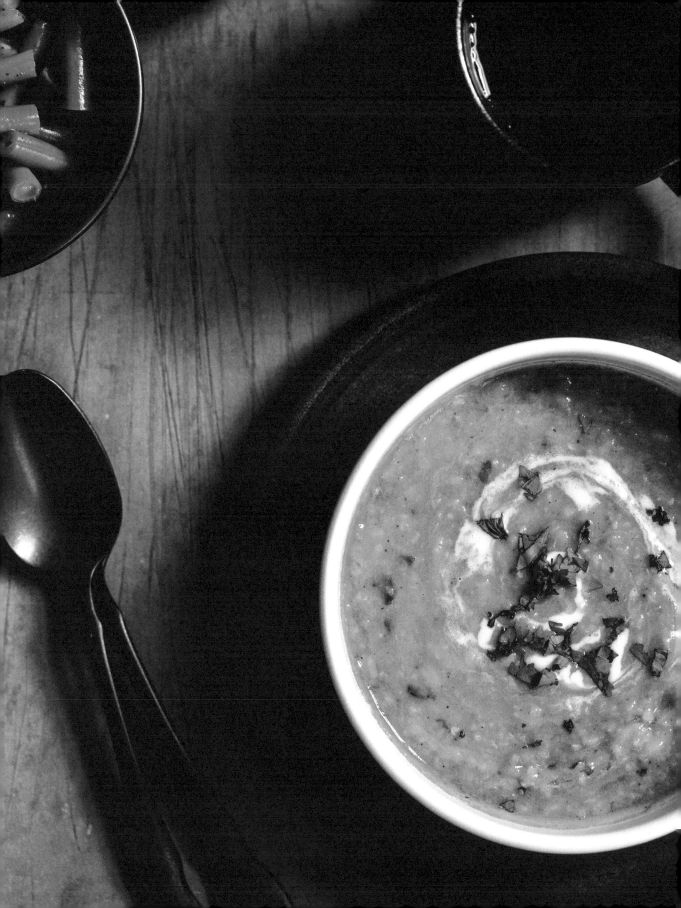

# Beets and Barley Stew

**SERVES 4–6**

This gingery one-pot meal is a purifying combo that is also filling and sweet. Barley and beets together tone the uterus and build the blood. The secret here is a little white rice. White basmati rice gives a creamy smooth texture to a whole-grain dish. I always add $\frac{1}{4}$ cup to whole-grain kicharis.

½ cup green mung beans, soaked overnight

½ cup barley, soaked overnight

4 cups water

¼ cup white basmati rice

¼ tsp hing powder

½ tsp ground turmeric

1 tbsp Essential Spice Mix (page 238)

2 tbsp ghee

1 tbsp grated fresh ginger

½ tsp ajwain or cumin seeds

½ cup chopped, peeled beets

1 cup chopped carrots

1 tsp salt

1 cup chopped parsley

Lemon quarters, to garnish

Drain and rinse the beans and barley.

In a large stockpot, bring the 4 cups of water, beans, and grains to a boil over high heat.

Add the hing, turmeric, and spice mix; reduce the heat to low and simmer covered for 45 minutes, until most of the water is absorbed.

About 15 minutes before the grains finish cooking, warm the ghee in a frying pan over medium heat.

Add the ginger and ajwain or cumin seeds, and fry for 2 minutes, until the seeds are golden brown and fragrant.

Add the chopped vegetables and toss to combine. Add 2 tbsp water. Cover and steam for 10 minutes or until soft. The smaller the vegetable pieces, the faster they will cook. Use a fork to test for doneness.

Add the cooked veg and salt to the grain mixture, and stir to combine. Remove from the heat and let stand for 5 minutes.

Ladle the stew into bowls. Pile a few tablespoons of parsley on top of each bowl just before serving and top with a lemon quarter to be squeezed and stirred in before eating.

**Pressure/slow cooker variation:** Rinse the soaked beans, barley, and rice, then pressure cook them, along with the hing and spices for 18 minutes in $4\frac{1}{2}$ cups of water.

Sauté the veggies as described above, and add them to the cooker; mix well. Cover and let stand for 5 minutes before serving with parsley and lemon.

# New Moon Kichari

**SERVES 4**

Light, simple, and formulated to reduce any gas or bloating, this is a great meal to sustain you on the heavy days of your period or during a cleanse. A traditional kichari, this makes a smooth, soft, comforting bowl. Increase the ratio of mung to rice if you need it heartier.

6 cups water

1 cup basmati rice

½ cup yellow split mung beans (ideally soaked for one hour or more)

1 tbsp Essential Spice Mix (page 238) or 1 tsp each thyme, oregano, and/or basil (fresh or dried)

Pinch of hing powder (optional)

1 cup coarsely chopped fennel bulb

1 cup chopped kale, stems removed

½–1 tsp salt

Chopped cilantro, for garnish

FOR THE TEMPERING

1–2 tbsp ghee

½ tsp each ajwain, coriander, and fennel seeds (optional; see note)

Bring 5 cups of the water to a boil in a large saucepan over high heat. Set the other cup of water aside to add during cooking as needed.

Rinse the rice and beans twice, or until the water runs clear.

Add the beans, rice, spice mix, and hing (if using) to the water in the saucepan and wait for it to boil on high. Immediately reduce the heat and simmer, with the cover ajar, for 15 minutes. Do not stir.

Add the fennel and kale on top to steam for 15 minutes. At this point, add more hot water if it is getting dry. Pour the water on top and do not stir.

Simmer 10 minutes more if the beans are still in their original shape; they should break up and be unrecognizable.

## Make the Tempering

Warm the ghee in a small skillet over medium heat; add the ajwain, coriander, and fennel seeds (if using). When the seeds pop, about 2 to 3 minutes, pour into the kichari.

Add salt, stir well, and let stand covered for a few minutes.

Kichari should have a soupy, soft consistency; serve it as you would a stew. Garnish with fresh cilantro.

**Note:** Omit the tempering spices if you're using thyme, oregano, and/or basil; simply stir in the ghee and top with the herbs before serving.

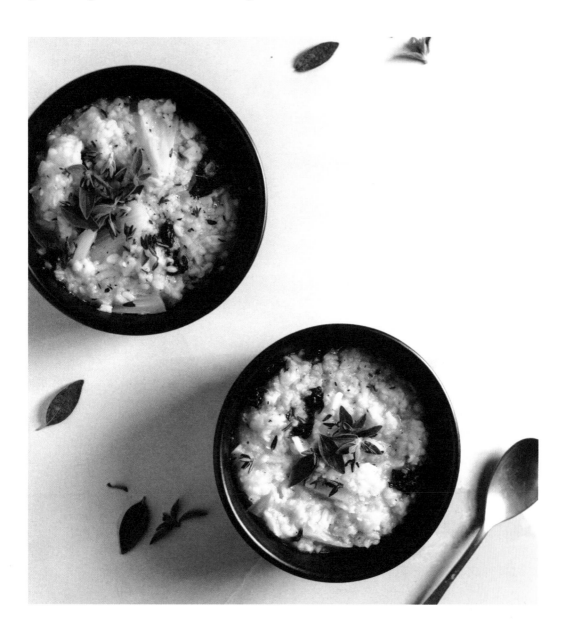

# Umami Kichari

This warming and savory stew contains onion and garlic, which ground the mind and support the libido and immunity in the cold months. Urad dal is said to strengthen the uterus, skin, and hair, as well as support lactation. This legume is usually used in small quantities and mixed with mung beans or rice, as in this kichari recipe. This soup will support you best when taken by itself as a meal—it has everything you need. If you are craving chocolate or calorie-dense snacks, work this builder into your diet.

½ cup urad dal

½ cup basmati rice

One 2-inch strip of kombu

5 cups water

1–2 tbsp ghee

1 clove garlic, minced

¼ cup chopped red onion

2 tbsp minced gingerroot

1 tbsp Essential Spice Mix (page 238)

1 cup chopped kale

2 tsp salt

1 tbsp apple cider or rice vinegar

Cilantro or parsley, to garnish

Rinse the dal and rice together until the water runs clear. Soak them, with the kombu, in the water overnight.

In a large saucepan, bring the soaked mixture to a boil over high heat, then reduce the heat to low and simmer while you fry the garlic and onion.

In a small frying pan, warm the ghee over medium-high heat.

Add the garlic and onion, and sauté for about 1 to 2 minutes, until they begin to brown. Add the ginger, give it a quick stir, and remove from the heat.

Remove the kombu from the rice and dal mixture. Add the ghee mixture, spice mix, and kale to the simmering pot. Do not stir; allow the kale to steam on top. Cover and cook for 30 minutes.

Remove from the heat; stir in the salt and vinegar. Add another ½ cup of hot water if the kichari is too thick.

Spoon into bowls and serve with a garnish of cilantro or parsley.

# Beet Love Two Ways: Gingered Beet Soup and Herbed Beet Pickles

Beets are one of those unique foods that both purify and build red blood. Beets mobilize agni with a sharp quality and build blood with sweet and astringent tastes.

Beets are messy, however, and I've created these two recipes to allow you to prepare a few pounds of beets at one time and work them into a couple of meals. I cook up the beets and pickle a week's worth, then make soup with the rest. In cold weather I eat beet pickles with a meal almost daily, and I enjoy beet soup when I'm on my moon cycle. The brightness of beets is especially welcome in late winter; they invigorate not just the agni but also the mind.

To prepare enough beets for both recipes, simply follow the instructions for boiling and peeling them, using about $2\frac{1}{2}$ pounds of beets total and enough water to cover them all.

## Gingered Beet Soup                                      SERVES 4

> **4 cups water**
>
> **1 lb beets (about 3 medium beets without tops)**
>
> **2 cups full-fat coconut milk**
>
> **1 cup vegetable broth**
>
> **1–2 tsp grated fresh gingerroot**
>
> **1 tsp salt**
>
> **Ground black pepper to taste**

In a large saucepan, bring the water to a boil over high heat.

Wash the beets and drop them into the water, untrimmed. Add more water if needed to cover the beets. Cover, and reduce the heat to simmer for 45 to 60 minutes, until soft. Check the softness with a fork or knife tip after 45 minutes.

Drain the beets and let them cool by submerging them in a bowl of cold water in the kitchen sink. When they are cool enough to touch, drain off the water, move them to a cutting board, and trim off the tops and tails. Under cold running water, slide the skin off the beets one at a time.

Cut the cooked beets into halves or quarters and place them in a blender.

Add the rest of the ingredients and blend to a smooth puree.

Return to the saucepan and heat to the desired temperature.

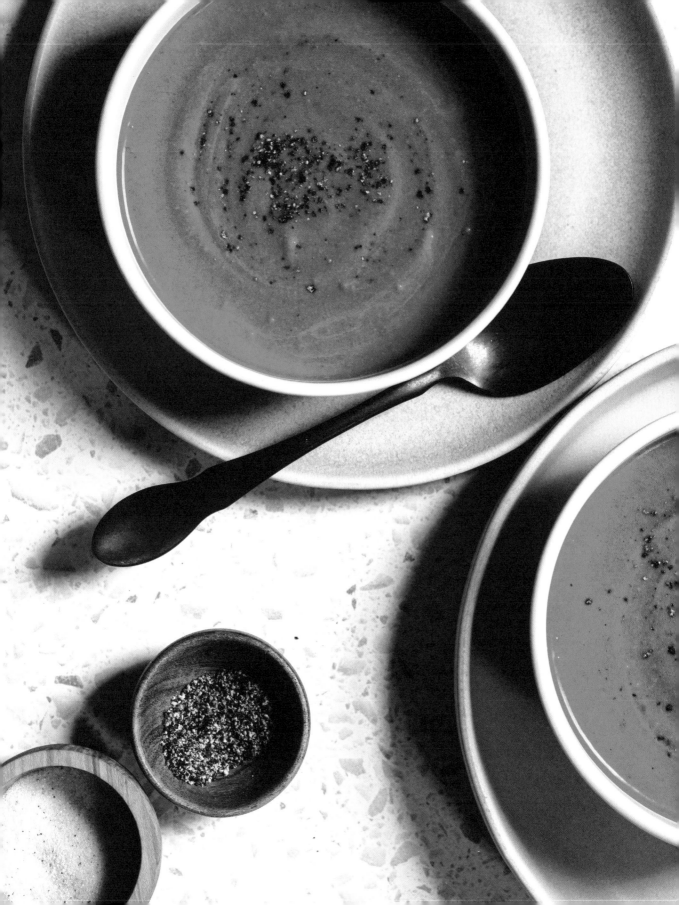

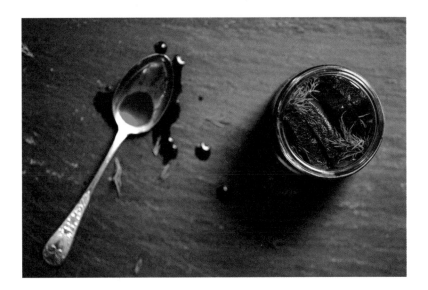

## Herbed Beet Pickles

**MAKE 1½ CUPS**

**About 1½ lbs beets (2 large or 3 medium), trimmed**

**½ cup apple cider vinegar**

**½ cup water**

**3 sprigs of fresh herbs, like dill, rosemary, or basil**

**½ tsp salt**

In a large saucepan, bring enough water to cover the beets to a boil over high heat.

Wash the beets and drop them into the water, untrimmed. Return to a boil. Cover, and reduce the heat to simmer for 45 to 60 minutes, until soft. Check the softness with a fork or knife tip after 45 minutes.

Drain the beets and let them cool by submerging them in a bowl of cold water in the kitchen sink. When they are cool enough to touch, drain off the water, move them to a cutting board, and trim off the tops and tails. Under cold running water, slide the skin off the beets one at a time.

Slice the cooked beets into ¼-inch rounds, then into half-moons or sticks. Place in a glass jar.

Mix the vinegar, water, herbs, and salt together in a bowl. Pour into the jar, making sure the beets are covered with the brining liquid by at least 1 inch.

Refrigerate in the jar overnight and shake before serving.

The pickles keep for two weeks in the fridge. Shake the jar every day for best results.

**Pressure/slow cooker variation:** To cook the beets, place them in the cooker with about 1 inch of water. Pressure cook for 20 minutes for large beets and 15 minutes for small. Allow the pressure to come down for 10 minutes, then release naturally. Follow the remaining recipe instructions for cooling, peeling, and preparing.

# Warm Arame and Kale Salad

**SERVES 4 AS A SIDE**

Arame, a dark and mineral-rich sea vegetable, is packed with blood builders. This recipe purifies with kale's bitter taste and nourishes with sweet, sour, and salty tastes. Sesame is another mineral powerhouse. Ayurveda considers sesame oil to be the best among vegetable oils because it is vata pacifying and easy to assimilate into the tissues. Be sure to purchase untoasted sesame oil to ensure it is fresh.

½ cup dried arame seaweed

1 tsp + 2 tbsp sesame oil

1 tbsp grated fresh ginger

1 head lacinato kale

2 tbsp water or broth

1 tbsp tamari, plus extra to taste

1 tbsp Triple Mineral Gomasio, (page 299) or toasted sesame seeds, for garnish

Ground black pepper to taste

Soak the seaweed in warm water for 7 to 10 minutes, then rinse and drain.

Toss the drained seaweed in a mixing bowl with 1 tsp sesame oil and the ginger. Set it aside to let the flavors meld as you work on the kale.

Strip the kale leaves off the stems and chop into 2-inch pieces. Set aside.

Whisk the water and tamari together; set aside.

In a frying pan, fry the seaweed mixture in 1 tbsp of the sesame oil. Sauté 1 minute, until warmed through, then transfer back to the bowl.

Add the last tablespoon of the oil to the same pan, and toss the kale in it until all pieces are coated. Add the tamari mixture to the kale and toss to coat.

Cover and steam over low heat for about 10 minutes, until the kale is soft and tender but still green. Add another splash or two of water if needed to keep the kale from sticking to the pan.

Remove the cover and add the seaweed to the pan. Toss the kale and seaweed until there is almost no water in the bottom of the pan, about 1 to 2 minutes. Kale should be tender but not mushy.

Garnish with Triple Mineral Gomasio and a bit of black pepper.

**Pro tip:** Top the salad with cubes of tofu fried in sesame oil, ginger, and tamari for a heartier meal.

# Pumpkin Seed Cilantro Pâté

**MAKES 2 CUPS**

Including a variety of seeds in the diet provides an array of blood- and bone-building minerals. Pumpkin seeds are sweet and oily, and they are used as an antiparasitic. Walnuts are highlighted in Ayurveda texts as an aphrodisiac. Combine this with cooling cilantro leaves for a balanced condiment that provides all six tastes to round out any meal. Serve a big spoonful with rice or atop kicharis and dals.

**1 cup pumpkin seeds**

**½ cup walnuts**

**3 cups water**

**One bunch cilantro**

**1 tsp salt**

**2 tbsp olive oil**

**Juice of ½ lemon**

**1 tsp raw honey**

**2 tbsp miso paste**

Soak the pumpkin seeds and walnuts together in the water overnight. Drain, rinse, and place in a food processor.

Rinse the cilantro, pat dry, and cut off the stems. Place in the food processor along with the rest of the ingredients and process until smooth.

Transfer to a small container and refrigerate. Use within seven days.

**Tips:** If you don't like cilantro, parsley works well in this recipe.

You can use either white or red miso. Red will have a stronger, soy sauce–flavor. White is very mild.

# Carrot and Green Bean Palya

**SERVES 2**

This method of steaming vegetables in spices with coconut is versatile and can be used for winter squash, cabbage, and beets, to name a few. This is a pleasing and colorful combination to have alongside dosa, dal, and grain dishes.

Hing, a gum resin with an onion-like taste, is used in Ayurveda to redirect apana downward and soothe gas and bloating. Use only a pinch, as its flavor is strong. Hing powder, the easiest form to cook with, can be purchased at Indian markets and suppliers listed in appendix C.

> **1 tbsp coconut oil**
>
> **1 tsp mustard seeds**
>
> **Pinch of hing powder (optional)**
>
> **1 cup green beans, trimmed and cut into 1-inch pieces**
>
> **1 cup diced carrots**
>
> **¼ cup finely shredded coconut**
>
> **1 tsp ground cinnamon**
>
> **½ tsp salt**
>
> **¼ cup water**

Warm the coconut oil in a large skillet over medium heat. Add the mustard seeds and hing (if using), and sauté in the oil for 2 to 3 minutes. Cover the pan so the seeds don't escape when they pop.

Add the green beans, carrots, and shredded coconut; cook for a few more seconds, stirring to distribute the oil and seeds throughout. Add the cinnamon and salt, then the water. Stir, cover, and reduce the heat to low. Simmer for 10 minutes.

Remove from the heat and serve warm.

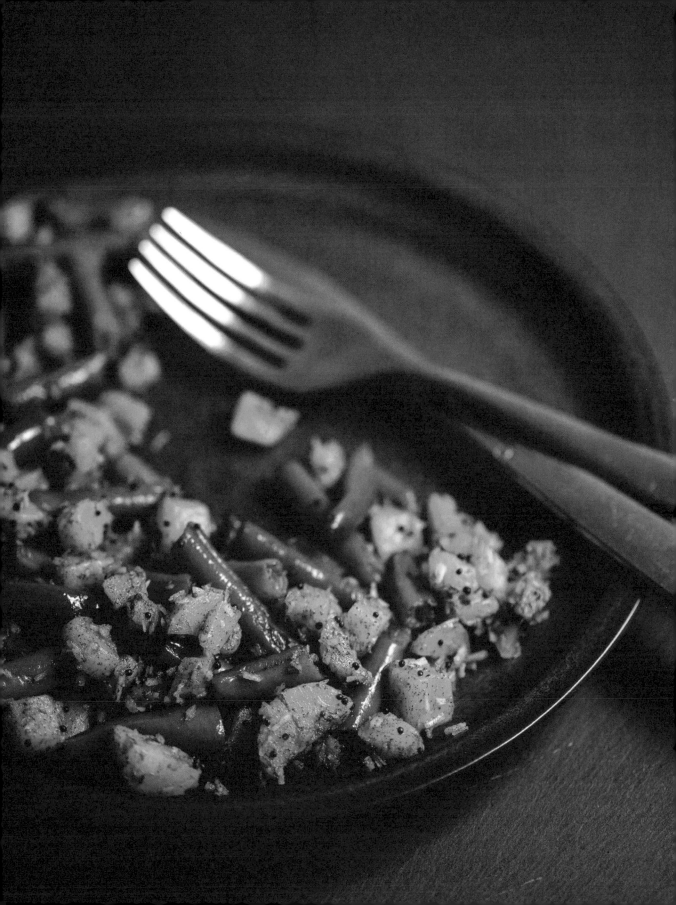

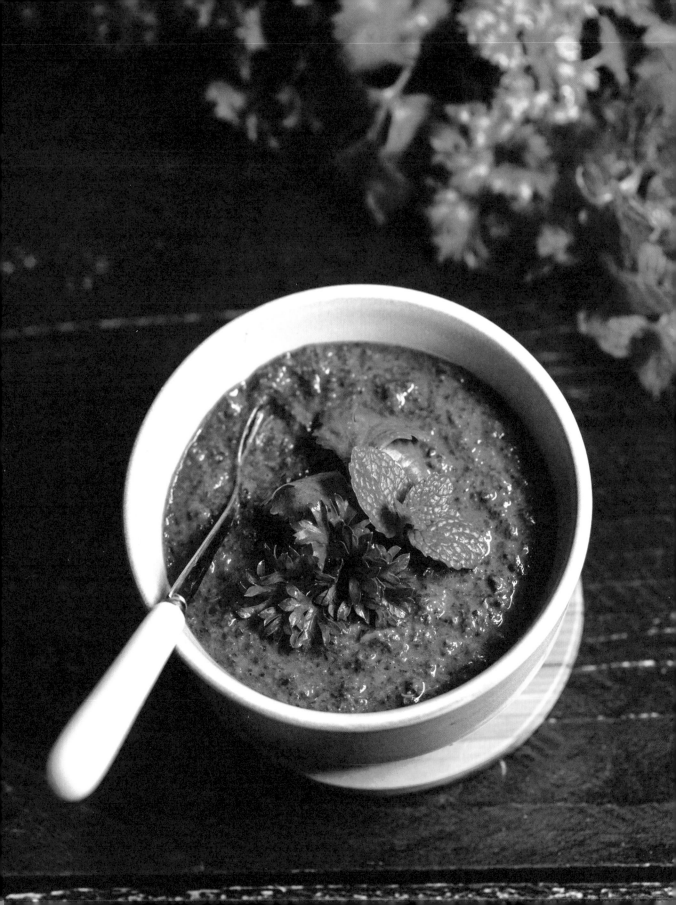

# Mixed Greens Chutney

**MAKES ABOUT 1 CUP**

Fresh garden herbs are a wonderful way to get the power of bitter herbs for blood cleansing in your diet! All those leafy culinaries that grow easily in your climate—dill, arugula, parsley, basil, and more—contain concentrated amounts of purifying tastes. Experiment with this balancing, colorful condiment to find your favorite combinations. A green chutney, like those served alongside dosa and samosa, is a versatile way to render the bitter and astringent tastes of your herbs atop builders like grains, kicharis, roasted vegetables, and meats.

> **4 bunches (double handfuls) of mixed greens**
>    (Cilantro, mint, arugula, parsley, basil, and dill all work well.)
> **1 green chili, or 1 tbsp minced gingerroot**
> **1 tsp coconut sugar, cane sugar, maple syrup, agave, or honey**
> **1 tsp coriander powder**
> **Juice of 2 limes**
> **4 tbsp olive oil**
> **1 tsp pink salt**

Add all ingredients to a blender or food processor in the order listed. Pulse until smooth. Add more lime juice if you need to loosen up the mixture. Season to taste.

Store in a glass vessel in the refrigerator for up to one week.

# Sesame Crunch Chutney

Sesame seeds are tops in Ayurveda because of their natural richness in five of the six tastes. As a food, they can nourish all the tissues. In the Western view, sesame has a high amount of calcium and is therefore recommended for bone health.

Sesame is most nutritious in a preparation where it is ground, like tahini or gomasio, because whole sesame seeds tend to pass through our bodies undigested. This example of a "dry" chutney can be sprinkled over moist dishes like cooked veggies, grains, and soups for a delightful crunch. Sesame chutney is a great savory addition to your kichari.

> 1 cup brown, raw, unhulled sesame seeds
> ¼ cup finely shredded dried coconut
> 3 tsp Essential Spice Mix (page 238)
> ½ tsp pink salt

Dry roast the seeds in a skillet over medium heat. Stir constantly, remove from the heat when they brown and begin to splutter. Transfer the seeds to a wide bowl to cool.

Roast the coconut in the same pan over medium heat, stirring constantly. When you can smell the coconut, stir in the spice mix and salt and remove from the heat. Add to the bowl of seeds and let cool. (This will just take a few minutes.)

Grind the mixture in a mortar and pestle, or pulse just halfway in a small food processor. Keep it a little coarse; do not overgrind or it will turn to butter.

Store in a glass jar on the shelf, and use within two weeks.

# Triple Mineral Gomasio

**MAKES ABOUT ¾ CUP**

I developed this recipe as a way to ensure I am getting my trace minerals and B vitamins, which are essential for the new production of menstrual blood each month. Gomasio is always on my table. I can tell when I'm not eating enough sea veggies because I begin to feel the wind come out of my sails.

This is a fancy addition to soups, vegetables, and kicharis that adds flavor and looks very pleasant sprinkled over foods. It is a vegetarian must. If you can't find all the different sea vegetables, forge ahead with what you can find; it's a very versatile recipe.

> **2 sheets nori seaweed**
>
> **½ cup unhulled sesame seeds**
>
> **2 tbsp black sesame seeds (optional)**
>
> **1 tbsp dulse flakes**
>
> **1 tbsp kelp powder**
>
> **1 tsp salt**

Toast the nori by waving it over a stovetop burner until it turns bright green and crispy, just a few seconds. If you put it too close to the heat, it will blacken, especially if you have a gas burner. Break the toasted sheets into quarters.

Roast the sesame seeds in a heavy-bottomed pan, such as a cast-iron one, over medium-low heat. Stir constantly until they begin to brown, just a few minutes. Remove from the heat and cool completely.

Crush the sesame seeds halfway by whizzing them briefly in a food processor. Pulse, and feed the nori pieces into the blade. Let the pieces get small enough to fit through a shaker top, but don't process to a powder or dust. Pulse in the dulse flakes, kelp, and salt.

Store in a shaker jar at room temperature for up to three months.

**Note:** Most health food stores carry dulse, kelp, and nori in the "international" food section. Kelp powder is often also found with bulk herbs and spices. See the resources in appendix C for where to find culinary seaweed.

Toasted nori can also be used as a crispy side or crumbled on top of a soup before serving.

# 24

# Nourishing Treats

Sweet treats are aphrodisiacs, made with whole foods in small amounts and gently spiced. The sweet taste as found in nature is the primary factor in juicing up the generative system and provides the grounding elements. Whether it's for libido, fertility, or creativity, use these recipes to amp up your shukra, or sexy juice.

Replace nutrients after your period or support pregnancy and breastfeeding with building treats made of natural sugars, ghee, sesame, and almonds. The unctuous nature of these treats is also a rasayana for aging. Forget about conventional sugary sweets, and reach for the nutritious ones instead. This will satisfy your body's true craving for physical and subtle forms of satisfaction that underlie a sweet tooth, and leave you feeling full power.

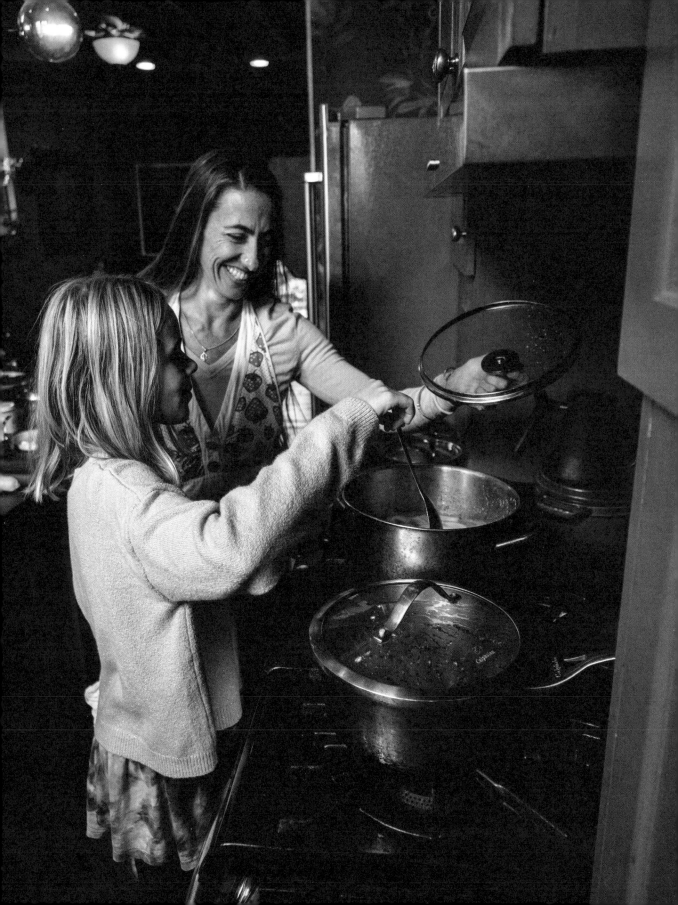

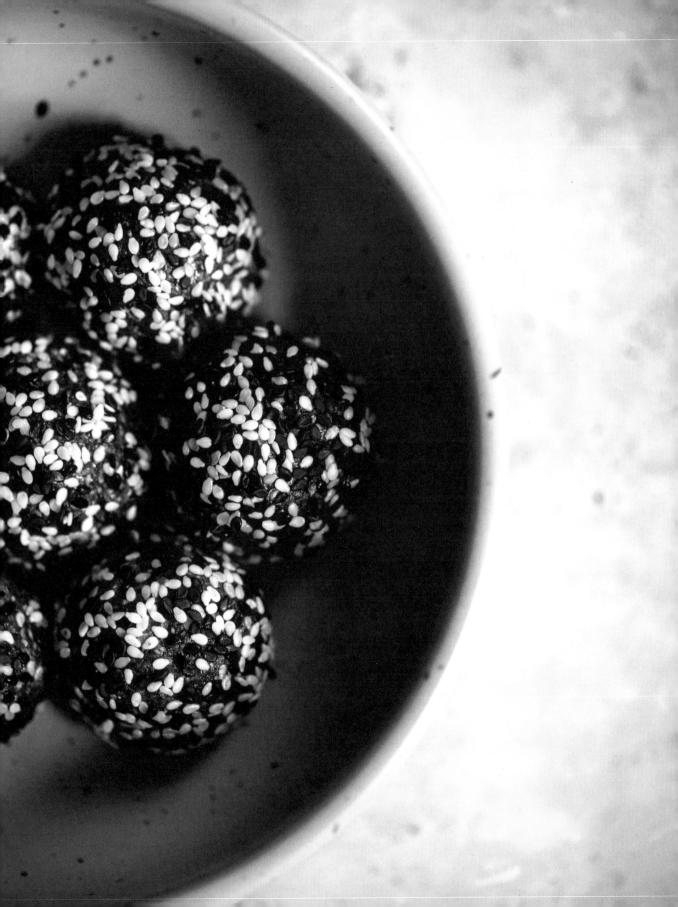

# Black Sesame Balls

This version of the black sesame ball is not as sweet as the traditional version made of sesame seeds ground with raw sugar, and better fits into my "treats as food" philosophy. The balls are warming and very earthy and satisfying when you've got a craving for you're-not-sure-what.

Black sesame is a powerful bone builder (as you can see in the box on page 304) and supports red blood and all the deep tissues. Its benefits are too many to name, but know that including it in your diet will bring deep strength in many ways.

    ¼ cup black sesame seeds
    1 cup dates, pits removed
    3 tbsp tahini
    ⅔ cup rolled oats
    ½ tsp ground cardamom
    Pinch of salt
    2 tbsp mixed black and white sesame seeds, for rolling

In a heavy-bottomed pan, toast the sesame seeds over medium heat until they pop. Remove from the heat and transfer to a plate or wide bowl to cool completely.

Grind the cooled sesame seeds in a coffee or spice grinder.

Process the dates in a food processor until they form a ball. If the dates are not moist, soak them in water for 5 to 10 minutes first, then drain.

Add the seeds and the rest of the ingredients to the food processor and process to combine. Allow the oats to break up for a smoother texture (unless you like it chewy). Add a little more tahini if needed to make the mixture sticky.

Place the sesame seed mixture in a small bowl. Roll 1–2 tablespoons of the mixture into a ball, then roll it in the black and white seeds to coat. Repeat until all of the mixture has been made into balls.

These sesame balls will keep in an airtight container on the counter for up to one week.

While visiting my friend Sahana Murthy, the founder of Mysore Rasayana Kitchen, I noticed a baggie of black sesame balls on her counter. She offered me one, telling me her aunt made them for her "for my periods." I knew enough about the benefits of black sesame to understand this but was struck by how women's food-wisdom was baked into the family unit. I imagined Sahana's aunt considering her niece's menstrual cycle, while preparing *ellu unde* (black sesame balls). I never forgot that, and I invited Sahana to share a story about women's wisdom in her family—and those black sesame balls I saw in the baggie.

One of the golden memories from childhood is my grandmother making black sesame balls. She not only made them delicious but also made sure we didn't binge on them. My parents/grandparents taught us the importance of eating everything in balance. Even today my dad tells me that "one should eat in moderation and be able to digest. That's good health."

In India when girls reach puberty, the first sixteen days are considered a vulnerable phase. There are various rituals conducted during this time. Some of the common rituals and lifestyle practices include oil massage every day, eating mostly *rasams* with garlic, consuming various rasayanas, and eating black sesame balls.

My grandmother used to insist that we eat black sesame, especially during menstruation and say, "This will turn your spine into a rock, eat it." However, she would never let us eat more than one as they are warming/heating in nature.

# Date Honey

**MAKES 1 CUP**

Dates are an aphrodisiac. Being both sweet and mineral-rich makes them a building food for both rasa and rakta dhatus. Making dates into a syrup, or molasses, is a practice that goes back millennia in India and the Middle East. Date honey can be used in the same way you use maple syrup or honey. Since Ayurveda is very clear about not using honey in heated preparations, this honey-like preparation can be used in hot tea or baking as a substitute. This is a great way to use up dates that aren't perfectly juicy and delicious on their own.

> **2 cup Medjool dates, pits removed**
> **3 cups boiling hot water**

Chop the dates into quarters.

In a large bowl or glass jar, pour the hot water over the dates just to cover, and soak for 2 hours (longer if you are using a dry date variety, like deglet noor).

Transfer the dates and water to a wide bowl; mash with a potato masher. The consistency should be like thin jam. Add more hot water, 1 tbsp at a time if needed to get it thin enough to strain.

Use a nut milk bag to squeeze the liquid out of the dates directly into a saucepan.

Place the pulp back in the bowl and add just enough hot water to cover it, about 2/3 cup.

Repeat the process once more: mashing the dates and water, then straining through the nut bag into the saucepan.

In the saucepan, bring the date juice to a boil, then reduce the heat and simmer, uncovered, for about 30 minutes. The syrup will reduce to the consistency of thin honey but will thicken as it cools.

Store in a glass jar in the refrigerator. Date honey stays fresh for several months.

**Variation:** If you want to use a different variety of date, like the commonly found deglet noor, you can. It may take a longer soak and more water to get a good mash and strain. I recommend soaking drier dates overnight. The honey will not be quite as sweet and flavorful, but it will still be amazing and nutritious.

# Almond Cardamom Diamonds

**MAKES 20 SQUARES**

Known as *burfi*, this fudge-style treat has only a few ingredients and is simple to make. Sure, it has a lot of sugar, but it also has building qualities and minerals from almonds and makes a wonderful celebratory treat. It's one of those meditative recipes that has you stirring for a while, immersed in the aromas and qualities of the ingredients as they roast to a fantastic golden color. To make this recipe ideal for the postpartum stage, add the optional ginger with the cardamom.

> **1 cup evaporated cane juice or less refined sugar**
>
> **⅔ cup water**
>
> **1 tsp ground cardamom**
>
> **1 tsp ground ginger (optional)**
>
> **2 cups almond flour (Blanched will have the skins removed, for digestion, and will make smoother fudge.)**
>
> **2 tbsp ghee**
>
> **2–3 tbsp slivered almonds**

Line an 8 × 8-inch glass dish with an extra-large piece of parchment paper, folded and pressed into the corners.

In a wide, heavy-bottomed saucepan, combine the sugar and water. Bring to a boil over high heat, stirring to dissolve. Reduce the heat to medium and boil for 10 minutes, stirring constantly.

Add the cardamom and ginger (if using); stir.

Add almond flour to the boiling mixture and mix quickly.

Keep stirring in a circular motion; the mixture will become thick. Soon the almond flour will absorb the liquid and become a paste.

Continue to cook, folding the mixture occasionally and not letting it burn. Collect any pieces off the sides. After about 6 or 7 minutes, the mixture will ball up.

Reduce the heat to low. Add the ghee and mix well, scraping the bottom of the pan.

Remove from the heat and transfer the ball to the paper-lined dish.

*(continued)*

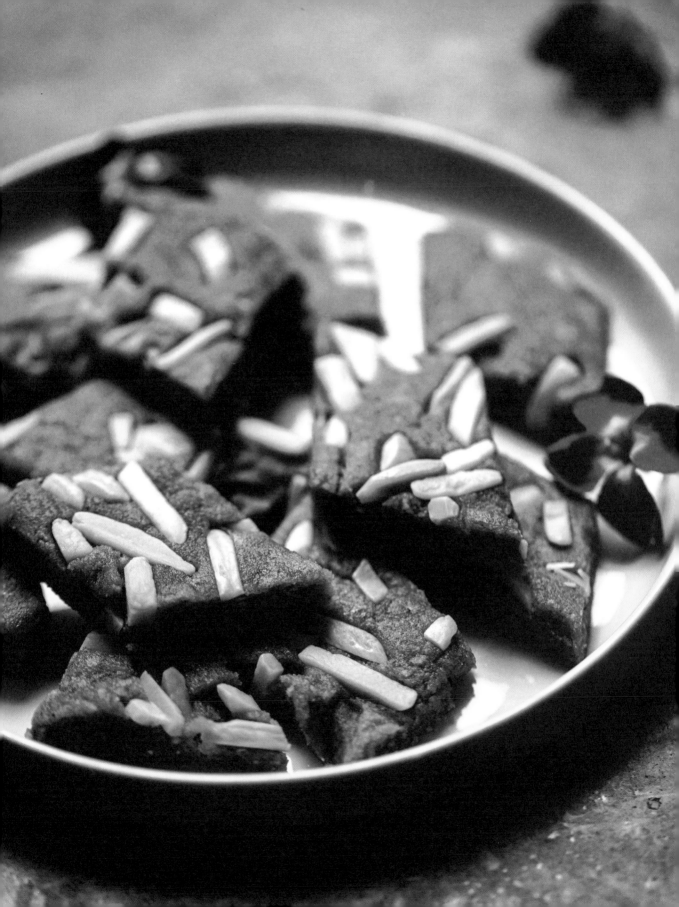

When it is cool enough to touch but still warm and pliable, use your hands to press it into the dish.

Sprinkle the top with almond pieces. Press them into the fudge by folding the parchment paper over and smoothing the top of the mixture.

If you want to get fancy, cover with parchment paper and roll smooth with a can of beans (or whatever you've got that fits in the pan).

Cool completely before cutting. Lift the parchment paper out of the pan and onto a cutting board to slice the bars into diamonds.

Pack in a glass storage container with parchment paper between the layers. Almond Cardamom Diamonds stay good on the counter for up to one week—if they last that long! If they are soft, keep them in the refrigerator.

**Note:** I store these out of view so I don't gobble them up.

# Kate's Tahini Treat

**SERVES 1**

I am a fan of made-to-order, single-serving treats. I whip up just enough and avoid the distraction of trying not to eat a whole batch. This is my go-to when I get big-time sweet cravings before my menstrual cycle, and it hits the spot every time, thanks to the deeply building qualities of sesame and the minerals of maple syrup. After much experimentation, I offer you the most satisfying and tasty combo of seed butter and sweetener out there.

> **2 tbsp tahini**
>
> **1 tbsp maple syrup or Date Honey (page 305)**
>
> **¼ tsp Sweet Rose Masala (page 236) or ground cinnamon**

Whisk together all the ingredients in a ramekin until smooth.

This can be spread on toast or a cracker. Personally, I lick it off the spoon—no middle (wo)man.

Remember to sit down to enjoy your treat.

**Variations:** The possibilities for variations to this recipe are endless. For another version, use Hibiscus Rose Cordial (page 312) instead of maple syrup. For yet another variation, add 2 tablespoons cacao powder and go choco. The thicker texture of this variation may require a little oil (sesame or coconut) or more maple syrup to thin it down.

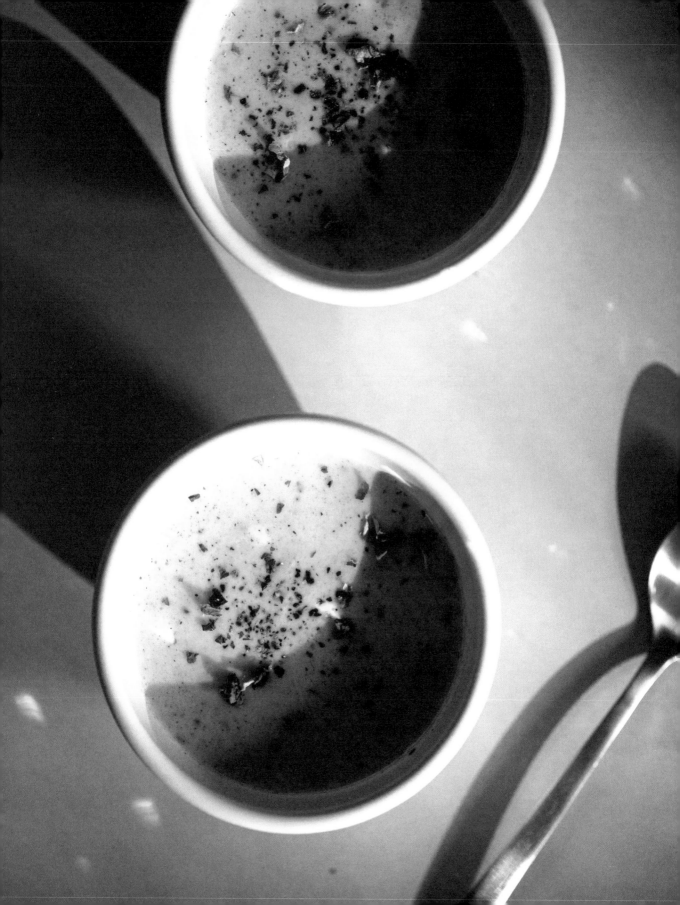

# Rasala Medicinal Yogurt

**SERVES 1–2**

Here, yogurt is transformed from sour and clogging to a sweet, nourishing treat. Rasala is a magical preparation that combines fresh yogurt with sugar and spices. The sour, heating quality of yogurt is balanced by sugar, and the heavy, moist nature of yogurt is balanced by spices. According to Ayurveda texts, such a recipe is nutritive and moistening, works as an aphrodisiac, and provides strength.

Many women are in the habit of grabbing yogurt on the go, as it is known to be high in protein and calcium. Ayurveda, however, suggests that to make yogurt tridoshic, it must be spiced and a little sweet, otherwise its moist and sour qualities are not good for everyone. Taking a few minutes to transform your yogurt also improves your digestion and appetite! Enjoy a small bowl after a meal as a digestive.

> **8 oz fresh, whole-milk yogurt**
> **1 tsp evaporated cane juice, honey, or coconut sugar**
> **Pinch of ground black pepper**
> **1 tsp Sweet Rose Masala (page 236)**

Let the yogurt come to room temperature, 20–30 minutes.

Combine all the ingredients in a small bowl. Use a fork or a whisk to vigorously whip together. Enjoy as an appetizer or a side dish with a simple meal.

**Tip:** If you are looking to lighten this up into a beverage, mix the ingredients together in a blender with 1–2 cups water and blend for 30 seconds to combine. Drink this diluted yogurt on an empty stomach to hydrate and balance agni. You'll love it.

# Hibiscus Rose Cordial

**MAKES 1 CUP**

This sweet and exotic cordial can be used as a flavoring agent in all kinds of ways. Mix it with water to make a refreshing drink, or add it to milk for a fragrant, creamy treat. Rose has bitter and sweet tastes, both cooling. For the perfect shade of pink, you have to use white sugar, but white sugar is nutritionally void. I am willing to sacrifice the vibrant color and use sweeteners with mineral content. Turbinado sugar, on special occasions, would make this a little more pink.

> 1 cup dried rose petals
> 3–4 hibiscus leaves
> 1 cup water
> 1 cup granulated sugar (jaggery, coconut sugar,
>     evaporated cane juice)

Place all the ingredients in a medium saucepan and bring to a boil over high heat.

Reduce the heat to low and simmer uncovered for 5 minutes. Do not overdo this step or the cordial will taste bitter.

Remove from the heat and strain the liquid through a fine mesh sieve to remove the flowers.

Return the liquid to the stove and simmer over low heat for 10 minutes, until it is the consistency of maple syrup.

Refrigerate in a glass jar for up to two weeks.

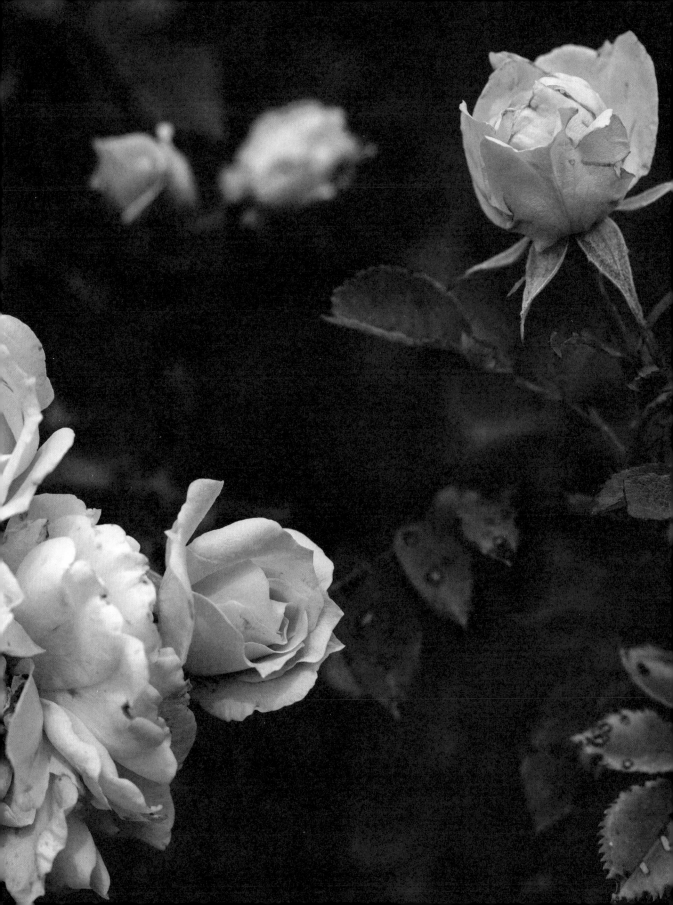

# Appendix A

## HEALING PRACTICES

Food and herbs are a tangible and ever-present part of our days, and they make a great starting place for healthy changes. Body therapies for tissues, skin, and yoni and subtle practices for restoring the free movement of energy, opening channels, redirecting vata, and balancing the mind require setting aside a little more time in your routine—and it's worth it. Chronic imbalances respond especially well to body therapy or breath practice. Often, causative factors that are etched into our energetic blueprint will require more than food for healing. A healing practice is likely to save the day.

Practices for healthy artava and apana restore the downward flow of apana and open the channels of the generative system through the use of steam, oil, and heat. Practices to support hormone balance calm solar energies and promote more lunar, soft, and cool energies. Practices for mind, sleep, and mood target the head, the channels of the mind, and the nervous system to foster calm.

Keep in mind that balance rarely comes overnight, and most practices will bear fruit with consistent, patient application over time. If you have any doubts about how to do any of these practices or if they are right for you, please consult a practitioner.

### Practices for Healthy Artava and Apana

Herbal Sitz Bath (page 316)

Castor Oil Packs (page 318)

Yoni Steaming (page 318)

Breast Massage (page 320)

### Practices to Support Hormonal Balance

Nadi Shodhana (Alternate Nostril Breathing) (page 321)

Abhyanga (Oil Massage and Dry Brushing) (page 323)

Sitali Cooling Breath (page 323)

Moonbathing (page 327)

### Practices for Mind, Sleep, and Mood

Shiro Abhyanga (Head Massage) (page 328)

Herbal Bath Ritual (page 329)

Sama Vritti Ujjayi (Rhythmic Breathing) (page 322)

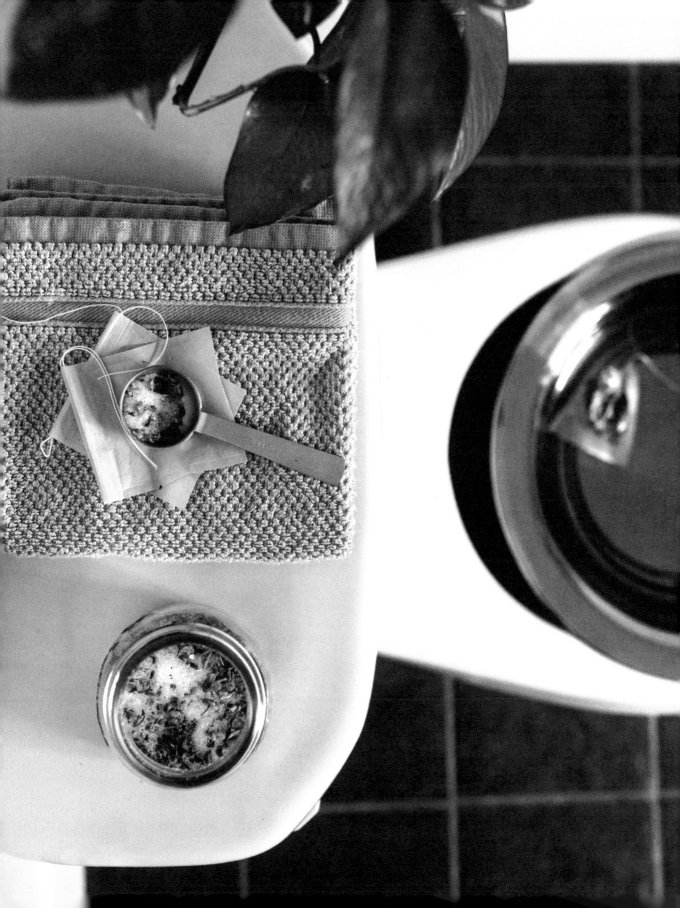

## HERBAL SITZ BATH

A sitz bath is done by submerging the pelvic area in warm water or a warm medicated solution for 15 to 20 minutes. Sitz baths relax the muscles of the perineum and clean the anus and vulva without any abrasion. They are used for pain relief and to heal and soothe swollen vaginal and labial tissues postpartum. Soothing, cooling, astringent, and antiseptic herbs, such as rose and lavender in their dried form, can be added to the water. Do not use essential oils, which may cause a burning sensation. Warm water increases blood flow, encouraging healing, while cooling herbs reduce inflammation. Sitz baths can also reduce the size of hemorrhoids, promote their healing, and relieve associated pain.

Prepared herbal mixes and stainless steel or plastic basins can be used, as can sitz bath kits. A small basin that inserts into the toilet seat is best if you're using an herbal solution. Filling a tub with about 5 inches of water, enough to cover the pelvic and perineal space, can also work but will use up a lot more of your herbs and requires you to clean the tub well before each bath to reduce any risk of infection. A small basin is much easier to sterilize.

Sitz baths must only be used when there are no signs of infection. When in doubt, consult your health care provider before using a sitz bath.

**Sitz bath tips:** Favor herbs that are cooling and astringent, and use a little salt for an antiseptic effect. Use warm water, not hot, which can be too drying. Adding a few drops of sesame oil can be soothing for dryness. Herbal solutions, such as the one below, can be brewed ahead of time and rewarmed.

# Epsom Salt Sitz

Place your basin on top of the toilet seat.

Fill the basin with warm water and add ½ cup Epsom salts. Stir to dissolve.

Submerge affected areas in the basin and relax for 15 to 20 minutes. Add more warm water if the water cools.

Dry the area well with a soft cloth.

Clean the basin well with dish soap, and rinse with hot water.

# Herbal Salts Sitz Recipe

**MAKES ABOUT 1½ CUPS**

**1 cup pink or sea salt**

**Use any combination of the following herbs:**

**2 tbsp dried lavender**

**2 tbsp dried rose petals**

**2 tbsp dried raspberry leaves**

**2 tbsp dried chamomile flowers**

**Natural unbleached tea bags**

Mix together the salt and herbs and keep in a glass jar, tightly covered.

For each sitz, fill a teabag with 2 tbsp of the herb and salt mixture.

Fill the basin with warm water and add the bag. Steep for about five minutes.

Submerge affected areas in the basin and relax for 15 to 20 minutes. Add more warm water if the water cools.

Dry the area well with a soft cloth.

Clean the basin well with dish soap, and rinse with hot water.

## YONI STEAMING

The ancient practice of vaginal steaming warms, softens, and opens the cervix, which aids in uterine cleansing and smooth downward flow. The practice can be done sitting on a pot of herbal steam with towels wrapped around your waist to trap the steam; it is a similar method to steaming your face when you have a sinus infection. Steam invites a smooth flow where there is stagnation, dryness, or constriction. This is a warming and moving practice, best for vata and kapha imbalances of the artava channels.

Due to the hot and moist qualities of steam, yoni steaming is contraindicated when there is a burning sensation, redness, intense menstrual bleeding, or any open cuts or sores on the vaginal or labial tissue. Steaming is also not appropriate during your period, when you're pregnant, or soon after birthing. If you have an IUD, you should not steam, as the practice could displace the device.

Yoni steaming can be done a day or two before ovulation to enhance the likelihood of pregnancy. Steaming can be healing for irregular or slow-onset periods; vaginal dryness; and premenstrual pain, cramping, and bloating. Steaming can also help completely release menstrual fluids, rejuvenate vaginal tissues during menopause, and in some cases increase libido and orgasm by "getting things moving." Herbs can be added to the steam water to support uterine cleansing or soothing and moisturizing.

Please consult a midwife, doula, or Ayurveda practitioner about whether yoni steaming can help you and when and how often to do it. Find a link to a how-to online course about yoni steaming in appendix C.

## CASTOR OIL PACKS

Castor oil packs are an effective way to alleviate painful periods, relieve constipation, and support uterine health.

Castor oil is warm and moist, which are the qualities used to relax and soften tissues and to open channels. Castor oil packs allow penetrating heat to break up physical and energetic blockages and move stagnation. Application over the lower abdomen opens the channels of artava, increasing blood flow to the uterus, and with regular use, it can break up fibroids as well as prevent their growth.

Castor oil packs also move apana vayu and free up the downward flow. This is an excellent remedy for constipation and low back pain at any time, as well as before your period. Expect to stick with it for at least three months, and practice anywhere from daily to three times weekly. More frequent applications will yield faster results. Castor oil packs can be integrated into an evening routine. To make practice more convenient, you can purchase a kit (see the resources in appendix C).

Do not use castor oil packs when you have your period. Take days off when there is red blood, and resume practice once your flow is finished.

**3 tbsp castor oil**
**Hot water bottle**
**Cotton flannel, at least 18 inches square, or a cut-up T-shirt or pillowcase**
**Plastic bag or plastic wrap (a shopping bag will do)**

Warm the castor oil by standing the bottle in a pan of hot water for 5 minutes.

Fill the hot water bottle two-thirds full with very hot water. Press a bit of the air out before screwing the cap on tightly. This will make the bottle less firm so it stays put.

Fold the cloth into a rectangle that covers the space between your navel and pubic bone, from one hip bone to the other.

Keep a cozy shirt on, fold it up over your breasts to protect it from the oil, and remove your pants.

Dampen one side of the cloth with castor oil. It should be moist but not dripping.

Place the cloth over your abdomen and cover with plastic (this is to protect your shirt as castor oil stains fabric).

Place the hot water bottle over the plastic and the cloth.

Rest with the pack on for 60 to 90 minutes. A longer application yields faster results. Afterward, take a hot shower and soap the area twice to remove all traces of oil from your skin. Swabbing with a solution of baking soda and water will also remove the oil.

**For constipation:** Use daily, until the flow gets going. Resume at the first signs of a slowdown. Over time, you will learn how to use the practice to nip constipation in the bud.

**For painful periods and overall uterine health:** Practice daily or three times weekly, depending on the severity of your symptoms for at least three cycles. You should notice less cramping within a few months. When stagnation clears, you may experience one or two heavy, painful periods. If these periods persist, see your doctor.

When there is no longer pain associated with your periods, taper off to weekly practice for a month or two. In some cases, the imbalance is healed, and periods will remain pain free; in other cases, painful periods may return after a while. Resume practice at the first signs of imbalance. Learn to be attentive to tension in your abdomen. This practice may support you in relaxing your abdomen, thereby improving digestion and elimination.

## BREAST MASSAGE

The armpit, chest, and throat are serially restricted for most women and require vigilant care. We spend a lot of time with our arms by our sides, reaching forward, or hunching. All these actions close off flow to the armpit. The tissue and the energy in this part of the body may feel hard to the touch, sunken, or immobile. Restriction to the flow of circulation to the breasts is physical as well as psychosomatic.

The armpit is the drainage site for the lymph that moves through the breast. Hormonal changes before menstruation can cause swelling that traps fluid in the breast, causing the tenderness, lumpiness, and increase in size of the breasts before your period. In the short term, increasing flow to the breasts reduces related PMS symptoms. In the long term, it may reduce the risk of cancer. Breasts are primarily composed of adipose tissue, which tends to hold toxins. The breasts attract endocrine disruptors (estrogen lookalike chemicals), and it is important to reduce the use of products that contain them. Breast massage helps keep a consistent flow of prana to the armpits and chest, so the lymph is free to flow through and take out the garbage. As we have seen, the body's waste exits through the digestive tract, so overall strong agni, a good diet, and regular elimination allow the body to clear out excess hormones and toxins from the breasts. It should be no surprise that breast health is related to digestive health.

Wear loose clothing around your breasts and armpits (avoid underwire bras). If you wear a sports bra for exercise, avoid keeping it on for the rest of the day. This will allow the circulatory benefits of your exercise to reach your breasts. And breathe. Breath is a primary healing factor in circulation.

## HOW TO DO A SELF-MASSAGE

Spending extra time on your breasts as you massage oil into the skin, even in the shower, is a great way to increase circulation to the area and get to know your breast tissue, which is likely to change at different stages of your menstrual cycle.

Castor oil, the most penetrating of the oils, is excellent for softening lumpy or swollen breast tissue, breaking up cysts, and increasing circulation. Apply it in the shower; it is very thick and requires soaping off after massage. Apply in a circular motion, firmly massaging it into the breast tissue and kneading the flesh where the breast meets the armpit. Take care, as your tub may get a bit slippery. A sprinkle of baking soda and a quick wipe after the shower will remove any residue.

Breast tissue becomes denser in the forties and fifties. Changes in the quality of the tissue with age is normal. Knowing your breasts well, through regular massage, sets you up to recognize abnormal changes. Be sure to talk with a health care provider about how to do a self-examination and what changes or irregularities to look for.

# Ditch the Antiperspirant

Antiperspirant—not deodorant—is an armpit product that is designed to block sweating, which blocks the natural flow of energy and should be avoided. If you use a deodorant (which doesn't block the sweat pores), please make sure it doesn't contain any toxins like phthalates, aluminum, or "fragrance," which should not be applied in close proximity to the breast. Whip up a Double-Duty Sage and Salt Deodorant Spritz (page 225) to ditch the poison.

## PRACTICES TO SUPPORT HORMONAL BALANCE

### NADI SHODHANA (ALTERNATE NOSTRIL BREATHING)

Alternate Nostril Breathing is the queen of practices for essential balance. This practice can calm hot flashes, normalize irregular periods, improve sleep and mood swings, and so much more due to its vata-pacifying nature.

The solar and lunar nadis, or energy channels, correspond to the right and left nostrils, respectively. Ideally the breath shifts constantly from one channel to the other in a rhythmic pattern, which balances our energy pathways. When our solar and lunar energies are out of balance, the shift between nadis may become disturbed, or vice versa, when imbalance in the energy pathways leads to other imbalances. This practice purifies the two major energy channels in the body, establishing and maintaining essential balance. Five minutes daily is a good starting place. I recommend setting a timer (do not use your phone!). Once 5 minutes becomes comfortable, consider working up to 20 minutes daily for the best results. Increase sessions slowly by a few minutes each week. To reach 20 minutes comfortably might take you three to six months.

First thing in the morning is an ideal time to practice and sets up the energy channels for the day ahead. If the morning is not available, evening practice is also beneficial and can help you slow down and get a good night's sleep.

Sitting in a comfortable position with a straight spine, gently close your eyes. If it is uncomfortable or not possible to sit in a simple cross-legged or kneeling position on a meditation cushion or blanket, sit on the edge of a chair.

Take a few natural breaths, and allow your mind to settle on your breath.

Fold the tips of the index and middle fingers of your right hand inward to your palm. You may also use your left hand if you cannot use the right.

With your elbow elevated so your arm is at a right angle with your body, close your right nostril with your thumb and inhale through your left nostril.

Use the ring and pinky fingers of your right hand to gently close your left nostril and release your right nostril. Exhale through your right nostril.

Keeping your left nostril closed, inhale through your right.

Release your left nostril and block the right one with your right thumb. Release your breath through your left nostril.

This completes one round. The same pattern continues for each additional round. It is important that the breath remains smooth and relaxed throughout the practice.

As you get the hang of the breath pattern, check in with the space between your eyebrows and your right shoulder. These are two places that tend to tense up during practice. Soften them, and keep up the breath pattern at your own pace. Take your time.

Close the practice with an observation of the qualities of your breath and mind space.

Once this practice becomes comfortable, you can experiment with doing the pattern as a visualization and keep your right hand relaxed on your lap. If you are unable to use either hand for the practice, do the visualization technique instead.

## SAMA VRITTI UJJAYI (RHYTHMIC BREATHING)

*Sama* means "balanced," *vrtti* means "fluctuation," and *ujaayi* means "victory." This breathing exercise makes one victorious over the fluctuations of the mind! Bringing the breath into rhythm also reduces the stress response, relaxes the channels, and calms the nerves. This is an excellent practice to try when you feel agitated, especially in the space between a trigger and your reaction. Often a few rounds of even breathing will create a centered space where your next move becomes clear.

Sit comfortably, where you won't be disturbed, and set a timer (not your phone!) for 5 minutes.

Close your eyes and take three breaths, just to settle in.

Begin to inhale and slowly count, "One . . . two . . . three . . . four," landing on the end of the inhalation at four.

Begin to exhale and slowly count, "One . . . two . . . three . . . four," completely emptying the breath at four.

Continue like this, counting rhythmically to 4 on each in-breath and each out-breath. Concentrate on making the in- and out-breaths the same length and strength. This may take some practice. Counting helps you keep the rhythm. Stick with it, pay attention, and keep going until the alarm goes off. With practice, you can increase the duration by 1 minute at a time, if you like. The more minutes you spend breathing in rhythm, the more stable and relaxed you will feel and the longer that feeling will stay with you.

## SITALI COOLING BREATH

This brief breath practice is very simple and works immediately. For hot flashes or overheating for any reason, such as after vigorous exercise, sit comfortably, and do Sitali Breath until your body cools down. The placement of your tongue literally cools the air as it enters your body. Keep your mind on the sensation of cool entering your body.

Open your mouth and form your lips into an O.

Curl your tongue and extend it slightly through your lips. If your tongue can't curl into a taco shape, simply breathe through the O shape of your lips.

Inhale through your tongue, slowly and smoothly. Feel the cool sensations of the air on your tongue and inner cheeks.

Exhale slowly through both nostrils.

Repeat for a total of at least three breaths. You may work up to ten breaths.

## ABHYANGA (OIL MASSAGE AND DRY BRUSHING)

The application of oil to the body is a longevity practice that nourishes and increases resiliency of the body and nervous system. Oil, followed by the application of heat, softens the channels and tissues, improves circulation, and detoxifies through the skin. *Abhyanga* means specific movements applied to the limbs. The practice involves applying oil to the skin, head, ears, and feet before showering and letting it absorb, then washing it off.

Massage is most effective for detoxification of the skin in the morning, as are all of the din-acharya methods. However, oil's stabilizing qualities can also induce good sleep, pain relief, and relaxation when used in the evening. A coconut oil massage can cool the body in hot weather or calm inflammation. Because the skin needs to digest the oil, massage is not recommended after eating, during your period, when you are sick, or when ama is present. Oil's heavy, dense, moist qualities can increase ama if the oil is not digested. Oil massage is fantastic during pregnancy, but keep the strokes gentle. If you start to feel itchy or develop a rash, take a few days off. When in doubt, work with a practitioner on how and when to use oil massage.

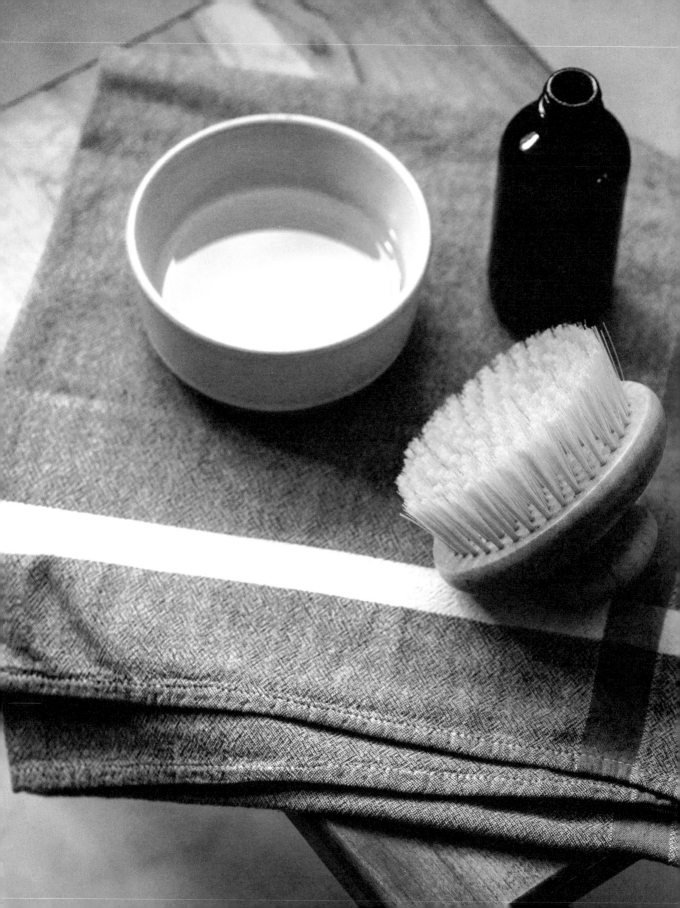

How you do self-massage is as important as when and what kind of oil you use. Some believe that simply applying the oil is the purpose, while others believe the massage itself is equally important. Pay close attention to your vibe. Make sure you are not rushing, approaching this activity as just a tedious chore. Consider what a treat it is to have this time to care for yourself, and imagine all the benefits you are promoting in your body and mind with this ancient practice. Self-massage in an act of love. Foster gratitude for all the functions your body carries out seamlessly all the time, without conscious effort. Reflect on how your attention pays off in the longevity bank every and any time you perform an act of self-care.

## HOW TO DO SELF-MASSAGE

Warm ¼ cup oil in a jar or squeeze bottle placed in hot water. Make sure the room is cozy and warm; use a space heater if necessary. Prepare the room and remove your clothes before you begin. Lay an old bath towel on the floor and sit down, or place a towel over the toilet seat or the side of the tub and sit there. Breathe deeply a few times and give thanks for the time and space for self-care.

First put a tablespoon of the oil in your palm and apply it to the crown of your head. (Read the Shiro Abhyanga section on page 328 for more about head massage. If you are not planning to wash your hair, do not oil your head.) Use your palms to make wide circles over your face; avoid getting oil in your eyes. Oil your ears and the area behind your ears; use your pinkies to put oil in your ears and nose. Rub oil into the sides of your neck and across the tops of your shoulders.

Place a few tablespoons of oil in your palms and rub it down your arms and legs, using more oil as necessary. First coat all four limbs, then firmly rub the oil into your arms with long, downward strokes; repeat with your legs. Use circular movements to massage your joints, and don't forget your fingers and toes. Apply more oil to your chest, abdomen, low back, and sides with large, clockwise circular movements. Be gentle on your abdomen. Massage your breasts well. Use an up-and-down stroke on your breastbone. Finish by massaging your feet well, using side-to-side strokes across the soles. I like to lace my fingers between my toes and massage circles around my ankles.

When you've finished, lie back on the towel and relax for 5 to 30 minutes, or lie in a moderately hot bath. The massage should take about 10 minutes, and aim for at least another 10 minutes of rest. Even 5 minutes of massage followed by a shower is beneficial. When you have more time, let it soak in longer for greater benefits.

Enjoy a hot shower, but wipe your feet first so you don't slip. Be careful! If there is any doubt about moving around when your feet are slippery or you have any history of balance issues, do not oil the soles of your feet. Oil your feet at bedtime instead. Use a natural lavender, sandalwood, or neem soap. Apply shampoo to your hair before wetting it to cut the oil. Pat yourself dry. Your skin may still seem slightly oily, but it will gradually be absorbed. Afterward, clean your shower floor of residual oil. I do this by spraying a little cleaner and rubbing it around with my feet. Baking soda, left on for a few minutes then wiped clean, will also absorb oil.

If you have access to a steam room or sauna, this is an excellent and very purifying addition. It is best to keep it to less than 10 minutes, about once a week, when used in conjunction with oil. To understand if more frequent heat and oil therapy is good for you, consult an Ayurveda practitioner.

**Note:** When your towel becomes very oily, it can create a fire hazard if you put it in the dryer after washing. Better to hang your abhyanga towels to dry and replace them periodically instead.

## Choosing a Massage Oil

Always use refined oils. This ensures that impurities have been removed, and you will notice refined oils do not have a strong smell. You may enjoy changing your massage oil with the seasons as indicated in the seasonal guidelines. Do a patch test with any oil before applying it to your entire body, to be sure you are not allergic to it.

**Sesame oil.** Traditionally sesame oil is favored for its ability to build strength and softness in the body. It is warming and indicated for those who run cold and experience dry skin.

**Sunflower and almond oil.** These two lighter oils are neutral (neither heating nor cooling) and are indicated for those who do not experience very dry skin or those who don't absorb sesame oil well. They can also be mixed with sesame oil.

**Mustard oil.** Mustard oil is light, heating, and stimulating for cool, heavy body types. This can be mixed with sunflower oil to reach a comfortable amount of warmth.

**Coconut oil.** Coconut oil is cooling and indicated for those who run hot or have sensitive skin.

Once a week is a minimum requirement for oil massage, unless your body is naturally moist. Anytime you practice abhyanga, it's money in the health bank. Frequency of oiling depends on how dry your body is, stress levels, season, and age. Vata imbalance, menopause, pre- and postnatal times, and high stress are all important indicators for frequent, if not daily, oil massage. If you notice more dry skin in winter, increase the frequency to several days a week; the same applies to periods of increased workload or stress or if you have difficulty sleeping. As you get used to the practice, you will notice its effects and become aware of when an oil massage is needed. Soon enough, you will know what factors in your life increase dryness, mobility, and stress, and this will become a tool to balance those factors.

## DRY BRUSHING

For those with heavy, moist kapha constitutions, or those working on getting rid of ama, dry brushing is a better choice than oiling, which can compound kapha qualities and exacerbate ama. This practice is useful in cases of excessive moisture in the body and heavy, dense qualities, which can bring on lethargy, weight gain, or water retention. Dry brushing stimulates the body and mind and increases circulation. When you are doing oil massages regularly, it is a good idea to do a gentle dry brushing to clear away dead skin once a week or so.

Use a natural bristle, dry brush (available in drugstores and health food stores) on dry skin. If your skin is sensitive to the bristles, use a rough washcloth or traditional *garshana* gloves, made of raw silk, on dry skin. Beginning at your ankles and moving up toward your heart, make small, brisk circles to exfoliate and stimulate the skin of your entire body, especially the armpits and chest, inner thighs and groins, and anywhere stubborn fat tissue likes to hang around. Take 3 to 5 minutes and be firm, but do not disturb the skin. Emphasize the upstroke. More pressure is not better; keep it gentle. Practice this technique anywhere from daily to once a week, before having your shower.

## MOONBATHING

Ayurveda texts describe walks in the moonlight as a summer routine for keeping cool. The light of the moon and soma are cool in nature and enhance the cool quality in the body and mind (since the moon and mind are *samanya*, or similar). Taking in lunar energy cools and calms the mind and optimizes rasa. From a hormonal perspective, moonlight balances stress hormones and promotes sex hormones, and it can even regulate the menstrual cycle. Moonbathing can be practiced outdoors in warm weather. If it's too cold outdoors for comfort, you can bask in a patch of moonlight through a window. (For more on lunar rhythms and routines, see chapter 9.)

# PRACTICES FOR MIND, SLEEP, AND MOOD

### SHIRO ABHYANGA (HEAD MASSAGE)

This technique is excellent for improving sleep quality, increasing the luster and volume of hair (especially when hair thins or dries during menopause), and relieving stress. Lean into this practice weekly as a remedy for anxiety, sleep problems, thinning hair, or dry scalp. Beginning at the first signs of imbalance will give you the best results.

Ayurveda body treatments for the mind generally focus on the head, mouth, ears, and nasal passages for their proximity to the brain and the activity of the sense organs. Head massage and oiling of the ears and nose can be used to calm the mind. Because oiling the scalp requires a thorough shampoo afterward, practice the head massage one or two times weekly when it is convenient for you to wash your hair after, such as a weekend morning. When your sleep is disrupted, head massage can be an excellent way to calm your mind at bedtime. To avoid going to bed with a wet head, you can wrap your oiled head in an old towel, scarf, or hat and shampoo it in the morning. Take care not to let your head get cold overnight. Head massage with oil is contraindicated in cases of congestion, illness, brain fog, or lethargy.

Melt 2 tablespoons coconut oil in a small vessel or ramekin. (If you run cold, sesame oil is a good choice.) Warm the oil slightly if it is cold out. Remove any hair ties and brush tangles out of your hair. Begin by gently kneading your shoulders and neck a few times with circular motions. Dip your fingers into the oil and distribute it evenly over your fingertips. Spread your fingers and work your hands into the hair on either side of your head, above your ears, your fingers pointing toward the crown. With a shampooing-like action, work your fingertips up to the crown of your head. Gently massage your scalp until the crown is covered with oil. This is the most important part of the scalp. Dip your fingers into the oil again and "shampoo" the rest of your scalp; this should take 5 minutes or more. Rub a bit of the oil entirely over each ear with small circular motions, and slide your pinky tips into your ears to coat the canal. Wrap your head if it's bedtime, or relax for 10 to 30 minutes with the oil on your head.

To clean your hair, apply shampoo first to dry hair and work it into the first 2 inches or so. Add a splash of water to create suds and massage it into a lather. Add more water as needed to build enough suds for your whole head. Those with thick hair may need to shampoo again to remove all the oil. Sesame oil may require more shampooing than coconut oil.

## HERBAL BATH RITUAL

Taking a solitary bath is an excellent new moon ritual to bring your energy inward. Use rose, lavender, sandalwood, and jasmine essential oils or dried flowers to make an herbal bath. These pitta-reducing plants, when used in an herbal bath, will slow you down and calm your mind, soothing pitta and vata—but be careful not to let the bath become too hot. A room temperature or cool bath can be used in hot weather.

Epsom salts dissolved in a hot bath relieve pain and tension from vata's hard and constricting qualities. Oil massage before an herbal bath also detoxifies and relaxes.

Create a ceremony, and take a few deep breaths before you sink into the bath.

Soak in the tub for at least 20 minutes, attuning your mind to sensations in your body, the sound of your breath, the texture of your skin and the water, and the aroma of the herbs and flowers. Listen to soft music or chanting, if you like.

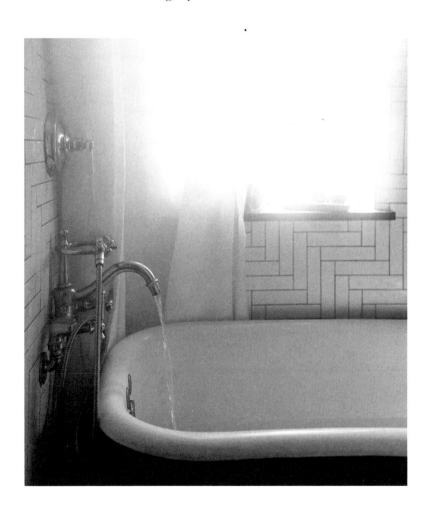

# Appendix B

## FOOD THERAPEUTICS REFERENCE CHARTS

These charts contain classifications of the foods and herbs mentioned in this book, which I have chosen based on their availability and efficacy. The lists are not exhaustive; they do not contain all the substances available in the pharmacopeia or all the substances mentioned in Ayurveda texts. (Note that there are many reliable, comprehensive herbal resources out there to pique your curiosity and a few listed in appendix C.) Over time, you will add your own experiential knowledge of the substances native to where you live to this foundation of knowledge.

## Digestive Actions of Spices

**Spices to balance a cold, bloaty, gassy gut and to relieve back pain and constipation related to the menstrual cycle**

| | | | |
|---|---|---|---|
| Ajwain | Cumin | Mustard seed | Rosemary |
| Basil | Garlic | Nutmeg | Thyme |
| Cinnamon | Ginger | Oregano | |
| Clove | Hing | Pepper | |

**Spices to reduce heat and acid, hot flashes, skin rashes, and acne**

| | | | |
|---|---|---|---|
| Cardamom | Fennel | Peppermint | Turmeric |
| Coriander | Lavender | Saffron | |

**Spices to reduce brain fog and painful, heavy periods and to increase appetite and digestive strength**

| | | | |
|---|---|---|---|
| Ajwain | Clove | Mustard seed | Rosemary |
| Basil | Cumin | Oregano | Thyme |
| Bay leaf | Fenugreek | Pepper | Turmeric |

# Anuloma to Redirect Apana Vayu

| | | | |
|---|---|---|---|
| Angelica/dong quai | Eggplant | Motherwort | Sage |
| Brahmi | Hing/asafetida | Musta | Urad dal |
| Burdock | Hot water | Raspberry | |
| Chamomile | Mint | Rose | |

# Rasayana to Rejuvenate and Build Ojas

| | | | |
|---|---|---|---|
| Almonds | Figs | Oat straw | Tulsi |
| Amla/amalaki | Ghee | Rose | Turmeric |
| Angelica/dong quai | Hemp seed | Sea moss | Walnuts |
| Ashwagandha | Licorice | Sesame | Vidari/wild yam |
| Brahmi | Meat | Shatavari | |
| Coconut | Milk | Sugar | |
| Dates | Nettle | Triphala | |

# Stanya to Increase Breast Milk

| | | | |
|---|---|---|---|
| Ajwain/caraway/ celery seed | Fenugreek | Raspberry | Vidari/wild yam |
| | Nettle | Urad dal | |

## Demulcent to Moisten and Protect Tissues

| | | | |
|---|---|---|---|
| Chia seeds | Kombu | Marshmallow | Slippery elm |
| Flaxseeds | Licorice | Sea moss | |

## Vajikarana for Aphrodisiac Qualities, to Strengthen Generative Tissues, and to Promote Fertility

| | | | |
|---|---|---|---|
| Ajwain | Dates | Ripe mango | Sweet rice porridge |
| Amla/amalaki | Licorice | Rose | |
| Ashwagandha | Milk | Shatavari | |
| Black grapes, prunes, and raisins | | | |

# Appendix C

## BIBLIOGRAPHY AND RESOURCES

## BIBLIOGRAPHY AND READING LIST

### CLASSICAL AYURVEDA TEXTS CITED

Agnivesa. *Charaka Samhita*. Translated by Ram Karan Sharma and Vaidya Bhagwan Dash. Varanasi: Chowkhamba Krishnadas Academy, 2009.

Joshi, Nirmala. *Ayurvedic Concepts in Gynaecology*. Delhi: Chaukhamba Sanskrit Pratishthan, 1999.

Shastri, A. *Sushruta Samhita of Sushruta*. Reprint, Varanasi: Chaukhamba Sanskrit Sansthan, 2010.

Usha, V. N. K. *Streeroga-Vijnan*. Delhi: Chaukhamba Sanskrit Pratishthan, 2019.

Vagbhata. *Ashtanga Hrdayam*. 6th ed. Translated by K. R. Srikantha Murthy. Varanasi: Chowkhamba Krishnadas Academy, 2009.

Vatsyayana. *Kamasutra*. Translated by Amal Shib Pathak. Delhi: Chaukhamba Sanskrit Pratishthan, 2015.

### BOOKS ON WOMEN'S HEALTH, HERBALISM, AND AYURVEDA

Bachman, Margo Shapiro. *Yoga Mama, Yoga Baby: Ayurveda and Yoga for a Healthy Pregnancy and Birth*. Boulder, CO: Sounds True, 2013.

de Fouw, Hart, and Robert Svoboda. *Light on Life: An Introduction to the Astrology of India*. Silver Lake, WI: Lotus Press, 2003.

Desai, Sharmila, and Anna Wise. *Sadhana for Mothers*. New York: Yoga Words, 2015.

Feit, Rebecca. *It Starts with the Egg*. 2nd ed. New York: FranklinFox Publishing, 2019.

Grzych, Heather. *The Ayurvedic Guide to Fertility*. Novato, CA: New World Library, 2021.

Joseph, Sinu. *Rtu Vidya: Ancient Science Behind Menstrual Practices*. Chennai, India: Notion Press, 2020.

Kodikannath, Jayarajan, and Alyson Young Gregory. *The Parent's Complete Guide to Ayurveda*. Boulder, CO: Shambhala Publications, 2022.

Kurdyla, Jennifer, and Amy Rodriguez. *Root and Nourish: An Herbal Cookbook for Women's Wellness*. New York: Tiller Press, 2021.

O'Donnell, Kate. *The Everyday Ayurveda Cookbook*. Boulder, CO: Shambhala Publications, 2014.

O'Donnell, Kate. *The Everyday Ayurveda Guide to Self-Care*. Boulder, CO: Shambhala Publications, 2020.

Ou, Heng. *The First Forty Days: The Essential Art of Nourishing the New Mother*. New York: Stewart, Tabori, and Chang, 2016.

Pole, Sebastian. *Ayurvedic Medicine: the Principles of Traditional Practice*. Philadelphia: Singing Dragon, 2012.

Romm, Aviva. *Hormone Intelligence*. New York: Harper One, 2021.

Welch, Claudia. *Balance Your Hormones, Balance Your Life*. Boston: Da Capo Lifelong Books, 2011.

Weschler, Toni. *Taking Charge of Your Fertility*. New York: William Morrow, 2015.

## WOMEN'S HEALTH PRACTITIONERS

This is a list of the practitioners who have contributed to this book:

**Adena Rose Bright**
Women's health education, consultations, fertility awareness coaching
www.adenaroseayurveda.com

**Paula Crossfield**
Vedic astrology resources and podcast
www.weaveyourbliss.com

**Brighid Doherty**
Community herbalist and founder of the Solidago School of Herbalism and *The Healthy Herb* podcast
www.solidagoherbschool.com

**Emily Glaser**
Ayurveda and Vedic astrology
www.tejasveda.com

**Heather Grzych**
Ayurveda practitioner and fertility specialist
www.heathergrzych.com

**Sahana Murthy**
Ayurveda cooking
www.rasayanamysorekitchen.com

### FIND A PRACTITIONER NEAR YOU

In the United States, National Ayurvedic Medicine Association directory: https://www.ayurvedanama.org/
In Canada, Ayurveda Association of Canada: https://ayurvedaassociation.ca/
In Europe, European Ayurveda Medical Association: www.ayurveda-association.eu

### SOURCING INGREDIENTS

These are all trusted suppliers of ghee, spices, herbs, and any specialty ingredients. You may also find good suppliers closer to home, which is even better.

**Banyan Botanicals** has Daily Swish pulling oil, dinacharya products, Ashwagandha Bala and other herbal massage oils, organic spices, and bulk herbs. Find a discount code at https://ayurvedicliving.institute/ayurveda-oils.
www.banyanbotanicals.com

**Farm True** sells small-batch ghee, herbal massage oils, spices and teas. Find a discount code at https://ayurvedicliving.institute/ayurveda-oils.

**Frontier Co-op** sells dried Western herbs and spices.
www.frontiercoop.com/

**Full Moon Ghee** offers ghee made on the full moon.
https://fullmoonghee.com

**Ironbound Island Seaweed** harvests a variety of seaweeds.
www.ironboundisland.com

**Maine Coast Sea Vegetables** provides different types of sea vegetables.
https://seaveg.com

**Mountain Rose Herbs** is a purveyor of dried Western herbs and spices.
https://mountainroseherbs.com

**One Mighty Mill** makes heirloom wheat products.
www.onemightymill.com

**Pukka Herbs** sells the closest thing to an herbal infusion in a teabag and makes herbal medicines available in the United Kingdom and Europe.
www.pukkaherbs.com

**Pure Indian Foods** is a source for herbal ghee, cultured ghee, spices, Best Hing Ever, red rice, and urad dal. www.pureindianfoods.com

**Queen of Thrones** has convenient Castor Oil Pack Kits. www.shopqueenofthethrones.com/

## PANCHAKARMA CENTERS

These are centers I have direct experience with, although there are many other excellent ones.

### INDIA

**Sitaram Beach Retreat**
https://sitaramretreat.com

**Vaidyagrama Healing Village**
www.vaidyagrama.com

### UNITED STATES

**The Ayurvedic Center of Vermont**
www.ayurvedavermont.com

**The Ayurvedic Institute**
www.ayurveda.com

## WOMEN'S HEALTH RESOURCES

**The Ayurvedic Living Institute** is an online school with topics including Ayurveda cooking, self-care, women's health, a yoni steaming course, and professional development for Ayurveda practitioners. https://ayurvedicliving.institute

*The Darkest Time of Year and the Return of the Light: An Infertility Ceremony* is an online article by contributor Anna Jefferson.
https://medium.com/@annavj/
the-darkest-time-of-year-and-the-return-of-the-light-an-infertility-ceremony-ab2e33a4eb05

**Environmental Working Group** can provide consumer guides on endocrine disrupting chemicals, organic food, and safe personal care products.
www.ewg.org

**Kripalu Center for Yoga & Health** is a retreat and education center that offers Ayurveda treatments, courses, and certification.
https://kripalu.org

**The North American Menopause Society** has information for both consumers and professionals about promoting women's health from midlife forward.
http://menopause.org

*Women's Health and Hormones* is an online video course presented by Dr. Claudia Welch. https://drclaudiawelch.com/courses/
womens-health-hormones-part-i

*Yoga for Women* by Emma Balnaves, is an eight-page booklet guiding women through the three main stages of life.
https://shadowyoga.com/wp-content/uploads/
2017/12/yogaforwomenarticle.pdf

# Acknowledgments

I would like to thank the following people who were instrumental in the process of creating this book:

All the folks at Shambhala Publications for the vision and its execution, especially Sara Bercholz, champion of the wisdom traditions.

Rochelle Bourgault, the book midwife 2.0.

Cara Brostrom, whose cultivation of good space shows in her work. Cara would also like to thank Jordan Brooks, Chris Okerberg, Hannah Jacobson-Hardy and Sweet Birch Herbals, Foxtrot Herb Farm, and Melissa Warwick.

The models: Jordan Brooks, Becky Wright, Mary Spencer, Evelyn Okerberg, and June Garres.

My bestie, Erin Casperson, for the Ayurveda expert edits—triple gold star as usual.

Dr. Elizabeth Bostock, Western medical expert editor.

Lauren Fenterstock and Aaron Stephan for the handmade location.

Carabeth Connolly, head recipe tester.

Great teachers, in order of appearance: Robert Moses, Nancy Gilgoff, Sharath Jois, Dr. Robert Svoboda, Dr. Claudia Welch, Dr. A. R. Ramadas, Dr. Scott Blossom, Dr. Anusha Seghal, and Emma Balnaves.

My partner, Rich Ray, for patiently putting up with me writing books.

My parents, for raising me to believe I can do anything I put my mind to.

Those who support my work from behind the scenes in ways that are obvious or not so obvious: The Kripalu Center, Melissa and Simon, Frank W. Smith, and the Portland Ladies Firepit Club.

My students, who bring out the best in me, and all those who attend my workshops in person and online.

All my readers, wherever you are. You bring the Shakti.

# Notes

1. Agnivesa, *Charaka Samhita*, trans. Ram Karan Sharma and Vaidya Bhagwan Dash (Varanasi: Chowkhamba Krishnadas Academy, 2009), chapters 3 and 12.

2. Agnivesa, *Charaka Samhita*, Chikitsasthana 15:34–35.

3. Nirmala Joshi, *Ayurvedic Concepts in Gynaecology* (Delhi: Chaukhamba Sanskrit Pratishthan, 1999), 20.

4. Agnivesa, *Charaka Samhita*, Chikitsasthana 30:115.

5. Vagbhata, *Ashtanga Hrdayam*, 6th ed., trans. K. R. Srikantha Murthy (Varanasi: Chowkhamba Krishnadas Academy, 2009), Sutrasthana 8:49.

6. Joshi, *Ayurvedic Concepts*, 33.

7. Romm, Aviva MD, *Hormone Intelligence* (New York: HarperOne, 2021).

8. Carla Dugas and Viola H. Slane, *Miscarriage* (Treasure Island, FL: StatPearls Publishing, 2022).

9. Agnivesa, *Charaka Samhita*, Sharirasthana 8:49.

10. Janice Dolk, "My Story of a Journey from Menarche to Post-Menopausal," *Elephant Journal*, October 14, 2022, www.elephantjournal.com/2022/10/my-story-of-a-journey-from-menarche-to-post-menopausal/.

# Index

**A**

abdomen, 39, 126, 147, 168, 174, 319

abhyanga (oil massage), 323–27
 in healing apana, 44
 how to do self-massage, 325–26
 in menopause, 191
 during new moon, 93
 overview and nature, 323
 postpartum, 168
 during pregnancy, 162
 qualities of, 17, 18
 self-massage, instructions, 325–26
 sleep and, 183
 when not to do, 59, 126, 162, 323
 when to do, 59, 87, 181, 182, 323, 329
 *See also* dry brushing; massage oils; shiro abhyanga

achara rasayana, 205–6

Adityas, 48. *See also* celestial bodies

adrenaline, 3, 5, 11

aging and old age, 54
 air element in, 196
 Ayurvedic/Vedic view of, 178–79, 187, 199
 meals and, 74
 moksha in, 117
 rasa and, 29
 *See also* longevity

agni, 31, 320
 ama and, 75, 76
 awareness of, 70
 cleansing and, 81, 82, 83
 foods supporting, 85
 hormones and, 3, 60
 imbalances in, 77
 low/weak, 69, 143, 230
 in menopause, 192

in menstruation, 119, 124, 126, 129
natural rhythms and, 74
postpartum, 168, 171
rasayana foods and, 202
samana vayu and, 40
sleep and, 63
strongest time for, 72
*See also* jathara agni

ahara rasa (food-juice), 28, 69, 70, 72, 228, 233

air element, 11, 58
 apana vayu and, 39
 balancing, 54
 in bones, 194
 in head, 50
 lunar rhythms and, 90
 in menstrual cycles, 137
 postpartum, 167
 in vata, 12, 20

ajwain, 173
 seeds, 232, 268, 273–74, 284–85
 therapeutic uses, 129, 330, 331, 332

alcohol, 34, 64, 85, 100, 127, 138, 140, 183

almond, 124, 214
 Almond Cardamom Diamonds, 306–8
 Basic Almond Milk, 240
 flour, 306–8
 full moon sprouted, 96
 milk, 14, 96, 193, 202, 243, 250, 260
 oil, 326
 therapeutic uses, 193, 201, 331

aloe, 151, 181, 201, 202

aloe juice, 195, 250, 254

Alternate Nostril Breathing. *See* Nadi Shodhana

ama
 agni and, 69

buildup, 75, 76, 143
cleanses and, 81
clearing, 75, 77, 228
dry brushing and, 327
fertility and, 156
massage and, 59, 323
undereating and, 77
weight gain and, 192

amenorrhea, 16, 146

amla/amalaki, 164, 201
 Chyawanprash Herbal Jam, 256–57
 therapeutic uses, 151, 331, 332

anabolic, 4, 15. *See also* building (*brmhana*)

anatomic terms, 27

angelica/dong quai, 331

animal products, 85, 195, 276

antiperspirant, 321

anuloma, 39, 331

apana vayu, 27, 44
 anuloma to redirect, 331
 generative health and, 38
 location and functions, 39, 40
 in postpartum, 43, 173–74
 supporting, 41, 128, 314, 317–20
 suppressing, 43
 while menstruating, 124, 125, 126, 130, 136

aphrodisiacs, 152, 156, 243, 293, 300, 305, 311, 332. *See also* vajikarana

appetite, 14, 69, 76, 128, 171, 330

arame, 215, 292

armpits, 320, 321

artava dhatu, 27
 cleansing and, 80
 conception and, 31, 155
 practices for, 181, 314, 317–20
 *See also* generative organs

artavavahasrotas, 26–27
 and apana, relationship of, 39

hormonal birth control and,
149
location and functions of, 38
menstruation and, 119
supporting, 69, 193
use of term, 31
artha, 106, 107, 113, 116
ashramas (four stages of life), 105
appetites and, 74
doshas and, 107
timing of, 108, 117
*See also individual stages*
*Ashtanga Hrdayam*, 80, 105,
136, 152
ashwagandha, 193, 244, 248,
331, 332
ashwagandha rasayana, 201
asthi dhatu, 26
astringent taste, 213, 214
avocado, 17, 181, 193, 260
Ayurveda, 3, 8
on body, 47
flow of life in, 54, 206
on food, 67
on grief, 154
historical context for, 178–79,
201
on human organism, 12, 50
on menstruation, 90
on mind, 185
on physiology, prioritizing, 25,
26–27
on substances and qualities,
211
terminology of, 23
Western medicine and, 4, 23,
83, 146, 153

**B**

back pain, 18, 38, 127, 318–19,
330
balance, 3, 54
cleansing and, 80
in diet, 8, 304
of lightening and building, 81,
202
of sex and stress hormones, 5

of solar and lunar, 4, 89
*Balance Your Hormones, Balance
Your Life* (Welch), 5
bananas, 17, 164, 201
barley, 17, 269, 284–85
basil, 286–87, 291, 297, 330
baths and showers, 17
herbal bath ritual, 329
in morning, 59
during new moon, 93
bay leaf, 272, 330
beans, 17, 18, 274, 294. *See also*
mung beans
beef, qualities of, 16
beers, yeasty, 19
beets, 114, 214, 294
Beets and Barley Stew, 284–85
Gingered Beet Soup, 289
Herbed Beet Pickles, 291
"belly binding," 168
birth control
hormonal, 149, 150
natural, 149–50
birthing
apana vayu and, 40, 161
artava and, 38
recovery from, 167–68, 175
bitter taste, 213, 214
bladder, 22, 38, 57, 137, 174, 254,
269, 279
blood, 11, 28, 33, 214. *See also*
menstrual blood; red blood
bodily urges, suppression of,
42–43, 76, 127, 136, 138,
143
body, 20, 62
Ayurvedic view of, 47
influence of sun and moon on,
49–50
natural energy flow of, 39
body weight, 82, 157, 191–92, 201
bones
elements and, 10, 12
nourishing, 28–29, 30,
193–95, 215
bowels, 57, 128, 137, 202
brahmacharya, 107, 109, 112

brahmi, 182, 193, 248, 253, 331
brahmi ghrita, 194
brain fog, 19, 75, 76, 328, 330
breakfast, 74
Creamy Coconut Breakfast
Kichari, 264
Yogurt Rice, 265–66
breast milk, 29, 69, 161, 166, 331
breastfeeding, 29, 82, 83, 162,
170, 171, 173, 300
breasts
fibrocystic, 6, 17, 30
massaging, 59, 320
nipples, 38
pitta aggravated in, 127
breath and breathwork, 17, 19,
39, 42, 57, 196, 205. *See also*
Nadi Shodhana; Sama Vritti
Ujjayi; Sitali Cooling Breath
Bright, Adena, 165
broccolini, 276–77
broth
bone, 129, 193, 194–95, 214
Chicken Bone Broth, 277
Essential Mineral Vegetable,
272
qualities of, 16, 17, 19
vegetable, 291
"bucket syndrome, the," 6
building (*brmhana*), 4, 6
aging process and, 179, 190
foods for, 85, 86, 128
in menstrual cycle, 122
in perimenopause, 181
qualities, 15
rasa and, 30
therapies, 87
burdock, 129, 222, 272, 331
burnout, mental and physical, 7
butter, 161, 164

**C**

cacao powder, 249, 260, 309
caffeine, 17, 71, 126
cane juice, 256–57, 268, 306–8,
311, 312
caraway, 173, 331

cardamom
  actions of, 330
  ground, 234, 235, 236, 247,
    303, 306–8
  pods, 256–57
carrots, 9, 272, 276, 284–85, 294
castor oil
  for breast massage, 59, 320
  for feet, 65
  packs, 17, 318–19
catabolic, 4, 15. *See also* lighten-
    ing (*langhana*)
celery seeds, 173, 331
celestial bodies, 47–48, 49, 50, 51
cereals, hot, 15
cervix, 11, 31, 149, 318
cesarean delivery, 173, 174
chamomile, 221, 317, 331
*Charaka Samhita*, 28, 29, 38,
    159, 211
chasteberry, 151, 186
cheese, 16, 17, 18, 19
cherries, 129, 214
chia, 193, 195, 259, 332
chicken, 276–77
chilis, 16
chocolate, 249
chyavanprash, 170, 202, 256–57
cilantro, 16, 265–66, 272,
    273–74, 293
cinnamon, 234, 236, 243, 244,
    256–57, 271, 294, 330
circadian rhythms, 48
clary sage essential oil, 225
cleansing
  Ayurvedic view of, 80
  contraindications, 83
  levels of, 78, 80, 83
  one-day, 92
  timing, 80
  *See also* detoxification; home
    cleansing
clear quality, 19
cloudy/slimy/sticky quality, 19
cloves, 236, 330
coconut, 16, 124, 201
  Basic Coconut Milk, 241

milk, 201, 239, 247, 264,
    276–77, 289
  shredded, 294, 298
  therapeutic uses, 331
coconut oil
  for massage, 87, 162, 170, 181,
    323, 326
  in soup, 276
  for tempering, 273–74, 294
coconut sugar, 85, 264, 268, 297,
    311, 312
coffee, 16, 85, 127, 138, 140
conception, 19, 67
  artava dhatu and, 31, 155
  preparing for, 156, 157–58
condiments
  Mixed Greens Chutney, 297
  Sesame Crunch Chutney, 298
  Triple Mineral Gomasio, 299
congestion
  chronic, 75, 76
  contraindications, 328
  dosha imbalance and, 14
  sleep and, 63
constipation, 20, 26, 76, 174,
    318–19, 330
cool quality, 16
coriander, 171
  actions of, 330
  ground, 273–74, 276, 297
  seeds, 231, 233, 235, 236, 238
corn and corn snacks, 17, 18
cortisol, 3, 5, 6, 11
crackers, 17, 18
cranberry juice, 254
cravings, 128, 130, 135, 137, 140,
    142, 162, 249
cream, heavy, 19, 281–82
creativity, 11, 31, 32, 69, 93, 95,
    130
cucumbers, 16, 19
cumin, 171
  actions of, 330
  ground, 269
  seeds, 231, 238, 273–74,
    284–85
curry leaves, 265–66, 273–74, 279

curry powder, 276
cysts, 16, 17, 19, 21, 146, 320

**D**
daily routines
  fertility tracking and, 149
  longevity and, 205
  making time for, 57
  menstruation and, 123
  *See also* dinacharya
dairy, 18, 19, 85
dal
  Every Body Dal, 280
  mung dal, 281–82
  Yellow Dal Supreme, 273–74
  *See also* urad dal
date sugar, 85
dates, 17, 201, 303
  Date Honey, 305
  Medjool, 171, 242, 243, 260
  therapeutic uses, 214, 331, 332
deglet noor, 260, 305
demulcents, 195, 218, 332
dense/solid quality, 17
deodorant, 225
depression, 6, 63
detoxification
  abhyanga for, 323–27
  body's natural, 78, 126
  celestial influences on, 48
  foods to favor and avoid, 85
  lightening (*langhana*) in, 80
  in morning, 55, 59
  order of, 83
  rasa and, 28
  *See also* cleansing
dharma, 106, 107, 112, 116
Dharmashastra, 112
dhatus, seven types, 25, 26
diarrhea, 21, 76, 135
digestion
  balance and, 30
  celestial influences on, 48
  hormones and, 4
  kapha imbalance and, 143
  ojas and, 32
  sleep and, 63

spices for, 330
digestive tract, 10, 11, 320
digestives, 210, 228, 236. *See also*
    spiced waters
dinacharya, 154, 323
    cleansing and, 84
    meaning of term, 55, 109
    *See also* daily routines
disease, causes of, 41
Doherty, Brighid, 226
dosha(s), 25
    aims of life and, 107
    determining, 9
    five elements and, 12
    imbalance in, 14
    life stages and, 105, 107
    locations and functions of, 22
    meaning of term, 12
    in menstruation, 120, 122, 130,
        131, 134, 136, 144
    perimenopause and, 181
    qualities of, 20
    seasonal fluctuation of, 60–61
    six tastes and, 213, 214
doulas, Ayurvedic-trained, 168
dravya rasayana, 201
dry brushing, 17, 87, 327
dry quality, 17
dryness, mitigating, 181
duality, 4, 8, 14
dulse, 215, 272, 299
dysmenorrhea, 146

**E**

ears, 10
    in morning routine, 58
    oiling, 65, 87, 171, 181
earth element, 12, 44, 109, 164,
    276
    aging and, 192, 200
    in bones, 193, 194
    building qualities of, 210, 213
    in kapha, 12, 21, 109
    perimenopause and, 179, 180
eating habits, 77
    best practices, 71–72
    overeating, 16, 19, 63, 69

timing, 72, 75
eggplant, 85, 128, 214, 331
elements, five
    body and, 9–12, 25
    in menopause, 187, 192
    in nourishment process, 28–29
    six tastes and, 214
elimination, 319
    apana vayu and, 40
    menstruation and, 127
    in morning, 55, 57, 63
    and qualities, signs of excess, 17
    regular, benefits of, 320
    suppressing, 136, 138
    urgency and frequency, 39
endocrine system, 3, 48
endocrine-disrupting chemicals
    (EDCs), 78, 81, 83, 320
endometriosis, 146
energy channels, 321, 322–23
Epsom salts, 93, 317, 329
estrogen, 3
    functions, 6
    in menopause, 190, 191, 193
    in menstruation, 121
    in perimenopause, 185
    "undetectable," 44
    water element and, 11
*Everyday Ayurveda Guide to*
    *Self-Care* (O'Donnell), 26,
    158, 194
exercise and activity, 8, 16–17
    during cleanses, 87
    competitive/aggressive, 18
    longevity and, 205
    during menstruation, 124,
        125–26, 130, 138, 141, 143
    moon cycles and, 95, 100
    postpartum, 174
    rakta and, 34
    seasonal shifts and, 62
exhaustion, 34, 63, 97, 137, 167,
    171
eyes, 11, 58, 59, 60, 97

**F**

fat tissue, 6, 12, 28–29, 190
fats, saturated, 16
feet, oiling, 65, 87, 171, 181
fennel, 171, 272
    actions of, 330
    bulb, 286–87
    seeds, 231, 235, 238, 256–57
fenugreek, 171, 173, 213, 281–82,
    330, 331
ferments, 34, 62, 140, 182
fertility
    cleansing qualities for, 156
    energy of, 153
    herbs for, 151
    moon and, 47, 95, 97, 123
    ojas and, 32
    overall health and, 158
    pitta and, 61
    rasa and, 67
    sex hormone depletion and, 7
    shukra and, 27, 31
    vajikarana for, 332
    water element and, 11
fetus, Ayurvedic view of, 159, 161
fibroids, 6, 16, 17, 19, 146, 318–19
figs, 93, 214, 261, 331
fire element, 11
    hormones and, 60
    in pitta, 12, 21
    rakta and, 33, 34
    solar energy and, 49, 51
fish, 17
flax milk, 242, 244
flaxseeds, 85, 192, 193, 195, 214,
    242, 260, 332
flours, 17, 138, 268
follicular phase, 121, 130
food and nutrition
    cleansing and, 80
    consistency in, 151
    for fertility, 152
    fried foods, 16, 30, 62, 140, 193
    during lunar cycles, 92, 93, 95,
        96, 100
    medicinal, 67, 210, 215, 262
    in menopause, 192–93

food and nutrition (*cont.*)
    menstruation and, 127–29, 130, 137, 138, 140–41, 143, 304
    nourishment process, 28–29
    optimizing, 32
    postpartum, 171–73
    during pregnancy, 162–63, 164–65
    prioritizing, 70
    raw food, 18
    sleep and, 64
    spicy, 15, 18, 34, 62, 130, 182
    tissue affinities of, 26
    for women's health, 214–15
fruits
    citrus, 16
    cooked, 18, 193
    raw, mixing with food, 85
    red and blue, 129

**G**

garam masala, 281–82
garbini parichaya, 161
garlic, 97, 213, 288, 304, 330
garlic scapes, 272
gas and bloating, 11, 14, 20, 127, 137, 166, 171, 228
generative juices. *See* shukra
generative organs, 25, 27
    artava and, 38
    Ayurvedic terms for, 23
    disorders of, 146–47
    toxins in, 78
    within vata territory, 22
generative system, 27
    circulation's role in, 26–27, 38–39
    doshas in, 14
    lunar rhythms and, 89
    nourishing, 29
    strengthening, 151
    vata and, 38, 54
generative tissues
    affinities for, 26, 214
    ahara rasa and, 69
    estrogen and, 6

kapha in, 22
nourishing, 29, 96, 213, 247
seasonal shifts and, 60
strengthening, 200, 332
*See also* dhatus, seven types
gestation, 38, 90, 155, 159, 161, 175
ghee, 124, 306–8
    for artava nourishment, 157
    making during full moon, 96
    medicated, 194
    postpartum, 171, 172
    during pregnancy, 164
    for rasayana, 201
    in soups, 268, 284–85, 288
    tempering with, 265–66, 286–87
    therapeutic uses, 32, 44, 80, 181, 185, 193, 331
    tissue affinities of, 26
    in tonics, 243
    *See also* shatavari ghee
ginger, 171
    actions of, 330
    fresh, 265–66
    ground, 16, 244, 249, 253, 260, 264
    in soups, 268, 269, 271, 284–85
    tea, 15
gingerroot, 234, 276, 288, 291, 297
gluten, 17, 164
goat milk, 215
gooseberries, 164
grains
    hard quality, 18
    rinsing, 274
    whole, 64, 85, 93, 140, 163, 171, 192, 214
grapes, 140, 164, 214, 332
green powders, 252
greens, 16, 19, 62, 171
    bitter, 15, 213
    cooked, 140, 143
    dark, 129
    leafy, 85

    Mixed Greens Chutney, 297
grief, 41, 154, 163
grihastha, 57, 107, 113, 114, 116, 159
gross/big quality, 19
growth hormones, 3, 31
gunas (qualities)
    in balancing body, 22
    characteristics, foods, activities, and signs of excess, 16–19
    imbalance in, 15
    seasons and, 61
    ten pairs, 14

**H**

hair
    lunar cycles and, 95
    in menopause, 190, 203
    nourishing, 213, 221, 288
    ojas and, 33
    and qualities, signs of excess, 17, 18
    rasa imbalance and, 30
    shiro abhyanga and, 325, 326, 328
hala hala, 274
hard quality, 18
haritaki, 202
health care practitioners, consulting, 75, 83, 145–46, 147, 174, 186, 200
heart, 32, 34, 40, 67
heavy quality, 16
hemorrhoids, 173, 174, 316
hemp, 85, 192, 331
herbal infusions, 210
    Cleansing, 222
    Cooling, 220
    Cool-the-Flash, 226
    Double-Duty Sage and Salt Deodorant, 225
    how to make and use, 217
    length of use, 223
    Nourishing, 218
    Raspberry Leaf and Nettle Brew, 223
    Refreshing Phanta, 221
    Triphala Tea, 224

herbal teas, 19, 64, 85
herbs, 19
    buying, 226
    parts of plants, 217
    therapeutic use of, 211
    *See also specific herbs*
hibiscus, 221, 312
hing/asafetida, 265–66, 279,
    281–82, 284–85, 330, 331
home cleansing
    foods for, 84–85
    preconception, 157–58
    preparing for, 82
    therapies and postcleanse
        period, 87
    three meal plans for, 86
    timing, 81, 82–83
honey, 85, 164, 252, 256–57, 293,
    297, 311
hormone replacement therapy
    (HRT), 178, 203
hormones
    balancing, 8, 60, 314, 321–27
    lunar cycles and, 51
    in menopause, 191
    as messengers, 3–4
    types, 3
hot flashes
    breathing practices for, 321,
        323
    in menopause, 190
    in perimenopause, 181, 182,
        183
    and qualities, signs of excess,
        16
    rakta and, 34
    reducing, 100, 182, 226, 330
    vata imbalance and, 43
hot quality, 16
householding stage. *See* grihastha
human growth hormone (HGH),
    3

**I**

ida nadi, 50, 321
imbalance
    consistency in treating, 141

fertility tracking and, 149
    during menstruation, 126
    PMS as, 134, 145
    postpartum, 168
    in rakta, 34–35
    six tastes for, 214
    *See also under individual
        doshas*
immunity, 27, 32, 47, 67, 200
"in the bhav," 153
indigenous wisdom traditions,
    51, 123
indigestion, 14, 21, 59, 173, 228
infertility, 154
inflammation, 7, 21, 75, 77,
    201–2, 228, 316, 323

**J**

jackfruit, 164
jasmine, 65, 161, 329
jathara agni, 69
jivana ("life-giving") function,
    33, 215
jivaniya, 32
joints, 11, 21, 22, 75, 192, 200,
    325
Joshi, Nirmala, *Ayurvedic Con-
    cepts in Gynaecology*, 131
journaling, 123, 135, 145, 147

**K**

kale, 272, 280, 286–87, 288, 292
kama, 106, 107, 115, 117
Kama Sutra, 107, 115
kapha, 30, 62
    aggravating, 282
    aging and, 179
    in brahmacharya, 107, 109
    daytime sleep and, 63
    dry brushing for, 327
    elements of, 12
    fasting and, 92
    in generative system, 14
    imbalances, 156, 318
    locations and functions of, 22
    massage and, 59
    in menstruation, 120, 122, 131

moon and, 93, 95
    in pregnancy, 114, 154, 161
    qualities, 21
    spring and, 61
Kaur, Emily Murphy, 114
kelp, 215, 276–77, 299
kichari, 171
    Creamy Coconut Breakfast
        Kichari, 264
    in home cleansing, 81
    during menstruation, 129
    at new moon, 92
    New Moon Kichari, 286–87
    Umami, 288
kombu, 195, 271, 272, 273–74,
    288, 332
Kurdyla, Jennifer, *Root & Nour-
    ish*, 44

**L**

labia, 27, 38, 316
lavender, 65, 93, 317, 326, 329,
    330
legumes, 62, 158, 192, 195, 280,
    281–82, 288
lentils, 85, 158, 280
lethargy, 21, 156, 327, 328
libido, 200, 318
    healthy, 151
    longevity and, 202, 203
    low, 76
    moon and, 97, 122
licorice, 193, 195, 201, 331, 332
light quality, 16
lightening (*langhana*), 4
    aging and, 190
    foods for, 85, 86
    in menstrual cycle, 122
    qualities, 15
    rasa, 30
    therapies, 87
limes, 16, 255, 273–74, 297
liquid quality, 17
liver, 34, 183, 233
longevity, 115, 193, 199, 200
    abhyanga, 323–27
    libido in, 202

longevity (*cont.*)
    mental attitudes in, 205–6
    ojas and, 32
lotus, 129, 151, 214, 217, 279
lunar cycles and rhythms, 90–91
    aligning with, 181
    awareness of, 50, 123
    cleansing and, 83
    effects of, 48
    girls and, 109
    menopause and, 191
    menstruation and, 49, 121, 122, 123–24, 130
    postmenopause and, 202
    *See also* moon
lunar energy
    balancing, 4
    channel of, 50, 321
    fertility and, 153
    qualities of, 47, 49–50
luteal phase, 121, 130
lymphatic system, 11, 27, 28, 76, 320

**M**

majja dhatu, 26, 185
mamsa dhatu, 26
mango, ripe, 17, 332
maple syrup, 85, 268, 297, 309
marshmallow, 62, 193, 195, 217, 218, 332
masala, making one's own, 236
massage oils
    ashwagandha bala, 168
    choosing, 326
    in menopause and, 191
    during pregnancy, 162
    qualities of, 17, 18
    while menstruating, pausing, 126
meals
    ama production and, 76
    balancing, 70–71
    celebratory, 73
    during detox, 85
    lunch as largest, 72, 74
    medicinal, 210

    rhythms of, 74
    two-meal flow, 75
meat, 15, 16, 17, 18, 19, 331
meat soup, 32, 129, 138, 164, 165, 171, 214
meda dhatu, 26
melatonin, 5, 48, 60
menopause, 6, 187
    apana changes during, 39
    Ayurvedic view of, 178–79
    body therapies for, 115, 190, 318–19, 327, 328
    bone health during, 193–95
    defining, 190
    meals and, 74
    as natural transition, 178, 197
    and qualities, signs of excess, 16
    supporting, 191–92
    vata and, 115, 190
menstrual blood, 27
    amount, 120
    collection methods, 125
    color and texture, tracking, 135
    fire element and, 11
    foods for building, 128
    heavy bleeding, 147
    in perimenopause, 186
    rasa and, 29, 34, 67
menstrual cycle, 27
    air element and, 11
    apana changes during, 39, 40, 43, 124
    artava and, 38
    Ayurvedic view of, 119–21
    breasts and, 320
    castor oil packs, 318–19
    cessation of, 44
    cramping during, 136, 142, 232
    disorders of, 145–47
    dosha effects on, 14, 136–44
    exercise and rest during, 125–26
    heavy periods, 34, 39, 330
    irregular periods, 7, 136, 147
    lunar rhythms and, 49, 121, 122, 123–24, 130, 327

    massage and, 59, 323
    moonbathing and, 327
    as natural detox, 78
    nutritional support, 127–29, 130, 137, 138, 140–41, 143, 304
    overall health and, 130, 134
    practices for, 130, 321, 381
    and qualities, signs of excess, 16, 17, 18, 19
    reducing symptoms, 100
    scanty periods, 30
    sex hormones and, 6
    timing of, 123
    tracking, 123, 135, 145, 147
    Western medical view of, 120, 121
metabolic hormones, 3
metabolism
    ama and, 75
    boosting, 232
    fire element and, 11
    jathara agni in, 69
    menopause and, 74, 192
    ojas and, 32
    perimenopausal changes, 183
    sleep and, 55
microcosm-macrocosm, 12, 48
migraines, 140
milk, 9, 15
    almond-coconut, 241
    cow, 214
    goat, 215
    in pregnancy, 164
    as rasayana, 201
    therapeutic uses, 32, 80, 214, 331, 332
    tissue affinities of, 26
    in tonics, 239, 243, 247, 248, 249, 253
mind, 11, 199
    and body, relationship of, 50, 51
    fertility and, 155
    lunar energy and, 51
    in perimenopause, 185
    practices for, 322–23, 328–29

prana and, 109
mint, 140, 255, 297, 331. *See also* peppermint
miscarriage, 163
miso, 18, 293
mobile quality, 18
moksha, 106, 107, 117
mood swings, 7, 43, 321, 328–29
moon
    full, 95–97, 122
    new, 92–93, 122, 123
    waning phase, 89–90, 100, 122
    waxing phase, 89–90, 93, 95, 122
moonbathing, 95, 124, 130, 153, 161, 327
moringa, 250–52
morning practices, 55, 57–59
motherwort, 331
mung beans, 85, 129, 164, 171, 214, 273–74
    in kichari, 286–87
    in soups, 279, 284–85
Murthy, Sahana, 304
musta, 156, 331
mustard oil, 326
mustard seeds, 265–66, 273–74, 279, 294, 330
"My Story of a Journey from Menarche to Post-Menopausal" (Dolk), 203

**N**

Nadi Shodhana (alternate nostril breathing), 44, 50, 174, 182, 196, 321–22
nadis, 27, 50
nails, 17, 18, 95
neem soap, 326
nervines, 93, 182, 218, 248
nervous system
    abhyanga for, 59, 323–27
    affinities for, 26
    breathing practices for, 322–23
    in perimenopause, 185
    stimulation of, 42
nettle, 173, 218, 222, 223, 331

nori, 215, 299
nose in morning routine, 58
nut and seed butters, 85, 129, 192, 309. *See also* tahini
nutmeg, 128, 236, 330
nuts, 17, 18, 85, 128, 138, 140, 210, 214. *See also* almond; walnuts

**O**

oat straw, 218, 223, 331
oats, 62, 92, 214, 218, 303
oily/unctuous quality, 17
ojas, 27, 31
    building, 32, 166, 200, 331
    depleted, 152
    good and depleted, signs of, 33
    location of, 32
    in perimenopause, 185
    soma and, 47
    stress and, 153
    supporting, 69, 95, 151
olive oil, 181, 193, 293
olives, 17, 62
onions, 97, 213, 279. *See also* red onion
oregano, 228, 272, 286–87, 330
osteoporosis, 178, 192, 200
ovaries, 3, 6, 38, 146, 190
ovulation, 121
    air element and, 11
    apana vayu and, 40
    artava and, 38
    celestial influences on, 48
    kapha and, 142
    practices for, 130, 318
    and qualities, signs of excess, 17
    when transitioning from hormonal birth control, 150
ovum, 27, 121, 155, 156, 157

**P**

panchakarma, 75, 156
parinama (transformation), 54, 105, 187
parsley, 272, 284–85, 293, 297
pelvic floor, 44, 173–74, 175

pelvic region, 38–39, 40, 41, 126, 147, 186, 316
pepper, black, 16, 269, 330
peppercorns, 256–57
peppermint, 221, 330
perimenopause
    Ayurvedic view of, 179
    irregularity in, 181
    length of, 178
    menstruation and, 186
    mental fluctuations in, 185
    ojas in, 185
    ovulation cycle awareness and, 150
    signs of, 180
    symptom management, 100, 181–83
    symptoms, amount of, 7, 18
    timing of, 179
perineum, 316
pineal gland, 3, 47, 48, 60
pingala nadi, 50, 321
pink salt, 225, 297, 298, 317
pistachios, 201
pitta
    aggravating, 282
    aging and, 179
    in digestion, 28
    elements of, 12
    in generative system, 14, 100
    in grihastha, 107, 113, 114, 159
    locations and functions of, 22
    in menstruation, 120, 121, 122, 130, 131
    in pregnancy, 166
    qualities of, 21
    rakta and, 34
    reducing herbs, 182, 329
    sleep and, 4, 63, 182–83
    summer and, 61
    times, 60, 72, 74, 183
pituitary gland, 3, 60
plasma, 25, 26, 27, 28, 30, 89
plums, 140, 214, 261
PMS
    ama and, 75
    Ayurvedic approach to, 145

PMS (*cont.*)
  breasts and, 320
  information from, 134, 135
  kapha imbalance and, 142
  relief from, 127
polycystic ovary syndrome, 19, 75,
  146, 156, 213
pomegranates, 85, 129, 214, 254,
  255, 265–66
postmenopause, 61, 203
postpartum
  apana vayu in, 43
  Ayurvedic view of, 167–68
  daily routine, 170–71
  heart nourishment during, 67
  nutrition, 171–73, 223
  pelvic floor during, 173–74
  premature delivery and, 170
  support during, 168, 175
potatoes, 18, 85, 272
prakriti, 22
prana
  apana and, 39
  circulation of, 26–27, 50, 205
  generative health and, 38, 145
  intention and, 109, 202
  during menstruation, 124, 126
  redirecting, 155
prana vayu, 40
  blocking, 42–43
  sense organs and, 41–42
pranic body, 51. *See also* subtle
  body
pregnancy
  cleansing and, 83
  foods for, 163, 164
  frequent eating, 162
  heart nourishment during, 67
  kapha and, 114
  massage during, 323, 327
  medicinal herbs/spices,
    amounts of, 166
  shukra and, 90
  vata's role in, 161–62
  and work, balancing, 114
prepuberty, 61
progesterone, 3, 6, 11, 121

prunes, 129, 164, 214, 332
pumpkin
  Pumpkin Seed Cilantro Pâté,
    293
  puree, 244
pumpkin pie spice, 244
pungent taste, 213
purification. *See* detoxification
purusartha (aims of life), 105,
  106, 107, 108, 117. *See also*
  *individual aims*

**Q**
qualities. *See* gunas (qualities)

**R**
raisins, 129, 164, 214, 235, 261, 332
rajah, 27. *See also* menstrual
  blood
rajonivrutti. *See* menopause
rakta dhatu, 26, 27, 215
  ama and, 75
  in childbearing, 90, 164
  imbalances in, 34–35, 69
  meaning of term, 33
  in menstruation, 120, 128
  tonics, 239
raktavahasrotas, 27
rasa dhatu, 26, 27
  aging and, 179, 191
  ama and, 75, 77
  bone health and, 193
  building, 28–29
  healthy, signs of, 29
  imbalances in, 30, 69
  lunar phases and, 89–90
  menstruation and, 35, 120
  moonbathing and, 327
  nourishment and, 262
  ovum and, 155
  in postpartum, 166
  in pregnancy, 159, 161, 164
  purifying, 156
rasavahasrotas, 27, 28
rasayana, 80, 200–201, 202, 239,
  331. *See also* rejuvenation
raspberries, 259, 260, 331

raspberry leaves, 173, 217, 220,
  222, 223, 317
red blood, 27, 33, 215
red clover, 156, 220
red onion, 276, 288
rejuvenation, 29, 32
  cleansing and, 80, 83, 87
  from doing less, 200
  foods and herbs for, 201–2
  postpartum, 167
reproductive hormones, 3, 4
reproductive organs. *See* generative organs
respiration, 11, 40, 42, 56
rest
  cleansing and, 82
  during menstruation, 125,
    126, 141
  as rasayana, 201
rice, 129, 164, 201
  basmati, 85, 264, 265–66,
    284–85, 286–87, 288
  protein, 85
  red, 214
  Red Rice Kanji, 271
rituals, 7, 47, 66, 96, 97, 153, 155,
  239, 304
ritucharya, 60
rose, 65, 93, 182, 331, 332
rose oil, 65, 329
rose petals, 220, 226, 234, 317
  Hibiscus Rose Cordial, 312
  Moon Milk, 247
  Sweet Rose Masala, 236
rosemary, 228, 291, 330
rough quality, 17

**S**
saffron, 256–57, 330
sage
  Cool-the-Flash Tea, 226
  Double-Duty Sage and Salt
    Deodorant, 225
  therapeutic uses, 65, 182, 331
salads, 292
salt, 18. *See also* Epsom salts;
  pink salt

saltwater gargle, 87
salty taste, 213, 215
Sama Vritti Ujjayi (rhythmic breathing), 174, 322–23
samana vayu, 40
sandalwood oil, 161, 329
sandalwood soap, 326
sannyasa, 107, 116, 199–200
scalp, 59, 60, 64, 83, 328
screen time, 57, 60, 63, 64, 66, 124
sea moss, 215, 260, 331, 332
sea vegetables, 129, 214, 215, 249, 272
seasonal affective disorder, 51
seasonal shifts
    apana changes during, 39
    basics of working with, 62
    bodily signs and, 61
    cleansing and, 83
    observing, 60
seaweed, 193, 214. *See also specific types*
sedentary activities, 16, 17
seeds, 17, 85, 124, 129, 192. *See also specific types*
self-care
    caring for others and, 159
    community and, 175
    consistency in, 63
    in grihastha, 116
    making time for, 57, 78, 152
    during menstruation, 124–27
    prepregnancy, 155
    stress and, 185
semen, 31, 35
sense organs, 41–42
    caring for, 55, 58, 59
    during new moon, 92
    resting, 66, 71, 126
sesame, 181, 192, 214
    black, 299, 303, 304
    in gomasio, 299
    Sesame Crunch Chutney, 298
    therapeutic uses, 331
sesame oil
    frying with, 292

for massage, 65, 87, 162, 168, 326
    tempering with, 265–66
sex, abstaining from, 156
sex hormones, 5
    decrease in, natural, 6, 181, 191
    depleted, 7
    functions of, 6
    in menstruation, 121
    shukra and, 31
shakti (cosmic generative energy), 119
Shakti (goddess), 25
sharp/intense quality, 16
shatavari, 151, 181, 193, 243, 249, 331, 332
shatavari ghee, 157, 158
sheeta virya, 152
shiro abhyanga (head massage), 64, 87, 181, 328
shodhana (cleanse), 80
shukra, 26, 27
    building, 156, 214, 300
    eyes and, 97
    fertility and, 31, 90, 130, 149, 153
    food as, 67
    lunar energy and, 49
    moon and, 93, 95, 96
    and ojas, relationship of, 32
    qualities of, 151
    supporting, 193
    uses of term, 23, 31
sinuses, 11, 50
Sitali Cooling Breath, 323
sitz bath, herbal, 174, 316–17
skin, 10
    cleansing, 59
    detoxifying, 55
    disorders, 34
    estrogen and, 6
    in morning routine, 58
    and qualities, signs of excess, 17, 18, 19
    rasa and, 29, 30, 67
    rashes, reducing, 330
    support for, 221

sleep
    celestial influences on, 48, 51
    detoxification during, 55
    eating and, 74
    good and bad, distinguishing, 63
    herbs for, 65–66
    hormones and, 4
    lack of, causes, 64
    oversleeping, 16
    in perimenopause, 182–83
    postpartum, 170
    practices for, 59, 64, 321, 323, 328–29
    problems affecting, 66
    and qualities, signs of excess, 16
    timing of, 63
    waning moon and, 100
slippery elm, 17, 193, 195, 218, 332
slow quality, 16
smoking, 16, 152
smooth quality, 17
snacking, 70–71, 85, 138, 162
soft quality, 18
solar energy and rhythms, 4, 48–49, 89
    channel of, 50, 321
    in modern culture, 51, 66, 80
soma, 47–48, 49, 51, 93, 95, 97, 123, 202
soups and stews, 17
    Beets and Barley Stew, 284–85
    Chicken Soup, 276
    clear, 15
    Gingered Beet Soup, 289
    Lotus Root Curry, 279
    Red Rice Kanji, 271
    Spiced Barley, 269
    Spicy Black Gram, 281–82
    Warming Wheat, 268
    *See also* meat soup
sour taste, 213. *See also* amla/ amalaki
soy products, isolated, 85
space element, 10

space element (*cont.*)
aging and, 190, 196
apana vayu and, 39
balancing, 54
lunar rhythms and, 90
in menstrual cycle, 137
postpartum, 167
in vata, 12, 20
sperm, 27, 155, 156
spice mixes
Essential, 238
Sweet Rose Masala, 236
spiced waters, 62, 85, 166, 228
Ajwain, 232
Basic, 230
Cooling Fennel Soft Drink, 235
Coriander, 233
Essential, 231
Soothing Rose Sweet Tea, 234
spices, 211, 228, 236, 330. *See
also specific spices*
spirituality, 89, 115, 187, 196, 199,
205, 206
spring, 61, 82, 93
sprouts, growing, 96
squash, 18
summer, 273–74
winter, 129, 244, 272, 280,
294
srotas (channels), 27
stable quality, 18
stages of life. *See* ashramas
stanya, 331
stevia, 85
stomach, amount of food in, 72
strawberries, 259
stress, 6
abhyanga and, 327
celebrations and, 73
chronic, 6, 41
fertility and, 153
menstruation and, 126, 136,
140
ojas and, 185
rakta and, 34
reduction, fundamental principles of, 7

sleep and, 66
stress hormones, 3
alcohol and, 183
hot flashes and, 182
increased, signs of, 7
in menopause, 190, 191
and sex hormones, balancing,
5, 6
subtle body, 41, 47, 49, 50, 161
subtle/minute quality, 19
sugar, 85, 138, 201, 312, 331
sugarcane, 164
sukha, 112, 199
summer, 15, 61, 82, 221, 230,
235, 273, 327
sun baths, 16, 60
sunflower oil, 326
sunflower seeds, 85, 96
sweating, 5, 17, 87, 183, 190, 213,
321
sweet potatoes, 85, 129, 214
sweet rice porridge, 332
sweet taste, 213, 300

T
tahini, 171, 303, 309
Tantra, 47, 50
taste, role of, 28
tastes, six, 211, 213
teas, caffeinated, 17, 85
tejas, 167
testosterone, 3
throat, 320
thyme, 228, 272, 277, 286–87,
330
thyroid, 6, 260
thyroid-stimulating hormone
(TSH), 3
tomatoes, 85, 281–82
tongue, 70, 76, 77
tongue scraping, 57, 58, 126, 170
tonics, 210, 239
Aloe-Pom-Cran, 254
Basic Almond Milk, 240
Basic Coconut Milk, 241
Best Medicinal PSL, 244
Chyawanprash Herbal Jam,

256–57
Date Shake, 243
Golden Mind Milk, 248
Homemade Flax Milk, 242
Longevity Bone Tonic, 253
Moon Milk, 247
Moringa Green Drink, 250–52
Pomegranate Lime Mocktail,
255
Raisin Mantha, 261
Raspberry-Ginger Secret
Smoothie, 260
Sexy Cacao, 249
Strawberry Rose Smash, 259
toxins, 69, 320, 321. *See also*
endocrine-disrupting chem-
icals (EDCs)
treats, 300
Almond Cardamom Dia-
monds, 306–8
Black Sesame Balls, 303
Date Honey, 305
Hibiscus Rose Cordial, 312
Kate's Tahini Treat, 309
Rasala Medicinal Yogurt, 311
tridoshic types, 22
triphala, 224, 331
triphala rasayana, 201
trividha karana, 41
tulsi, 156, 202, 222, 331
turmeric, 236, 238, 248
in soups, 269, 273–74, 279,
281–82, 284–85
therapeutic uses, 171, 201, 330,
331

U
udana vayu, 40, 44
urad dal, 265–66
in kichari, 264, 288
in soup, 281–82
therapeutic uses, 173, 193, 214,
331
urination, 22, 38, 39, 40, 137,
161
uterine fibroids, 17, 146
uterus, 6, 10, 35, 146, 318–19

**V**

vaginal dryness of, 17, 181, 203, 318
vaginal opening, 27
vajikarana, 31, 151, 156, 200, 332
vanaprastha, 107, 115, 179, 186, 197
vata, 182–83
   aggravating, 78, 215
   apana and, 39, 41
   balancing, 137–38
   blood and, 119
   calming, 64, 65, 329
   elements of, 12, 58
   energy crashes and, 71
   five vayus and, 40
   generative system and, 14, 38, 54
   imbalances, 27, 38, 41, 43, 64, 66, 136–37, 318, 327
   locations and functions of, 22, 42, 194
   in menopause, 115, 190
   in menstruation, 120, 122, 123, 124, 126, 131
   pacifying practices, 93, 129, 321
   postpartum, 167–68, 174
   in pregnancy, 161–62
   qualities of, 20
   sannyasa and, 107, 116
   sleep and, 182–83
   in vanaprastha, 107, 115, 196
   winter and, 61
vayu
   disorders, 38
   five types, 40
   meaning of term, 39

Vedic astrology, 47, 48
vegetable juice, 85
vegetables
   cooked, 129
   raw, 17
   root, 15, 62, 93, 163, 171
   steamed, 15
   watery, qualities of, 16, 19
   *See also* specific types
vegetarian diets, 164, 165, 195
vidari/wild yam, 173, 193, 331
vinegar, 16
   apple cider, 288, 291
   rice, 288
vitamin D absorption, 48
vridha. *See* aging and old age
vulva, 25, 35, 181, 316
vyana vayu, 40

**W**

waking, timing of, 63
walnuts, 201, 293, 331
wasabi, 16
water, 19
   digesting, 230
   sparkling, 18, 255
   warm, 57, 58, 72, 140, 170
   *See also* spiced waters
water element, 11, 12
   in kapha, 12, 21, 142
   lunar energy and, 49, 51, 89–90
   perimenopause and, 180
   rakta and, 33, 34
water retention, 6, 21, 30, 61, 135, 156, 230, 327
watermelon, 15
weather, 61, 62, 74, 75

weight gain, 6
   dry brushing for, 327
   kapha imbalance and, 21, 63
   in perimenopause, 181
   sex hormone depletion and, 7
   sleep and, 63
Welch, Claudia, 5, 6
Weschler, Toni, *Taking Charge of Your Fertility*, 149–50
Western medicine and science
   on female anatomy, 25
   on infertility, 154
   on inflammation, 77
   on menopause, 178, 197
   on menstruation, 120, 121
   on perimenopause, 179
   on postpartum, 168
   *See also under* Ayurveda
wheat, 19, 62, 85
   heirloom, 164, 214
   Warming Wheat Soup, 268
whey protein, 85
wild yam. *See* vidari/wild yam
winter, 15, 60, 61, 82, 230, 256, 289, 327

**Y**

yams, 93, 114, 164, 214. *See also* vidari/wild yam
yoga, 16, 18, 19, 47, 50
Yoga philosophy, 50
yogurt, 164, 265–66, 311
yoni, 27, 316
   meaning of term, 25
   steaming, 18, 174, 318
   as symbol, 119

# About the Author

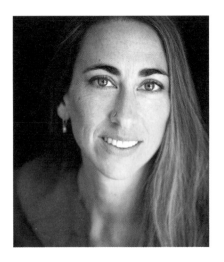

Kate O'Donnell is the author of four Ayurveda books published in seven languages, as well as an international presenter, Ayurveda practitioner, and mentor. She is the founder of the Ayurvedic Living Institute, https://ayurvedicliving.institute/, an online community space for self-transformation. She lives in Portland, Maine, and can be reached at hello@ayurvedicliving.institute.

## ABOUT THE PHOTOGRAPHER

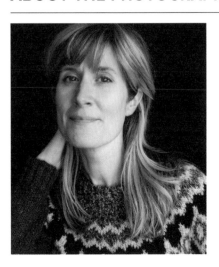

Cara Brostrom is an editorial and field photographer. Her work has been exhibited throughout Europe and North America and published in the *Boston Globe*, *Origin Magazine*, and *Yoga Journal* among others. She is the cocreator and photographer of *The Everyday Ayurveda Cookbook* and *Everyday Ayurveda Cooking for a Calm, Clear Mind*. Cara lives down a long dirt road in the forests of western Massachusetts.